Conceptual issues in psychological medicine

Conceptual issues in psychological medicine

Collected Papers of Michael Shepherd

Second edition

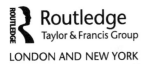 Routledge
Taylor & Francis Group

LONDON AND NEW YORK

For Margaret – '…un amas de fleurs étrangères,
m'ayant fourni du mien que le filet à les lier' (Montaigne).

First published 1990
by Routledge
27 Church Road, Hove, East Sussex, BN3 2FA

Simultaneously published in the USA and Canada
by Routledge
711 Third Avenue, New York, NY 10017

Routledge is an imprint of the Taylor & Francis Group, an informa business

Second edition 1998

Transferred to digital printing 2011

British Library Cataloguing in Publication Data
Shepherd, Michael, *1923–96*
    Conceptual issues in psychological medicine
    I. Title
    616.89

Library of Congress Cataloguing in Publication Data
Shepherd, Michael, 1923–96
    Conceptual issues in psychological medicine/Michael Shepherd. – New ed.
        p. cm.
    Includes bibliographical references and index.
    1. Psychiatry.   I. Title
    RC 458.S4   1998
    616.89–dc21   97–18007

    ISBN 978–0–415–16530–3

Publisher's Note
The publisher has gone to great lengths to ensure the quality of this reprint
but points out that some imperfections in the original may be apparent.

Contents

List of figures   vii
Foreword to the first edition, 1990   viii
Foreword to the second edition   xi
Acknowledgements   xiii

1 Sherlock Holmes and the case of Dr Freud   1

2 Formulation of new research strategies on schizophrenia   27

3 Morbid jealousy: some clinical and social aspects of a
   psychiatric symptom   39

4 Changing disciplines in psychiatry   69

5 Psychological medicine *redivivus*: concept and communication   91

6 The sciences and general psychopathology   107

7 Sir Aubrey Lewis – an Australian psychiatrist   122

8 The legacies of Sir Aubrey Lewis   134

9 The origins and directions of social psychiatry   152

10 Healing in perversion   157

11 The case of Arise Evans: a historico-psychiatric study   160

12 Epidemiology and clinical psychiatry   172

13 Karl Jaspers: *General Psychopathology*   187

14 John Ryle   192

Contents

15 Urban factors in mental disorders: an epidemiological approach 201

16 The only metaphysical man: a re-examination of Otto Rank 212

17 What price psychotherapy? 217

18 Two faces of Emil Kraepelin 221

Select bibliography 239
Name index 247
Subject index 249

List of figures

1.1   The death of Professor Moriarty   2
1.2   Typical forms of ears, according to Morelli   10
1.3   Ears and hands of Botticelli, according to Morelli   10
1.4   Sir Arthur Conan Doyle   13
2.1   Interactional model for factors possibly affecting the
      onset, course, and outcome of schizophrenia   32
2.2   Five-year follow-up of schizophrenics: course of illness   34
2.3   Meehl's causal chain   36
5.1   Forbes Winslow   93
12.1 Transmission of heroin abuse in Crawley New Town   181
12.2 Relation between trend of battle injury and neuropsychiatric
      admissions, Fifth US Army   182
12.3 Coverage of sickness continuum achieved by the
      major sources of morbidity statistics   183
15.1 Areas of residence (shaded areas) in the city of Chicago
      with high first-admission rates to hospital for schizophrenia in
      persons aged 15–19 years by 1930 census tract   204
15.2 Areas of residence (shaded areas) in the city of Chicago
      with high first-admission rates to hospital for manic-depressive
      psychoses in persons aged 15–64 years by 1930 census tract   205
15.3 Per cent of schoolchildren with neurotic or conduct
      disorders (deviance) in the Isle of Wight (IOW) and an Inner
      London borough (ILB), 1975   207
15.4 Numbers of children per 10,000 referred to child guidance
      clinics by school and election ward within a London
      borough, 1962–1966   208

Foreword to the first edition, 1990

Leon Eisenberg

Discriminating readers who purchase this volume, and those fortunate enough to receive it as a gift, are in for an uncommon intellectual adventure: an encounter with a first-rate mind. The essays in it are marked by rare intelligence, remarkable lucidity, and unusual erudition. After all, in how many books written by a psychiatrist does one find references to Voltaire's *Zadig*, Morelli's *Italian Painters*, Nadeau's *Histoire du Surréalisme*, Virginia Woolf's *The Death of the Moth*, Mumford's *The City in History*, and James's *The Varieties of Religious Experience*?

Many of the chapters reprint articles I read when they first appeared. Rereading them has proved just as rewarding as the reading in the first instance, though occasionally disconcerting, as when I discovered that I misremembered an important point or had so far forgotten another that it seemed a new discovery. Perhaps most unexpectedly, the wit has remained fresh. And wit, as Hazlitt once wrote, 'is the rarest quality to be met with among people of education.'

To physicians on our side of the Atlantic, Shepherd epitomizes the very best of English empiricism applied to psychiatry: in his resolute insistence on ascertaining the facts, when there are any to be had, in his unwillingness to go very far beyond those facts, and in his creativity in designing and implementing studies to add to the facts. Such traits may seem less remarkable to his British colleagues than they do to an American. Although we in the US clearly must bow to our French confrères when it comes to preference for theory over fact, we do have a distressing capacity for tolerating woolly-minded generalizations. Not so, Professor Shepherd and his pupils! I have come away from every encounter with Michael Shepherd, whether literary or personal, the wiser for it, even if I have at times felt a bit chagrined when his mordant comment let the hot air out of a pompous statement I had unwisely ventured in his presence.

The essays in this volume stand on their own; they need no exegesis here. To those whose careers are more or less contemporaneous with his, no introduction to the author is necessary because he will be well known to those who read at all (and those who don't are unlikely to begin now!). For students and young professionals, however, a brief biographic note may be useful because many of Shepherd's ideas, novel as they were at the time he set them forth, have become so much part of standard wisdom that they are no longer associated with his name and others are now principally known through the work of his pupils.

Michael took his medical education at the University of Oxford and his psychiatric training at the Maudsley in London. His doctoral thesis (required in the UK for a Doctor of Medicine degree) was a scholarly study of the hospitalization rates for major psychoses in the county of Buckinghamshire between 1931–3 and 1945–7. Most often, theses are exercises designed to enable students to demonstrate their mastery of the methods of a field, but Shepherd's work stands out as an important original contribution. His database enabled him, after he returned to the field for a third sample for the 1950s, to demonstrate that the decline in the hospital population during the most recent of the three periods antedated the introduction of psychotropic drugs; it had resulted from a more effective organization of psychiatric services rather than what was being hailed as the 'pharmacological revolution'. Had his point been recognized, the UK and the US might have been spared some of the inhumanity associated with precipitous deinstitutionalization in the absence of provision in the community for discharged patients.

He was the first to undertake the systematic study of psychiatric morbidity in general practice. It is by now so widely recognized that primary health care physicians constitute the 'de facto mental health service system' in the US that few recall Shepherd and his colleagues recognized that fact a dozen years before the phrase was coined in the US. Shepherd insisted that the therapeutic role of the family doctor must be strengthened if there is to be any realistic hope of providing mental health care to the population. His wisdom continues to be ignored on this side of the Atlantic where official spokesmen for psychiatry fight for specialist hegemony. In addition Shepherd has been a leading contributor to the refinement of psychiatric classification and diagnosis as a key consultant to the Division of Mental Health of the World Health Organization.

Although Michael is generous with the credit he gives to John Ryle, late Professor of Social Medicine at Oxford, and to Sir Aubrey Lewis, late Professor at the Institute of Psychiatry and head of the Maudsley, for his own intellectual development, he can justly be termed one of the two originators of psychiatric epidemiology in the UK, along with John Wing (another of Sir Aubrey's pupils).

Rereading Shepherd has also reminded me of a bit of sage advice a graduating student gave me 40 years ago when I arrived at medical school as an anxious freshman. Be sure, he said, to select medical books written by British authors when you have a choice; they're clearer, they have less filler, and they are far more interesting to read. As I floundered about, uncertain and insecure in the new environment, I clung to his advice, eager for anything that promised to help me survive. What he said, I must confess, did seem to me a stereotype, no more likely to be true than other overgeneralizations; surprisingly, it continued to bear up when I ventured to test it. Forty years later, on rereading Shepherd, I face another exemplar of my mentor's thesis.

Conceptual Issues in Psychological Medicine typifies what is best in British medical books. It is marked by a grace of style rare even in the best of British medical writing. Those who have been offended by the convention of referring to medical articles and books as the 'literature' will be comforted by Shepherd's essays. I envy the reader who will encounter these essays for the first time. The experience is one to be savoured.

Leon Eisenberg, M.D.
Harvard Medical School
Boston, Massachusetts

Foreword to the second edition

This reissue of Michael Shepherd's papers enables us to look back on the academic contributions of our first professor of epidemiological psychiatry. His written work is in the tradition of his great teacher, Aubrey Lewis, in combining the results of reading that goes well beyond the confines of psychiatry, with a pleasing elegance of style. He was the last of a generation of psychiatrists who was deeply versed in the European literature, which he was able to read mainly in the original languages.

We have taken the opportunity of removing some of his more ephemeral papers, as well as most of the case histories that follow his paper on morbid jealousy, in order to make way for some other papers that deserve to be collected, as each of them expresses something important that he wished to say.

'Epidemiology and Clinical Psychiatry' is a better statement of the contribution of his chosen specialty than the paper that appeared in the earlier collection, and the principles that he describes will all stand the test of time.

In the last years of his life Michael turned his attention to Emil Kraepelin, and considered the man and his ideas in the context of political ideas that were then current in Germany. He delivered this lecture with a passion that he had never previously allowed himself, and it is with pleasure that we reproduce it here. Many of Kraepelin's less desirable beliefs have been airbrushed away by his respectful proselytes: the picture Michael draws shows another, more disturbing side.

'Aubrey Lewis – an Australian Psychiatrist' appeared in a volume that is not generally available, and is an unusual addition to the published record about a remarkable man. The contrasting early lives of Howard Florey, Hugh Cairns and Aubrey Lewis – all originating from Adelaide – are fascinating, even if not altogether surprising. The revelation came later: the man who had been a loner in one environment flowered in another, and left behind him one of the world's great research establishments in psychiatry.

In his paper on Aubrey Lewis, Michael writes of the four legacies left behind by Sir Aubrey, and it is of interest to use the same framework when assessing Michael's contribution to the subject. The first is the general legacy, and this includes the mass of Michael's published work. In addition to these later papers one must include the previous collection *The Psycho-social Matrix of Psychiatry* as well as the many books and chapters listed in the select bibliography. His range was wide, and he brought the same critical intelligence and wide erudition to bear on them all.

His main specific legacy is the importance now granted to epidemiology as a tool for studying aetiological problems and for taking a public health stance towards mental health services. Both the World Psychiatric Association and the Association of European Psychiatrists now have flourishing sections of epidemiology: Michael made a massive contribution to bringing about such a happy state of affairs. The essays included in *The Scope of Epidemiological Psychiatry* (Routledge, 1989) allowed social scientists from across the world to honour his contribution to their chosen subject. His subsidiary specific legacy is the journal *Psychological Medicine*, which continues to uphold the high standards that he set as its founding editor.

When describing Sir Aubrey's demonstrative legacy Michael referred to his personal qualities, and here there are points of both similarity and contrast. Michael described Aubrey's 'courage to be unpopular', and comments 'clearly, he lived a life apart'. Both of these applied equally to Michael, although those who knew him only in his professional role may well not have appreciated the warmth and spontaneity that he displayed in social situations. He had a sardonic wit that sometimes contributed to unpopularity, but also gave great pleasure. The reader of 'Sherlock Holmes and the Case of Dr Freud' will get a hint of this mischievous side of a man who was capable of making one ache with laughter by imitating his colleagues. This was a quality completely absent in Sir Aubrey.

His residual legacy is the large number of his former students who now practise skills learned on his unit in many parts of the world. Many of these contributed chapters to the memorial volume already mentioned. We number ourselves among the many who learned a great deal from him.

David Goldberg
David Watt

Acknowledgements

We wish to thank the following publishers for permission to include previously published material in this work:

'The case of Arise Evans: a historico-psychiatric study', *Psychological Medicine*, vol. 6, no. 10, copyright Cambridge University Press, 1976 (ch. 11);
'Changing disciplines in psychiatry', copyright *British Journal of Psychiatry*,
1988 (ch. 4); 'Epidemiology and clinical psychiatry', copyright *British Journal of Psychiatry*, vol. 133, 1978 (ch. 12); 'Formulation of new research
strategies on schizophrenia', first published in *Search for the Causes of
Schizophrenia*, copyright Springer-Verlag, 1987 (ch. 2); John Ryle, introduction to *The Natural History of Disease*, copyright BMA/Keynes Press, 1988
(ch. 14); Karl Jaspers: *General Psychopathology*, copyright *British Journal of
Psychiatry*, vol. 141, 1982 (ch. 13); 'The legacies of Sir Aubrey Lewis',
Psychological Medicine Monograph, Supplement 10, copyright Cambridge
University Press, 1986 (ch. 7); 'Morbid jealousy: some clinical and social
aspects of a psychiatric symptom', copyright *The Journal of Mental Science*,
vol. 107, no. 449, July 1961 (ch. 3); 'The only metaphysical man: a re-
examination of Otto Rank', copyright *Encounter*, 1988 (ch. 16); 'The origins
and directions of social psychiatry', reprinted by permission of the publisher
from *Integrative Psychiatry*, September-October 1983, copyright 1983 Elsevier Science Publishing Co., Inc. (ch. 9); 'Psychological medicine *redivivus*:
concept and communication', copyright *Journal of the Royal Society of
Medicine*, vol. 79, November 1986, (ch. 5); 'The sciences and general psychopathology', introduction to the *Handbook of Psychiatry*, copyright Cambridge University Press, 1983 (ch. 6); 'Sir Aubrey Lewis – an Australian
psychiatrist', first published in D. Copolov (ed.) *Australian Psychiatry and
the Tradition of Aubrey Lewis*, copyright National Health and Medical
Research Council, Australia, 1991 (ch. 7); 'Two faces of Emil Kraepelin',
copyright *British Journal of Psychiatry*, vol. 167, 1995 (ch. 18); 'Urban
factors in mental disorders: an epidemiological approach', *British Medical
Bulletin*, vol. 40, no. 4, copyright Churchill Livingstone Publishers, 1984
(ch. 15).

Chapter one

Sherlock Holmes and the case of Dr Freud

Freud and Holmes

It has become a truism to maintain that most physicians, and all psychiatrists, can benefit professionally from some familiarity with the world of fiction. The works of such major artists as Balzac, Dickens, Shakespeare, and Ibsen, and those of many lesser writers, contain a host of characters depicting various morbid states of mind encountered in clinical practice. For this reason they illustrate, and often supersede, most textbooks of abnormal psychology and psychopathology.

But there is more to fiction than the portrayal of character. Writing of the art-form which he did so much to create Balzac observed that the province of the novel is the history of human manners, the nature of man's perception of himself, and the embodiment of ideas. One of these embodied ideas introduces my theme and does so, modestly enough, in the form of a detective story. The story in question is Nicholas Meyer's *The Seven Per Cent Solution*, a best-seller in several languages, winner of the Crime Writer's Golden Dagger Award, and the basis of a successful film.[1] The book purports to be a reprint from the reminiscences of Dr John H. Watson, the trusty friend and companion of the prince of detectives, Mr Sherlock Holmes. In it Watson recounts the true story of what happened after Holmes's disappearance and supposed death near the Reichenbach Falls, following a struggle with the infamous Professor Moriarty (see Figure 1.1).

On his surprising reappearance three years later Holmes claimed originally to have been travelling incognito, using the pseudonym of a Norwegian explorer called Sigerson. According to *The Seven Per Cent Solution* the facts were very different. Sherlock Holmes, it appears, was suffering from a severe mental disorder with delusional ideas concerning the machinations of Professor Moriarty, who was in reality a harmless teacher of mathematics. Tricked by Watson's ruse to provide him with medical care, Holmes travels

Based on a Squibb History of Psychiatry lecture to the Institute of Psychiatry, London, June 1984.

Figure 1.1 The death of Professor Moriarty

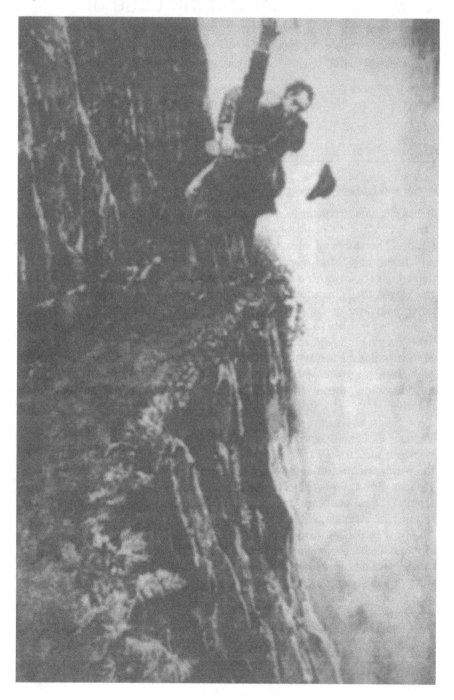

to Vienna for treatment by a young physician specializing in nervous diseases, who cures him by hypnosis and succeeds in identifying the roots of his long-standing malaise. The two men then join in a successful hunt for a local villain who is attempting to precipitate a world war.

Exciting as it is, however, the narrative is less relevant than the identity of the doctor, who is none other than Sigmund Freud. At their first meeting Freud is bowled over by his patient's ability to provide him with an accurate biographical sketch after no more than a brief glance round the consulting-room:

'Beyond the fact', says Holmes 'that you are a brilliant physician who was born in Hungary and studied for a time in Paris, and that some radical theories of yours have alienated the respectable medical community so that you have severed your connections with various hospitals and branches of the medical fraternity – beyond the fact that you have ceased to practise medicine as a result, I can deduce little. You are married, possess a sense of humour, and enjoy playing cards and reading Shakespeare and a Russian author whose name I am unable to pronounce. I can say little besides that which will be of interest to you.'

Freud stared at Holmes for a moment in utter shock. Then, suddenly he broke into a smile...

'But this is wonderful' he exclaimed.

'Commonplace', was the reply.

As the tale unfolds it becomes apparent that the connection between the two men depends on more than a literary device bringing together a fictional detective with personal problems and a well-known psychiatrist. The force of the story would clearly be lost if the protagonists were substituted by, say, Emil Kraepelin and Lord Peter Wimsey. The affinity between the two principal characters becomes increasingly apparent to Dr Watson, as it had to me years earlier when reading Freud's case histories. The very names of those memorable patients – the Wolf Man, the Rat Man, Anna O, Little Hans – conjure up Sherlockian overtones. Take, for example, the Wolf Man, or Sergei Konstantinovich Pankeyev, to give him his true name. His condition has baffled many other specialists, including Kraepelin, before he undergoes psychoanalysis by Freud who gradually traces the neurosis to its source in the primal scene.[2] In the process the patient is 'cured', the mystery is dispelled, and the truth revealed by a detached individual of superior ability who alone sees what lesser men fail to comprehend, and who draws quite unexpected conclusions from his observations. The whole pattern of presentation recalls G. K. Chesterton's description of the true object of an intelligent detective story – 'not to baffle the reader, but to enlighten him in such a manner that each successive portion of the truth comes as a surprise. In this, as in much nobler types of mystery, the object... is not merely to mystify but to illuminate.'

Psychoanalysis has, of course, been compared to detection by several observers, including Freud himself, who defended his activities in the *Introductory Lectures* by asking:

Suppose you are a detective engaged in the investigation of a murder, do you actually expect to find that the murderer will leave his photograph with name and address on the scene of the crime? Are you not perforce content with slighter and less certain traces of the person you seek?[3]

Still more to the point is a passage in the Wolf Man's personal recollections, in which he discusses his therapist's choice of literature:

Once when we happened to speak of Conan Doyle and his creation, Sherlock Holmes, I had thought that Freud would have no use for this type of light reading matter, and was surprised to find that this was not at all the case and that Freud had read this author attentively. The fact that circumstantial evidence is useful in psychoanalysis when reconstructing a childhood history may explain Freud's interest in this type of literature.[4]

As if to confirm the connection, in one of his letters to Jung on a delicate personal matter Freud refers explicitly to his activities: 'I make it appear as though the most tenuous of clues had enabled me, Sherlock Holmes-like, to guess the situation.'[5]

Here, then, is a curious association. To his admirers Freud tends to be either a nonpareil or a scientific giant comparable to the likes of Kepler, Copernicus, and Darwin. Abram Kardiner's opinion may serve as representative:

This adventure of self-discovery, recorded in *The Interpretation of Dreams*, has, to my mind, been equalled in human history only a few times. It is an odyssey of far greater intensity than is recorded in *Confessions* of St Augustine, and much more sincere and modest than those that are contained in the *Confessions* of Rousseau. *The Interpretation of Dreams* is restrained; yet it ranks in intensity with the kind of inner self-encounter and honesty that must have preceded the creation of Kant's *Critique of Pure Reason* and Einstein's general theory of relativity.[6]

What can such a man have in common with any fictional character, however prominent? In the *Timaeus* Plato remarks that: 'It is impossible that two things be joined without a third. There must be some bond to bring them together.' The nature of that bond is the theme of this essay.

Cocaine

One obvious pointer to its nature is contained in the title of Meyer's book. *The Seven Per Cent Solution* refers to the drug cocaine, which figured prominently in the careers of both Holmes and Freud. As early as 1887 we know from Dr Watson that his friend had been 'alternating from week to week between cocaine and ambition', and the journey to Vienna was undertaken because of Freud's published work on cocaine.

Several other physicians and pharmacologists have since interested themselves in the nature of Holmes's drug-dependence. Nearly fifty years ago *The Lancet* carried an anonymous article entitled 'Was Sherlock Holmes a drug addict?', arguing that when the great detective told Watson that he was injecting himself with cocaine he was pulling the worthy doctor's leg.[7] The nature of the substance was later disputed by Miller, who asserted that the drug in question must have been a belladonna alkaloid because of the moral and physical deterioration associated with the use of cocaine.[8] This view was in turn contested by Grilly,[9] citing no less an authority than Goodman and Gilman's *The Pharmacological Basis of Therapeutics*, in which it is stated that 'Sherlock Holmes took advantage of the central effects of cocaine, much to the perturbation of Dr Watson'.[10] Another eminent pharmacologist, Walter Modell, remarks that 'Although habit-forming, cocaine is not tenaciously so, and since it is not psychologically addictive, strong personalities like Freud and Sherlock Holmes had no trouble in controlling the habit.'[11]

The facts were rather different. Sherlock Holmes's creator, Sir Arthur Conan Doyle, carried out a number of experiments with a self-administered drug, but the substance in question was the relatively harmless gelsemium.[12] Freud's experiences with cocaine, on the other hand, were altogether more unfortunate. Ernest Jones's biography provides an outline of events: the early work with and enthusiasm for the 'magical drug'; the under-emphasis on its dangers, culminating in the suicide of a friend whom he persuaded to substitute cocaine for morphine; the failure to appreciate the significance of its properties as a local anaesthetic; and the ultimate disillusionment, without full acceptance of responsibility.[13] Even the hagiographic Jones is compelled to admit that many observers 'must at least have regarded him as a man of reckless judgement'. Others have gone further, seeing in this episode a microcosm of Freud's career, while Thornton has even suggested that the influence of cocaine played a much longer-lasting part in Freud's outlook than has been recognized.[14]

It is the effects of the drug on Sherlock Holmes, however, which are more relevant to our theme, for in 1966 an American psychiatrist, David Musto, first suggested that Holmes was suffering from a delusional illness associated with chronic cocainism which he called *paranoia moriartii*.[15] Musto's paper, which appeared in the *Journal of the American Medical Association*, was followed by letters of rebuttal, some affirming that Holmes was manic-depressive,[16] others that he merely suffered from occupational inertia.[17] In 1968 Musto elaborated on his notion in a paper entitled 'A study in cocaine', pointing out that the drug had stimulated the careers of two brilliant investigators, Sigmund Freud and Sherlock Holmes.[18] He suggested that between 1891 and 1894 Holmes had been recuperating under treatment, perhaps in Switzerland, but possibly in 'a pleasant sanatorium in the Viennese suburbs'. This would, of course, eliminate the pseudonymous Sigerson, though not without a reminder that this was the name of the neurologist who translated Charcot into English, shortly after Freud had translated him into German.[19] Musto's suggestion is also, of course, the origin of *The Seven Per Cent Solution*.

Zadig's method

But it is the enticing speculation which Musto derives from his theory to which I would draw particular attention:

> His ideas and especially his methods must have influenced those to whom he spoke. We are accustomed to the attention Holmes paid to the unusual fact, the unravelling of a complicated problem from the noting of a small slip or characteristic. This style of reasoning may have been the gift of Holmes to those who treated him for his temporarily inefficient mental processes.

To illustrate Holmes's 'style of reasoning', here is an early sample. The trusty Dr Watson has just arrived unexpectedly at 221B Baker Street, hoping to persuade the great man to accompany him on holiday. Before he can open his mouth Holmes tells him of the purpose of his visit:

> 'Knowing you as I do, it's absurdly simple', said he. 'Your surgery hours are from 5 to 7, yet at 6 o'clock you walk smiling into my rooms. Therefore you must have a locum in. You are looking well though tired, so the obvious reason is that you are having, or are about to have, a holiday. The clinical thermometer peeping out of your pocket proclaims that you have been on your rounds today; hence it's pretty evident that your real holiday begins tomorrow. When, under these circumstances, you come hurrying into my rooms – which, by the way, Watson, you haven't visited for nearly three months – with a new Bradshaw and a timetable of excursion bookings bulging out of your coat pocket, then it's more than probable you have come with the idea of suggesting some joint expedition.'

According to Musto, it is the mode of thought underlying passages of this type which constitutes the link that we have been seeking. This consists in the use of a method. And in *The Seven Per Cent Solution* this is acknow-ledged when Holmes responds to Freud's comment that his professional outlook is akin to medical observation by remarking: 'You have succeeded in taking my methods – observation and inference – and applied them to the inside of a subject's head.'

In the original canon Holmes is too concerned with demonstrating the value of this method to discuss its theoretical implications. Fortunately, we can turn to his real-life prototype for the purpose. Sherlock Holmes was modelled partly on Edgar Allan Poe's C. Auguste Dupin and partly on one of Conan Doyle's teachers, Joseph Bell, the Edinburgh surgeon whose powers of observation and diagnostic acumen were legendary. Conan Doyle made no secret of his debt to Bell, a man with 'sharp, piercing grey eyes, eagle nose, and striking features',[20] who could

> diagnose people as they came in, before even they had opened their mouths. He would tell them their symptoms, he would give them details of their lives, and he would hardly ever make a mistake. 'Gentlemen', he would say to us students standing around, 'I am not quite sure whether this man is a cork-cutter or a slater. I observe a slight callus, or hardening on one side of the forefinger, and a little thickening on the outside of his thumb, and that is a sure sign he is either one or the other.'[21]

In a letter to his old teacher, Doyle says of Holmes:

> I do not think that this analytical work is in the least an exaggeration of some of the effects which I have seen you produce in the out-patient ward. Round the centre of deduction and inference and observation which I have heard you inculcate I have tried to build up a man who pushed the thing as far as it would go.[22]

Bell responded modestly to the compliment:

> The only credit I can take to myself in what Holmes says is that appertain-ing to the circumstances that I always impressed over and over again upon all my scholars – Conan Doyle among them – the vast importance of little distinctions, the endless significance of trifles.[23]

In his critique of the stories, Bell acknowledged the growing interest by the public in detective fiction, and the narrative skill of the author who had created a 'shrewd, quick-sighted, inquisitive man, half doctor, half virtuoso'. But at the core of the achievement he identified a method:

> There is nothing new under the sun. Voltaire taught us the method of Zadig, and every good teacher of medicine or surgery exemplifies every

day in his teaching and practice the methods and its results. The precise and intelligent recognition and appreciation of minor differences is the real essential factor in all successful medical diagnosis. Carried into ordinary life, granted the presence of an insatiable curiosity and fairly acute sense, you have Sherlock Holmes as he astonishes his somewhat dense friend Dr Watson; carried out in a specialized training, you have Sherlock Holmes the skilled detective.[24]

Bell's reference to Zadig compels us to go back to Voltaire's wonderful fable, whose eponymous hero furnishes a detailed description of a horse which he has never seen, giving his reasons as follows:

In the lanes of this wood, I observed the marks of a horse's shoes, all at equal distances. This must be a horse, said I to myself, that gallops excellently. The dust on the trees in a narrow road that was but 7 feet wide was a little brushed off, at the distance of 3 feet and a half from the middle of the road. The horse, said I, has a tail 3 feet and a half long, which being whisked to the right and the left has swept away the dust. I observed, under the trees that formed an arbour 5 feet in height, that the leaves of the branches were newly fallen; from whence I inferred that the horse had touched them, and that he must therefore be 5 feet high. As to his bit, it must be gold of 23 carats, for he had rubbed its bosses against a stone which I knew to be a touchstone, and which I had tested. In a word, from the marks made by his shoes on flints of another kind, I concluded that he was shod with silver eleven deniers fine.[25]

Even Holmes could not have done better! It may be remarked, parenthetically, that this passage is itself derivative, being based on a translation of a sixteenth-century collection of stories about the travels of the three sons of the king of Serendippo, a book which prompted Horace Walpole to coin the term 'serendipity' in 1745. More than a century later Zadig's method came into its own as the cornerstone of what is sometimes called 'conjectural science'. Zadig is mentioned by name in George Cuvier's monumental study of palaeontology and the method receives detailed attention in an influential essay by T. H. Huxley, published in 1881 and entitled 'On the method of Zadig: retrospective prophecy as a function of science'.[26] Huxley concludes that:

The rigorous application of Zadig's logic to the results of accurate and long-continued observation has founded all those sciences which have been termed historical or palaetiological, because they are retrospectively prophetic and strive towards the reconstruction in human imagination of events which have vanished or ceased to be.

Huxley is here echoing William Whewell's famous exposition of the logic of induction.[27] Though his primary concern with 'retrospective prophecy' was related to his view of Darwinism as a scientific procedure dealing with unrepeatable causes which had to be deduced from their consequences, the method of reasoning, as he emphasized, is common to several physical sciences, including archaeology, palaeontology, astronomy, geology, and the semiotics of medicine. And, he might have added, to the scientific study of the humanities in the fields of literature (as stylometrics) and of the history of the visual arts, where scientific connoisseurship dates from the work of the Italian physician, Giovanni Morelli (1816–91).

Morelli

Attribution in painting, as Morelli demonstrated, could be established only by detailed study of the work itself, and in distinguishing the work of a master from that of a copyist he emphasized the necessity of concentrating on what had hitherto been regarded as trivial details. In his own words:

> As most men who speak or write have verbal habits and use their favourite words or phrases involuntarily and sometimes even most inappropriately, so almost every painter has his own peculiarities which escape him without his being aware of them.... Anyone, therefore, who wants to study a painter closely, must discover these material trifles and attend to them with care.[28]

The successful application of the Morelli method (see Figures 1.2 and 1.3), through retrospective prophecy, has been clearly analysed by modern art critics:

> Morelli's real contribution to the study of art was that he devised a method whereby (according to him) the gap between attribution and work of art could be so effectively bridged that we could talk of its being virtually certain that a particular painting was the work of a particular artist. Morelli's contention was this: every true artist is committed to the repetition of certain characteristic forms or shapes. If we want to determine the authorship of a work of art, we can do so only via recognizing the fundamental forms, the *Grundformen* of the artist to whom it is due. To identify the characteristic forms of an artist, we must go to the parts of the painting where these conventional pressures are likely to be relaxed; even if this means that we shall have to consider what to an educated aesthete of the last century could only have seemed 'trifles'. We must take seriously the depiction of the hand, the drapery, the landscape, the ball of the thumb, or the lobe of the ear.[29]

Figure 1.2 Typical forms of ears, according to Morelli

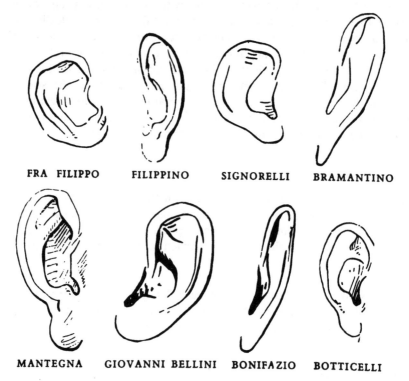

FRA FILIPPO   FILIPPINO   SIGNORELLI   BRAMANTINO

MANTEGNA   GIOVANNI BELLINI   BONIFAZIO   BOTTICELLI

Source: G. Morelli, *Italian Painters: Critical Studies of the Works,* trans. L.M. Richter, London, G. Bell & Son, 1883.

Figure 1.3 Ears and hands of Botticelli, according to Morelli

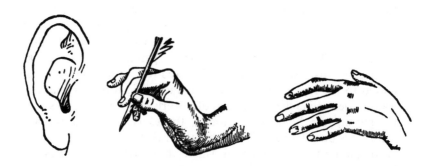

Source: Morelli, op. cit.

It is not always recalled that Conan Doyle's Uncle Henry was Director of the Dublin Art Gallery and an admirer of Morelli, who in turn referred to him as 'the splendid Mr Doyle'. Whatever the significance of their contacts may have been, the parallels between the teachings of Morelli and Sherlock Holmes are apparent and have been noted by several scholars. The art historian Arturo Castelnuovo has drawn attention to the resemblance between their methods;[30] Edgar Wind refers pointedly to the 'characteristic trifles by which an artist gives himself away, as a criminal might be spotted by a fingerprint';[31] and Carlo Ginzburg brings Holmes and Morelli together, 'each discovering, from clues unnoticed by others, the author in one case of a crime, in the other of a painting'.[32]

Not many physicians, though, might have been expected to be aware of Morelli's work. There was, however, one eminent exception. After his self-confessed 'discovery of art' in 1883 Sigmund Freud became keenly interested in art history and in his essay on 'The Moses of Michelangelo' he made a striking admission:

Long before I had an opportunity of hearing about psychoanalysis I learnt that a Russian art-connoisseur Ivan Lermolieff had caused a revolution in the art-galleries of Europe by questioning the authorship of many pictures, showing how to distinguish copies from originals with certainty and constructing hypothetical artists for those works of art whose former authorship had been discredited. He achieved this by insisting that attention should be diverted from the general impression and main features of a picture and by laying stress on the significance of minor details, of things like the drawing of the fingernails, of the lobe of an ear, of halos and such unconsidered trifles which the copyist neglects to imitate and yet which every artist executes in his own characteristic way. I was then greatly interested to learn that the Russian pseudonym concealed the identity of an Italian physician called Morelli, who died in 1891. It seems to me that his method of inquiry is closely related to the technique of psychoanalysis. It, too, is accustomed to divine secret concealed things from despised or unnoticed features from the rubbish-heap, as it were, of our observations.[33]

As if to confirm the point Freud further spells out the message in the *Introductory Lectures*:

It is true that psycho-analysis cannot boast that it has never occupied itself with trifles. On the contrary, the material of its observations is usually those commonplace occurrences which have been cast aside as all too insignificant by other sciences, the refuse, so to speak of the phenomenal world.[34]

His comment may be placed alongside Wind's observation:

> To some of Morelli's critics it has seemed odd 'that personality should be found where personal effort is weakest'. But on this point modern psychology would certainly support Morelli: our inadvertent little gestures reveal our character more authentically than any formal posture that we may carefully prepare.[35]

Commenting on the common ground between Morelli and Freud, Wollheim makes the connection directly:

> For Morelli a detail was important, if, first, it is free from conventional pressures and, secondly...it has a significance for the artist; just as, in Freudian analysis, a trait must first have acquired a meaning for the person...before it can do so for the analyst.[36]

And Arnold Hauser goes still further:

> Psychoanalysis tries to detect stylistic character from accessories, from unobvious yet revealing details rather than from essentials. Being a kind of psychology of exposure, it follows up clues rather than plain and direct forms of expression and expects the artist to give himself away, more or less as a neurotic patient does, neglecting, however, the fundamental difference, that the meaning of a style is not a puzzle, but a guide. In accord with the spirit of his detective work, Freud was deeply impressed by Morelli's method in art history as an attempt to establish the identity of stylistic trends, above all from those features of a work of art which had least to do with the artist's conscious and deliberate ways of expression. That is to say, the fashion in which a painter has drawn an ear or formed a finger, the character of his handwriting, of which he might not even have been aware, was, Morelli claimed, more revealing than the features by which the meant to express himself most clearly.[37]

So far, so good. But if Zadig's method of retrospective prophecy helps bridge the gap between our doctor and our fictional detective, it remains to enquire why this particular piece of fiction? To answer this question it becomes necessary to look more closely at the phenomenon rather than at the stories and the character of Mr Sherlock Holmes.

The phenomenon of Sherlock Holmes

Holmes first appeared in 1887 in a story published in *Beeton's Christmas Annual* by an unknown young physician, Arthur Conan Doyle (see Figure 1.4). Success was instantaneous and prolonged. The six stories that were

Figure 1.4   Sir Arthur Conan Doyle

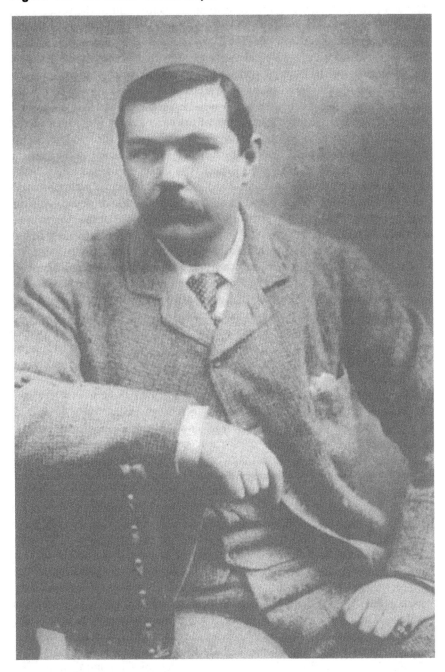

Source: BBC Hulton Picture Library.

originally commissioned eventually extended to sixty. They made Conan Doyle a rich man, enabling him to give up medicine, and in the process the character began to overshadow its creator. As early as 1893, when the *Strand Magazine* announced the impending death of Sherlock Holmes, public reaction was evident: mourning bands were worn in the City and the event was headline news in the foreign press. Holmes's resurrection led to an even greater mass response and many thousands of letters asking for help were addressed to 221B Baker Street. Nor was the interest confined to anglophonic readers. In 1895 an Arabic translation of the early stories was said to have been issued to the Egyptian police force as a textbook. France underwent an outbreak of 'Sherlockitis' inspired by a M. Herlock Sholmès, and a rash of medico-legal studies based on the canon. The Germans coined a new verb, 'sherlockieren' (to deduce or track down), and 'Sherlockismus' was compared with Werthermania. In Spain and Latin American Sherlockholmistos spread rapidly and the Russian, Turkish, and Romanian versions of the stories were rapturously received; in the Soviet Union they were to be recommended to the Red Army as a model of 'magnificent strength and great culture'.

As early as 1902, furthermore, the *Cambridge Review* carried an open letter to Dr Watson concerning the dates given in *The Hound of the Baskervilles*. This was the forerunner of a huge secondary literature which has included scholarly essays, journals, parodies, plays, and filmscripts. To date Holmes has been the subject of some three hundred films, a ballet, and several books, including eight full-scale biographies. Three bibliographies of Holmesiana have been published, each containing more than six thousand items.

For the most part Conan Doyle was both mystified and irritated by these developments. As early as 1896 he announced that Holmes was 'dead and damned' and that he felt towards him as he would to an overdose of *pâté de foie gras*. The success of Sherlock Holmes, he maintained, overshadowed his more original writings and his major work on spiritualism. None the less, after Doyle's death in 1930 a metempsychosis occurred and the reputation of the character has continued to grow steadily. Except for the Bible, no other writings have been published in as many different languages and editions as the tales of Sherlock Holmes. Visitors to London today who consult their *Michelin Guide* will find the entry for Baker Street beginning: 'The wide thoroughfare was 100 years old when Sherlock Holmes in the 1880s went to live at 221B.' In 1941 *The Times* carried an obituary commenting on the fiftieth year of Holmes's first demise. The British Society of Sherlockians meets regularly to dine at the Law Society and discuss the master and his exploits. The Japanese have a society, a magazine, and a pub in Tokyo, the 'Sherlock Holmes', with artificial fog on the ceiling. Other prominent associations perpetuating the legend include the 'Baker Street Irregulars', the 'Speckled Band of Boston', the 'Creeping Men of Cleveland', and 'The Wisteria Lodge Confederates of the Eastern Deep South', all with their individual rituals and apparel, and mostly containing a strong representation of physicians, especially medical historians. Much speculation has been devoted to particular diagnostic issues. What was the nature of Dr Watson's war wound? Did Holmes suffer from Marfan's Syndrome? And, as we have seen, was he dependent on cocaine?

From even these bare facts, then, it is apparent that in less than a hundred years the character of Sherlock Holmes has come to transcend time and space. As recently as July 1984 *The Times* could carry a letter entitled 'Greatly Exaggerated', by a reader complaining that he was

> disturbed to read in your columns . . . a reference to 'the late Mr Holmes'. I trust that since Mr Sherlock Holmes's death has not been confirmed in your obituary columns you will request your excellent Executive Editor not to spread such unjustified rumours of the loss of one of England's greatest men in future.[38]

As Orson Welles has observed, he is a man who never lived but will never die. He has, in short, left the world of fiction to enter the realms of myth.

Myth and mythod

Mythological characters are of central importance to creative writers and can be subdivided into two categories: those which are apocryphal (e.g. Faust, King Arthur, Don Juan), and those which are the products of an individual author's imagination (e.g. Frankenstein, Don Quixote). The capacity to create such characters, furthermore, is often independent of artistic merit, a point made with some authority by the poet, W. H. Auden:

> All characters who are products of the mythopoeic imagination are instantaneously recognizable by the fact that their existence is not defined by their social and historical context. . . . In consequence, once they have been created, they cease to be their author's characters and become the reader's; he can continue their story for himself. Anna Karenina is not such a character, for the reader cannot imagine her apart from the particular milieu in which Tolstoi places her or the particular history of her life which he records; Sherlock Holmes, on the other hand, is: every reader, according to his fancy, can imagine adventures for him which Conan Doyle forgot, as it were, to tell us. Tolstoi was a very great novelist, Conan Doyle a very minor one, yet it is the minor not the major writer who possesses the mythopoeic gift. The mythopoeic imagination is only accidentally related, it would seem, to the talent for literary expression.[39]

The phenomenon of Sherlock Holmes becomes comprehensible only if the character is viewed as the representation of a method embedded in a myth.

Then it also becomes possible to appreciate the force of a central paradox, namely that the presentation of Zadig's method is a counterfeit, a simulacrum of the real thing, what might be termed neologistically a 'mythod'. As a contemporary physician has remarked, the Sherlockian mode of procedure, 'although labelled as deductive and logical, is really intuitive and illogical, but it is so appealingly human that it is enjoyable in contrast to the tedium of a true analytic detective story'.[40] Thus in the example quoted earlier, a moment's reflection makes it apparent that there are several other explanations for Watson's irregular conduct. 'Therefore', 'obvious', 'evident', 'more than probable', says Holmes, but what he describes as 'absurdly simple' might as well have been termed 'simply absurd'. Hugh Kingsmill characterized Sherlock Holmes as an 'inspired imbecile', and Joseph Bell himself referred to the 'cataract of drivel for which Conan Doyle is responsible'. Christopher Isherwood drew the irreverent but inescapable conclusion when he described him as 'one of the truly great comic characters in our literature ... the classic caricature of the Amateur Detective in whose person the whole art of detection is made ridiculous ... [this] is what makes Holmes lovable and immortal'.[41]

Lovable and immortal, perhaps, but more a model of dogmatic assumption than of scientific detection. As one of Doyle's biographers remarks of the Holmes stories: 'It is only deduction if the reader can be made to believe that it is, by suspending his critical faculties.'[42] Within the protective carapace of a myth, however, reality assumes a different meaning. We enter another sphere of logic and it is only in these terms that we can at last approach the case of Dr Freud in its broader historical context.

Psychoanalysis and myth

In his 1908 preface to *The Interpretation of Dreams*, Freud commented sourly on its neglect by the three professional groups for whom it was written, attributing the demand for a second edition principally to what he termed the 'wider circle of educated and curious-minded readers'.[43] This was the circle which was to expand so greatly that in the preface to a subsequent edition Freud admitted candidly that: 'Just as formerly I was unwilling to regard the neglect of my book by readers as evidence of its worthlessness, so I cannot claim that the interest which is now being taken in it is a proof of its excellence.'

With the passage of time the significance of his verdict has become increasingly apparent. Freud himself attached prime importance to his scientific method, to having discovered what James Strachey calls 'the first instrument for the examination of the human mind'.[44] The three groups for whom his work was intended were the clinicians, the scientists, and the philosophers, but after more than three generations it is apparent that for the most part none of these groups has endorsed either his method or its application. The reasons for their refusal to do so are now so well known as to qualify for what Sherlock Holmes would have called the 'commonplace', and call for no more than a brief mention. For the clinicians it is chiefly the therapeutic claims of psychoanalysis which have been eroded, leading to a sharp decline in its prestige, even in the United States where it was most widely incorporated in clinical practice.[45] In his searching and lucid critique of the topic Sir Peter Medawar places particular emphasis on this issue as 'the only independent criterion by which the acceptability of psycho-analytic notions can be judged'.[46] For the biological scientist, he continues, the subject-matter of psychoanalysis is essentially unbiological and is rarely susceptible to experimental examination; and for the philosopher of science it fails to meet the fundamental criteria of refutation. The evidence marshalled by Fisher and Greenberg testifies to the effort invested in attempts to evaluate the theory and practice of psychoanalysis, the difficulties attendant on such an enterprise, and the ambiguity of the findings.[47]

What distinguishes Medawar's negative critique from that of most other scientists, however, is his further insistence that in as much as psychoanalysis merits consideration it does so not as a science but as a form of mythology which 'brings some kind of order into incoherence; it ... hangs together, makes sense, leaves no loose ends, and is never (but never), at a loss for explanation. In a state of bewilderment it may therefore bring comfort and relief'.[48] Medawar does not mean this as a compliment. As a scientific rationalist he favours Voltaire's view of all myths as fairy stories for savages, in this case forms of science fiction which echo the Romantic syllogism that lies can be myths which may in turn represent forms of truth. As far as it goes, his argument is watertight, challenging the dictionary definition of a myth as a story invented as a veiled explanation of a truth. For Medawar and like-minded critics there is no truth since: 'Freudian and other quasi-scientific psychologies are getting away with a concept of truthfulness which belongs essentially to imaginative literature, that in which the opposite of truth is not falsehood but another truth.' In this context the scientific/rational and the literary/mythical approaches to knowledge are profoundly opposed: 'Science tends to expel literature, and literature science from any territory to which they both have claims.'

Imaginative understanding

There is, however, another approach to mythology which has tended to fall outside the narrowly scientific thought-collective. In its modern form this is widely attributed to the Italian philosopher, Giambattista Vico (1668–1744), whose outlook has been summarized with admirable clarity by Isaiah Berlin:

> Vico looks at myths as evidence of the different categories in which experience was organized – spectacles, unfamiliar to us, through which

early man and remote peoples looked at the world in which they lived: the purpose is to understand whence we come, how we came to be where we are, how much or how little of the past we still carry with us. His approach is genetic, for it is only through its genesis, reconstructed by fantasia, guided by rules which he thinks he has discovered, that anything can be truly understood: not by some intuition of timeless essences, or empirical description or analysis of an object's present state.[49]

And, he continues:

This kind of knowledge is not knowledge of facts or of logical truths, provided by observation or the sciences of deductive reasoning; nor is it knowledge of how to do things; nor the knowledge provided by faith.... It is more like the knowledge we claim of a friend, of his character, of his ways of thought or action.... To do this, one must possess imaginative power of a high degree, such as artists, and, in particular, novelists require.

Vico's fantasia, or imaginative understanding, was the forerunner of what was to go by various names – empathy, intuitive sympathy, *Verstehen, Einfühlung* – and enable so critical a thinker as Emile Durkheim to put 'mythological truths' alongside 'scientific truths'. In his suggested typology of mythical functions G. S. Kirk distinguishes between the narrative-entertaining, the operative-valedatory, and the speculative-explanatory.[50] Of these it is the explanatory myth, representing an imaginative response to real problems, which is more closely related to scientific thinking. 'The value of myth for science', according to a contemporary assessment:

lies in providing a change of metaphor that creates a fresh focus, a new set of terms for dealing with intellectual material, and thus serves both to explain mental logjams and to provide a source of creativity in the search for answers. Solutions to scientific problems often require metaphors that may not yet be conceptualized.[51]

Viewed in this perspective, psychoanalysis as myth or 'mythod' can lay claim to scientific consideration, provided, first, that its metaphors are recognized for what they are and, second, that belief in the system as a whole be suspended. For the most part neither condition has been met, so that little headway has been made with its less sympathetic critics. Meanwhile, however, it has become clear that the declining reputation of the system in medical and scientific circles, disciples apart, impinges hardly at all on Freud's 'educated and curious-minded readers' for whom its mass appeal depends precisely on its imaginative rather than on its scientific character.

George Steiner, who may be taken as a polymathic representative of these readers, makes no bones about the matter. Conceding that much of classical psychoanalysis has lost any pretence to scientific status and that psychiatrists do not encounter patients who fit the Freudian paradigms, he concludes:

> Freud is one of the great mythologists, one of the great writers and imaginers of an arching metaphor of ordering myth and ritual (the analytic seance). His fantastic overvaluation of the sexual, the archaic alphabet of dreams which he put forward with such stylistic genius, his stoic agnosticism, are fading fast in the sumptuous mausoleum of the central European, middle-class, patriarchal *belle époque*.
>
> No less than Marxism, Freudian psychoanalysis remains one of the feats of the messianic Judaic vision for man after his emancipation from religiosity. Myth, be it that of an Oedipus complex, be it that of an Arcadia of human 'adulthood', is of its essence.[52]

Literature and mythology

A host of imaginative artists have responded gratefully to the metaphors, the language, and the allusions of Freudian theory, whose influence on the visual, literary, and musical arts of the twentieth century has been profound, as the history of the surrealist movement illustrates *par excellence*.[53] Some writers have repaid that debt by an emphatic understanding of its source, no one more searchingly than Thomas Mann, for whom: 'The mythical interest is as native to psychoanalysis as the psychological interest is to creative writing.'[54] This was, of course, fully recognized by its founder, who expressed his belief on more than one occasion that the roots of neurosis were to be found in mythological sources, and predicted to Carl Jung that together they would conquer the whole field of mythology. The historian of science, Frank Sulloway, concludes his massive study of Freud's thought with a catalogue of the twenty-six major myths which have contributed to the Freud legend.[55] And, significantly, since every narrative myth requires its hero, Sulloway pays special attention not only to the mythic content of Freud's ideas but to the personalization of his role in his own mythology, echoing Jung's perceptive comment of seventy years earlier: 'Like Heracles of old, you are human hero and demi-God, wherefore your dicta unfortunately carry with them a sempiternal value.'[56]

The dicta also carry literary overtones. Thus D. M. Thomas, introducing his remarkable novel *The White Hotel*, speaks explicitly of Freud and the 'discoverer of the great and beautiful myth of psychoanalysis', incorporates him as one of the *dramatis personae*, and includes a wholly convincing clinical case history, supposedly written by Freud himself, to present his heroine.[57] In justifying the procedure Thomas goes still further, claiming that:

In his case-studies Freud was often fictionalizing.... These are white hotel stories that Freud was writing...I suspect that for Freud it was just as important to get a good story, a well-shaped classical Greek story, as to get at the truth.[58]

Recalling Karl Popper's description of *The Interpretation of Dreams* as a collection of Homeric tales, Thomas's comment brings us back to the case histories, the keystone of the whole edifice. The few published accounts of Freud's personal cases usually render it difficult, if not impossible, to ascertain their veracity, but there is one exception. Anna Freud has acknowledged that the Wolf Man 'is the only one able and willing to co-operate actively in the reconstruction and follow-up of his case'.[59] Freud's original paper[60] purported to trace the sources of the subject's obsessional symptomatology back to childhood sexual experience, and on these retrospectively prophetic foundations there is constructed an ingenious set of theoretical causes relating to anal eroticism, castration fears, the primal scene, and the psychodynamics of obsessions. At the termination of the four-and-a-half-year-long analysis Freud regarded the patient as 'cured'. Some years later, however, he relapsed with a full-blown psychotic disorder, diagnosed by his second psychoanalyst as 'the hypochondriacal type of paranoia',[61] of which no trace had been detected by Freud. Again he was deemed to have been cured, but for the rest of his long life the Wolf Man remained intermittently unwell and dependent on psychiatric support, and in his final years, as alert and introspective as ever, he was persuaded to discuss his life in a series of talks with an independent interviewer. His personal affection for Freud remained undimmed but he was not uncritical of the way in which his doctors had employed Zadig's method, as the following example reveals:

w: In my story, what was explained by dreams? Nothing as far as I can see. Freud traces everything back to the primal scene which he derives from the dream. But that scene does not occur in the dream. When he interprets the white wolves as nightshirts or something like that, for example, linen sheets or clothes, that's something far-fetched, I think. That scene in the dream where the windows open and so on and the wolves are sitting there, and his interpretation, I don't know, those things are miles apart. It's terribly far-fetched.
o: But is it true that you did have that dream?
w: Yes it is
o: You must have told him other dreams.
w: Of course, but I no longer remember the dreams I told him.
o: And that didn't impress you when he interpreted dreams?
w: Well, he said it doesn't matter whether one takes note of that or not, consciously. The effect remains. I think that assertion would have to be

proven. I prefer free association because there, something can occur to you. But the primal scene is no more than a construct.

o: You mean the interpretation Freud derives from the dream, that you observed the coitus of your parents, the three acts of coitus?

w: The whole thing is improbable because in Russia, children sleep in the nanny's bedroom, not in their parents'. It's possible, of course, that there was an exception, how do I know? But I have never been able to remember anything of that sort.

In logic, you learn not to go from consequences to cause, but in the opposite direction, from cause to consequences. When, where we have an *a*, we also have a *b*, I must find a *b* when *a* recurs. If one does it the other way around, and concludes from effects to cause, it's the same thing as circumstantial evidence in a trial. But that's a weak argument isn't it? He maintains I saw it, but who will guarantee that it is so? That it is not a fantasy of his? That's one thing. We had best begin with the theory, and, secondly, when one makes something conscious that was in the subconscious, it doesn't help at all. Freud once said, 'I am a spiritual revolutionary'.... Well, I also have to look at psychoanalysis critically, I cannot believe everything Freud said, after all. I have always thought that the memory would come. But it never did.[62]

A striking 'white hotel' story, indeed, and one which may serve as a reminder of how closely this attempt to unravel the Platonic bond between Sherlock Holmes and Sigmund Freud involves the aspects of creative narrative which correspond to the mythic process and whose literary history, as Ricoeur observes, 'is a part of the long tradition emerging from the oral epic tradition of the Greeks, the Celts, and the Germans'.[63] It remains to identify the particular nature of the myth, and in his recently published study of the culture of psychoanalysis the Freudian literary scholar, Professor Steven Marcus, provides a helpful clue:

A few years before Freud began his great work, another physician-writer made his appearance in London. The work that he began to describe as being conducted at 221B Baker Street, makes for an interesting anticipation of the activities that would shortly begin in the Berggasse. The 'methods' of dealing with the material which is brought before the investigator this writer represented are well known ... Holmes believes that somehow all these stories actually and eventually make sense, and that he with his special skills can help bring overt and explicit sense to them and therefore to the reality to which they refer and whose structure they elliptically and fragmentarily represent ... although not everyone can tell it unaided.

It is worth noting, however, that the secrets and puzzles and ellipses in these stories always refer to outer reality – to sleeves, thumb-nails, boot-laces, and footprints; to wigs and paint and cobbler's wax; to thefts, frauds, lies, plots, and murders. The world is made coherent by solving these external mysteries.

When a few years later in Vienna, the physician-writer-detective with whom we are all familiar began to bring his work to the reading public he would base that work upon a strikingly similar set of assumptions and would present the world with a strikingly similar set of mysterious accounts. What the Viennese Holmes was going to do, however, was to take almost all the mysteries and secrets, and all the incoherent narratives, and place them inside. This shift from outer to inner reality marks a great historical transformation. On the one hand there seems to be something ironic in this circumstance that the detective story as a genre begins to flourish at just about the same moment in history when the locus of the mystery is in the course of dramatic change. On the other hand, the flourishing of the detective story (along with psychoanalysis, one might say) in the modern era does tell us something about the growth of a widespread and popular consciousness that the world has become an increasingly problematical place; that its structure is not immediately apprehensible; that we need help in understanding it; and that there may not be very much about the settled social or psychological order that we can take for granted. One way or another, it appears, we all need a detective. Whether he is a private eye or a third ear, we need him to help us get our lives and their stories straight.[64]

Detective fiction

With the detective story, therefore, we reach the point of our departure after following a trail which has led through cocaine, Zadig's method, the mytho-poeic faculty, and imaginative literature. The spectacular success of the detective story as a literary genre over the past 150 years has given rise to several historical studies,[65] and the typology and structure of detective fiction have been analysed with subtlety and erudition by Todorov.[66] In sociological terms it has been argued that 'what crime literature offered to its readers...was a reassuring world in which those who tried to disturb the established order were always discovered and punished'.[67] Psychological attempts at explanation have included several psychoanalytical interpretations. Thus Rycroft sees the criminal as personifying the reader's unavowed hostility to the parent,[68] while Pederson-Krag has asserted that the origins of the genre are to be found in the primal scene, the murder representing parental intercourse, the reader *qua* detective indulging in infantile curiosity, and Dr Watson supplying 'a safe defence, for should the punishing super-ego threaten, the reader can point to this character and say, "This is I. I was simply standing by." '[69] A more poetic and profound exposition is offered by Auden:

The fantasy... which the detective story addict indulges is the fantasy of being restored to the Garden of Eden, to a state of innocence, where he may know love and not as the law. The driving force behind this day-dream is a feeling of guilt, the cause of which is unknown to the dreamer. The fantasy of escape is the same, whether one explains the guilt in Christian, Freudian, or any other terms.[70]

This fertile suggestion has been tellingly extended by Brigid Brophy in her essay on the detective story as secular mythology.[71] In a secularized era which is short of myths, she argues: 'The cause in which the modern detective employs his method and his skills remains the same as that in which the Greek hero uses his magic powers and talismans – the deliverance of the population from a threat.' In detective stories, she continues, 'the only ones which laid down the pattern of a myth, it is guilt which is rationally understood and traced to its source'. On such foundations Sherlock Holmes and Sigmund Freud – the archetypical detective and the prototypical mental healer – are twinned as the contemporary heroes of an ancient legend. They take their place, furthermore, in the wake of the most prophetic myth-maker of the nineteenth century, Friedrich Nietzsche, who anticipated so much of Freud's thinking. It was Nietzsche who proclaimed the quietus of religious belief, equated truth with a new psychology, and predicted the substitution of the old gods by the *Ubermensch*, the new man, detached, quasi-omniscient. When Carl Jung described Nietzsche and Freud as 'answers to the sickness of the nineteenth century', he saw them as Joseph Bell's 'half doctors, half virtuosi'. And much of Holmes's appeal, as Julian Symons observes, is that: 'Far more than any of his later rivals, he was so evidently a Nietzschian superior man.'[72]

Perhaps this is the most fitting note on which to take leave of our two heroes, basking in mutual admiration in the pages of *The Seven Per Cent Solution*, two magi meeting appropriately in the no-man's-land between fact and fiction. The last word should surely go to Dr Watson, moved to bid farewell to his Viennese colleague with the highest compliment in his repertoire: 'Freud, you are the greatest detective of them all.'

References

1 N. Meyer, *The Seven Per Cent Solution*, London, Hodder & Stoughton, 1975.
2 S. Freud, 'From the history of an infantile neurosis', *The Standard Edition of the Complete Psychological Works of Sigmund Freud*, vol. 17, London, Hogarth Press and the Institute of Psycho-analysis, 1918 [1914], p. 7.
3 S. Freud, *Introductory Lectures on Psychoanalysis*, trans. J. Rivière, 2nd edn, London, Allen & Unwin, 1943.
4 S.K. Pankeyev, 'My recollections of Sigmund Freud', in M. Gardiner (ed.) *The Wolf Man and Sigmund Freud*, London, Hogarth Press, 1972, p. 135.

5   S. Freud, 'Letter to C.G. Jung', in W. McGuire (ed.) *The Freud/Jung Letters*, London, Hogarth Press and Routledge & Kegan Paul, 1974, pp. 234–5.

6   A. Kardiner, 'Freud – The man I knew, the scientist, and his influence', in B. Nelson (ed.) *Freud and the Twentieth Century*, London, Allen & Unwin, 1958, p. 46.

7   Occasional Correspondent, 'Was Sherlock Holmes a drug addict?', *Lancet*, 1936, ii: 1,555.

8   W.H. Miller, 'The habit of Sherlock Holmes', *Transactions and Studies of the College of Physicians of Philadelphia*, fifth series, 1978, 45: 252.

9   D.M. Grilly, 'A reply to Miller's "The Habit of Sherlock Holmes"', *Transactions and Studies of the College of Physicians of Philadelphia*, fifth series, 1978, 45: 324.

10 L. Goodman and A. Gilman, *The Pharmacological Basis of Therapeutics*, 5th edn, New York, Macmillan, 1975, p. 302.

11 W. Modell, 'Mass drug catastrophes and the roles of science and technology', *Science*, 1967, 156: 346.

12 A.C. Doyle, 'Gelsemium as a poison', *British Medical Journal*, 1879, 2: 483.

13 E. Jones, *Sigmund Freud: Life and Works*, London, Hogarth Press, 1953–7.

14 E.M. Thornton, *Freud and Cocaine*, London, Blond & Briggs, 1983.

15 D.F. Musto, 'Sherlock Holmes and heredity', *Journal of the American Medical Association*, 1966, 196, 1: 45.

16 B.M. Astrachan and S. Boltax, 'The cyclical disorder of Sherlock Holmes', *Journal of the American Medical Association*, 1966, 196, 12: 142.

17 G. Vash, 'The states of exhaustion of Mr Sherlock Holmes', *Journal of the American Medical Association*, 1966, 197, 8.

18 D.F. Musto, 'A study in cocaine', *Journal of the American Medical Association*, 1968, 204, 1: 27.

19 H.L. Klawans, 'The Norwegian explorer', in *The Medicine of History*, New York, Raven Press, 1982, p. 19.

20 H. How, 'A day with Dr Conan Doyle', *Strand Magazine*, 1892, 4: 186.

21 R. Blathwayt, 'A talk with Dr Conan Doyle', *Bookman*, 1892, 2: 50.

22 A.C. Doyle, quoted in R.L. Green (ed.) *The Uncollected Sherlock Holmes*, Harmondsworth, Penguin, 1983 [1892], p. 18.

23 J.M. Saxby, *Joseph Bell: An Appreciation by an Old Friend*, Edinburgh, Oliphant, Anderson & Ferrier, 1913.

24 J. Bell, 'The adventures of Sherlock Holmes: a review', *Bookman*, 1892, 2: 73.

25 Voltaire, 'Zadig', in *Candide and Other Tales*, trans. T. Smollett, London, Dent, 1937 [1748], p. 12.

26 T.H. Huxley, 'On the method of Zadig: retrospective prophecy as a function of science', in *Science and Culture, and Other Essays*, London, Macmillan, 1881 [1888], p. 128.

27 W. Whewell, *The Philosophy of the Inductive Sciences*, London, J.W. Parker, 1847.

28 G. Morelli, *Italian Painters: Critical Studies of the Works*, trans. L.M. Richter, London, G. Bell & Son, 1883.

29 R. Wollheim, 'Giovanni Morelli and the origins of scientific connoisseurship', in *On Art and the Mind: Essays and Lectures*, London, Allen Lane, 1973, p. 177.

30 E. Castelnuovo, 'Attribution', in *Encylopaedia Universalis*, vol. II, Paris, Pubs. Encylopaedia Universalis, 1968.

31 E. Wind, *Art and Anarchy*, London, Faber & Faber, 1963, p. 32.

32 C. Ginzburg, 'Morelli, Freud and Sherlock Holmes: clues and scientific method', *History Workshop*, 1980, 9: 5.

33 S. Freud, 'The Moses of Michelangelo', *The Standard Edition of the Complete Psychological Works of Sigmund Freud*, vol. 13, London, Hogarth Press and the Institute of Psycho-analysis, 1914, p. 222. Originally published in *Imago*, 3, 1: 15–36.
34 Freud, *Introductory Lectures*, op. cit.
35 Wind, op. cit.
36 Wollheim, op. cit.
37 A. Hauser, *The Philosophy of Art History*, London, Routledge & Kegan Paul, 1959.
38 J.A.C. Wilson, 'Greatly exaggerated', Letter to *The Times*, 19 July 1984.
39 W.H. Auden, 'Dingley Dell and the Fleet', in *The Dyer's Hand and Other Essays*, London, Faber & Faber, 1975, p. 407.
40 C.F. Kittle, 'Sir Arthur Conan Doyle – Physician and Detective', *Proceedings of the Institute of Medicine*, Chicago, Ill., 1981, 34, p. 7.
41 C. Isherwood, ' "The Speckled Band", by Arthur Conan Doyle', in *Exhumations*, Harmondsworth, Penguin, 1969, p. 106.
42 R. Pearsall, *Conan Doyle: A Biographical Solution*, London, Weidenfeld & Nicolson, 1977.
43 S. Freud, 'The Interpretation of Dreams', trans. J. Strachey, *The Standard Edition of the Complete Psychological Works of Sigmund Freud*, vols 4 and 5, London, Hogarth Press and the Institute of Psycho-analysis, 1953.
44 J. Strachey, 'Sigmund Freud: a sketch of his life and ideas', in *Two Short Accounts of Psychoanalysis*, Harmondsworth, Pelican, 1962.
45 J.H. Conn, 'The decline of psychoanalysis', *Journal of the American Medical Association*, 1974, 228, 6: 711.
46 P.B. Medawar, 'Further comments on psychoanalysis', in *The Hope of Progress*, London, Methuen, 1972, p. 57.
47 S. Fisher and R.P. Greenberg, *The Scientific Credibility of Freud's Theories and Therapy*, Brighton, Harvester Press, 1977.
48 P.B. Medawar, 'Science and literature', *Encounter*, 1969, 32, 1: 15.
49 I. Berlin, 'The divorce between the sciences and the humanities', in *Against the Current*, London, Oxford University Press, 1981.
50 G.S. Kirk, *Myth: Its Meaning and Function in Ancient and Other Cultures*, Cambridge, Cambridge University Press, 1970.
51 W.D. O'Flaherty, 'Inside and outside the mouth of God: the boundary between myth and reality', *Daedalus*, 1980, Spring: 93.
52 G. Steiner, 'Review of J.M. Masson's *Freud: The Assault on Truth*', *Sunday Times*, 27 May 1984.
53 M. Nadeau, *Histoire du Surréalisme*, Paris, Éditions du Seuil, 1964.
54 T. Mann, 'Freud and the future', in *Essays of Three Decades*, New York, Knopf, 1937.
55 F. Sulloway, *Freud, Biologist of the Mind*, London, Burnett Books, 1979.
56 C.G. Jung, 'Letter to Freud, 14.12.09', in W. McGuire (ed.) *The Freud/Jung Letters*, London, Hogarth Press and Routledge & Kegan Paul, 1974, p. 275.
57 D.M. Thomas, *The White Hotel*, London, Gollancz, 1981.
58 D.M. Thomas, 'Freud and "The White Hotel" ', *British Medical Journal*, 1983, 287, ii: 1,957.
59 A. Freud, 'Foreword', to M. Gardiner (ed.) *The Wolf Man and Sigmund Freud*, London, Hogarth Press and the Institute of Psycho-analysis, 1972, p. ix.
60 Freud, *Introductory Lectures*, op. cit.
61 R.M. Brunswick, 'A supplement to Freud's "History of an Infantile Neurosis" ', *International Journal of Psychoanalysis*, 1928, 9: 439.

62 K. Obholzer, *The Wolf Man Sixty Years Later*, Routledge & Kegan Paul, 1982.
63 P. Ricoeur, 'The question of proof in Freud's psychoanalytic writings', *Journal of the American Psychoanalytic Association*, 1977, 25: 835.
64 S. Marcus, *Freud and the Culture of Psychoanalysis*, London, Allen & Unwin, 1984.
65 J. Barzun, *A Catalogue of Crime*, New York, Harper & Row, 1971.
66 T. Todorov, 'The typology of detective fiction', in *The Poetics of Prose*, trans. R. Howard, Oxford, Blackwell, 1977, p. 42.
67 J. Symons, *Bloody Murder*, London, Faber & Faber, 1972.
68 C. Rycroft, 'A detective-story', *Psychoanalytic Quarterly*, 1957, 26: 229.
69 G. Pederson-Krag, 'Detective stories and the primal scene', *Psychoanalytic Quarterly*, 1949, 18: 207.
70 W.H. Auden, 'The guilty vicarage', in *The Dyer's Hand and Other Essays*, London, Faber & Faber, 1963, p. 146.
71 B. Brophy, 'Detective fiction: a modern myth of violence', in *Don't Never Forget*, London, Cape, 1966, p. 121.
72 Symons, op. cit.

Chapter two

Formulation of new research strategies on schizophrenia

I should begin by defining my terms of reference. When Professor Häfner first invited me to look into a crystal ball and formulate new research strategies in schizophrenia, I asked him whether my contribution was to be delivered in a session devoted to astrological psychiatry. He replied, with characteristic discretion, that he preferred to think in terms of astronomical psychiatry, exemplified by a star-studded symposium. Eventually, however, he returned to earth to explain that my contribution might serve to bridge the gap between the two general introductory reviews and the more specific papers to follow. A transitional paper of this type should allow for both a backward glance to where we have come from and an anticipation of where we are going without trespassing on the areas to be cultivated in this symposium. To try and achieve this objective I propose to subdivide my paper into three sections: definition, outcome, and causation.

In presenting this conspectus, however, I am conscious of the fact that any visitor who speaks about schizophrenia in Germany, particularly in Heidelberg, must choose his words with care. In his *Die Pathologie und Therapie der psychischen Krankheiten*, the book that Ludwig Binswanger justly called the Magna Carta of psychiatry, Wilhelm Griesinger comments that 'mental illness is only a symptom ... our classification depends on the symptomatological method by which alone can any classification be effected'.[1] Some of the fruits of the symptomatological method in respect to the schizophrenias were demonstrated to me at an early stage of my career by the late Wilhelm Mayer-Gross, to whom I turned for guidance concerning information about the disorder. He advised me to read the ninth volume of Bumke's handbook and learn about what he called 'Heidelberg schizophrenia'. In this volume, I came to realize, resides the evidence of how much of the groundwork of our knowledge of the schizophrenic syndrome was laid in Heidelberg, associated with such names as Karl Jaspers, Hans Gruhle, Kurt Schneider, and, of course, Emil Kraepelin.

Originally published in H. Häfner, W.F. Gattaz, and W. Janzarik (eds) *Search for the Causes of Schizophrenia*, Berlin, Springer Verlag, 1987.

Since the publication of that volume in 1932, however, the preoccupations of psychiatrists in Germany appear to have changed. Ten years ago Professor Janzarik's paper, 'The crisis in psychopathology', mentioned the 'disinterest and insecurity in tune with the spirit of modern times',[2] and last year, in his retrospective survey of the past forty years of German psychiatry,[3] Professor J.E. Meyer has identified seven themes as dominant during this period: (1) the era of 'shock' treatment, (2) the introduction of psychotropic drugs, (3) *Daseinsanalyse*, (4) the separation of psychiatry from neurology, (5) the Enquête Commission report, (6) psychiatry and psychotherapy, and (7) psychiatry and National Socialism. It is noteworthy that several of these topics are primarily of German national interest and that Professor Meyer mentions schizophrenia only twice, once in relation to insulin coma therapy and once in relation to neuroleptic drugs. If this may be taken as an overview of the situation during a difficult period of destruction and reconstruction, the situation in other countries was very different, much of it being concerned with the first of my three categories, namely definition.

Definition

From the late 1930s the torch of the German tradition was carried elsewhere, and helped light the fires of investigation throughout Europe and North America. By the early 1950s Manfred Bleuler was able to publish a massive review article of some 1,100 articles, most of them published in the UK, the USA, France, or Italy, which he entitled 'Research and changes in the study of schizophrenia, 1941–1950'.[4] The great majority of these studies, however, paid little regard to the need for agreement on terminology, concepts, or communication, and, significantly, the principal factor prompting Bleuler to undertake this daunting task was the First International Congress of Psychiatry held in Paris in 1950, when, as he pointed out, there emerged 'the realisation of the dangerous fact that we can no longer understand one another'.

The justice of this verdict was endorsed in 1957 at the Second International Congress, which was devoted entirely to schizophrenia. The foyer of the conference building was dominated by a large pyramid of books with one enormous volume entitled *Schizophrenia: New Knowledge* at the apex. Laying hands on it was no easy task, but one day I managed to ascend the biblio-mountain and bring the book down to ground level. It proved to be a pre-publication copy whose cover enclosed several hundred pages of blank paper! This mighty volume – impressive in appearance but empty of content – symbolized much of the meeting. A glance at the proceedings shows why this was so, for many disputations among the eminent clinicians on the subject of diagnosis was conducted in a manner reminiscent more of a medieval school of theology than of a scientific meeting. Indeed, one the symposia was devoted appropriately to the concepts of St Thomas Aquinas and Aristotle. The divine rights of the *Ordinarius* were stoutly defended and an outspoken participant reflected the spirit of the occasion as follows: 'You say this is a case of schizophrenia. Do you mean schizophrenia as Dr *X*, my chief, uses it or are you referring to schizophrenia as construed by your chief, Dr *Y* ?'[5]

This state of affairs was evidently no longer good enough, even for Heidelberg schizophrenia. One year later, in 1958, the WHO invited Erwin Stengel to examine the Tower of Babel which housed the schemata of classification in use at the time. Looking to the future, Stengel pointed out that while a scientifically based nosology depends ultimately on causal knowledge, communication can be greatly improved by widespread use of operational concepts and definitions, which, in turn, demand a common language and an acceptable nomenclature. With regard to the schizophrenias Stengel was explicit:

> Schizophrenia, then, as an operational concept, would not be an illness, or a specific reaction type, but an argued operational definition for certain types of abnormal behaviour .... The question, therefore, which a person or group of persons trying to reach agreement on a national or international classification ought to answer is not what schizophrenia ... is, but what interpretation should be placed on these concepts for the purpose of communication.[6]

If this seems a modest objective it does no more than echo Kraepelin's own retrospective assessment of his own system: 'I should like to emphasise that some of the clinical pictures outlined are no more than attempts to present part of the material observed in a communicable form.'[7]

It was against this background that in the early 1960s the WHO initiated a large-scale programme to standardize the psychiatric diagnosis, classification, and statistics, aiming to obtain international agreement on the use of one public system rather than on a multiplicity of private systems. This became known as Programme A, for which I must bear some responsibility as the organizer of the initial study of schizophrenia in 1965 which served as the prototype for the series. In the light of subsequent developments, incidentally, it is worth recalling that there were no American psychiatrists at that meeting, an invitation having failed to attract a single senior psychiatrist with sufficient interest in nosology to attend. It would have been difficult then to predict the appearance of DSM-III only fifteen years later.

The original WHO study, based on videotapes and written case histories, was focused on observer variation in the assessment of schizophrenia.[8] The findings demonstrated that the factors leading to disagreement and difficulty in communication derive from three principal sources, namely (1) variations in clinical observation and perception, (2) variations in the inferences drawn from these data, and (3) variations in the individual classificatory schemata employed. By the same token, it became apparent that variation in the first two of these categories could be reduced substantially by the introduction of a multidimensional system of classification which was recommended for public statistical purposes so as to do justice to the multifactorial nature of the condition. These objectives became more urgent as a result of the surge of biological investigations that followed the introduction of psychotropic drugs. The report of a WHO Scientific Group on 'Biological research in schizophrenia' at about the same time made the point explicitly:

> If it is possible to obtain an accurate detailed description of the patient's behaviour and present state and of changes in these factors over a period of time, it would appear to be unnecessary to insist on obtaining rigid agreement among different investigators on a precise diagnostic classification. The main requirement is that collaborating investigators in different centres should establish empirically that, despite theoretical differences, they can use the same clinical measuring instruments and arrive at similar quantitative conclusions concerning aspects of a patient's present state.... Given a sufficient number of reliable indices of this kind, correlations can be sought between individual clinical symptoms and syndromes and biological data. Agreement on a system of clinical diagnosis can then become a goal rather than pre-condition for collaborative... studies of schizophrenia.[9]

The past fifteen years have witnessed the flowering of this approach, resulting in a plethora of studies which make use of clinical data, computer-derived syndromes, numerical taxonomy, and ingenious statistical analysis. No doubt this acknowledgement of the need for numeracy represents a form of progress; there are very few tables and figures in the 783 pages of the ninth volume of Bumke's handbook. Far more of this concern, however, has to do with *reliability*, that is the consistency with which a measure assesses a given trait, than with *validity*, that is the extent to which the measure actually measures the trait. Bartko and Carpenter identified the importance of this distinction ten years ago:

> Establishing validity of a concept such as schizophrenia might be achieved by finding that patients so diagnosed can be distinguished from other patient groups by certain genetic, biochemical, psychological, course or treatment variables. However, to the extent that schizophrenic patients cannot be reliably diagnosed, one cannot expect to find a consistent set of validating data. Hence, even if a concept is valid, reliability in its use is required to assure communicative value and to provide the foundation for scientific evaluation.[10]

Underlying this approach, then, is the assumption that the schizophrenic syndrome can be defined provided that a satisfactory method of dealing with its phenomenological heterogeneity can be devised. Dr Carpenter and his colleagues have neatly summed up the sources of the confusion in astronomical terms (though in a manner quite different from that of Professor Häfner) by identifying four categories.[11] First comes the anti-matter approach, whereby heterogeneity is reduced through the annihilation of all causes failing to meet predetermined criteria. Second, the black-hole approach, which consigns all annihilated cases to the black hole of affective illness. Third, the satellite approach, assuming the existence of the two Kraepelinian planets and defining atypical disorders as satellites of uncertain provenance. Finally, the nova approach, assuming the possibility of more than two major stars and of heterogeneity as a mode of discovery in its own right.

A host of investigators are now employing their telescopes and space probes in the universe of phenomenology to try and decide between these alternatives, a choice which must influence research strategy. Relatively few of these workers, however, focus their attention on outcome, to which I now turn as my second category.

Outcome

The importance of outcome as the natural history of disease was emphasized by Griesinger as part of his argument against the notion of an ontological theory of illness. 'The nature, the concept of disease', he wrote, 'emerges only from the entire history of the disease ... i.e. the gradual progression of qualitative dysfunction ... In this way a *natural history* of the process of a disease will be observed, but in an entirely different sense from that given by the natural history school.'[12]

Not the least of the advantages attaching to this standpoint is that it lends itself to empirical clinical research. Richard Warner's interactionist model, adapted from that of Strauss and Carpenter, incorporates the prodromal phase of illness in its natural history (see Figure 2.1).[13]

Most of the individual items specified in this model are either clinical, psychological, or social. As individual beads on an interactionist thread they are discussed in some detail in this symposium. Their potential significance has become more evident with the growing awareness that the diagnosis of schizophrenia is not synonymous with a poor prognosis. Eugen Bleuler wrote in 1908: 'As yet I have never released a schizophrenic in whom I could detect signs of the disease; indeed, there are very few in whom one would have to search for such signs.'[14] None the less, less than thirty years later Ødegaard pointed out that subsequent follow-up studies have indicated that the picture had changed.[15] To date, however, these studies have been bedevilled by defects which have rendered the findings ambiguous.

Figure 2.1 Interactional model for factors possibly affecting the onset, course, and outcome of schizophrenia

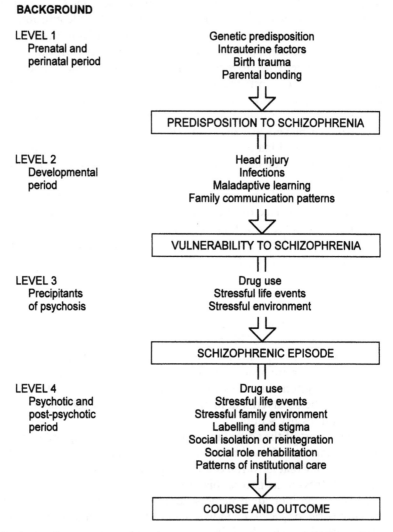

BACKGROUND

LEVEL 1
  Prenatal and
  perinatal period

Genetic predisposition
Intrauterine factors
Birth trauma
Parental bonding

PREDISPOSITION TO SCHIZOPHRENIA

LEVEL 2
  Developmental
  period

Head injury
Infections
Maladaptive learning
Family communication patterns

VULNERABILITY TO SCHIZOPHRENIA

LEVEL 3
  Precipitants
  of psychosis

Drug use
Stressful life events
Stressful environment

SCHIZOPHRENIC EPISODE

LEVEL 4
  Psychotic and
  post-psychotic
  period

Drug use
Stressful life events
Stressful family environment
Labelling and stigma
Social isolation or reintegration
Social role rehabilitation
Patterns of institutional care

COURSE AND OUTCOME

Source: R. Warner, *Recovery from Schizophrenia*, London, Routledge & Kegan Paul, 1985.

It is now clear that the design of a study aiming to elucidate the natural history of schizophrenia must take account of at least four factors: (1) the identification of all cases in a defined population during a fixed period of time; (2) the application of standardized diagnostic procedures with criteria of known reliability; (3) prospective follow-up procedures, preferably from the onset of first attachment for at least five years, with interim as well as end-point assessments and, preferably, uniform treatment regimes throughout the follow-up period; (4) standardized and independent clinical and social measures of outcome.

Of these criteria, the first remains the most difficult to satisfy. The identification of schizophrenia is traditionally made by hospital contact, on the assumption that in conditions of adequate medical care the patients suffering from the disorder will make contact with the mental health services. It may be recalled, however, that Kraepelin, in the fifth edition of his textbook, pointed out that there were probably many people who had suffered an attack of dementia praecox which had not been sufficiently severe to bring them to specialist attention.[16] In this context, particular interest attaches to Watts's virtually unique report on the long-term fate of a cohort of schizophrenics in his general practice population of 15,000 over the period 1946–83.[17] The diagnosis of all patients was confirmed by referral to a psychiatric institution, and there was a sharp fall in such referrals over the five years. Overall, furthermore, the outcome was much better than is generally assumed.

No hospital-based investigation has so far met all four specified criteria, but we have gone some way to doing so in a five-year prospective clinical and social follow-up study carried out on a representative cohort of 121 patients living within a stable, delimited population of an English county. An outline of this study has already been published,[18] and here I would make only a few points relevant to this symposium.

The first of these relates to clinical outcome which, again, belies the uniformly gloomy prognosis recorded by the early workers (see Figure 2.2). So marked a variation between good and poor prognostic groups raises questions in its own right, and a multivariate analysis was carried out to try and account for the differences. In the event, most of the variance could not be satisfactorily explained in terms of the variables included. Here is clearly a challenging area for new research strategies, whether they be focused on more complex psychosocial factors like 'expressed emotion' or biological factors like the immunoglobulin concentrations studied by Pulkinnen in relation to outcome.[19]

Mention may also be made of two striking sex differences. The first of these was the more favourable outcome enjoyed by females, a finding which has been confirmed by several other workers.[20] Most obviously, twice as many women experienced complete five-year remission, while more than twice as many men underwent a deteriorating course. Further, the average period of hospital care was three times longer among men than women over the quinquennium, though the same proportion of both sexes (35 per cent) displayed a relapsing course. Social functioning was consistently better among women on all variables.

The other sex difference relates to the age of onset of schizophrenic symptoms. By the age of 30 approximately 70 per cent of the men had

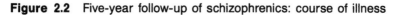

Figure 2.2 Five-year follow-up of schizophrenics: course of illness

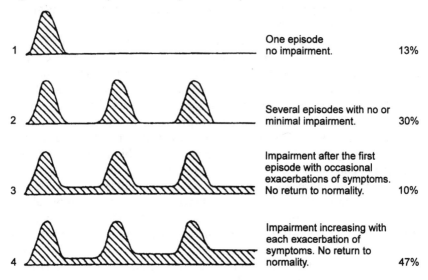

1   One episode no impairment.   13%

2   Several episodes with no or minimal impairment.   30%

3   Impairment after the first episode with occasional exacerbations of symptoms. No return to normality.   10%

4   Impairment increasing with each exacerbation of symptoms. No return to normality.   47%

Source: D.C. Watt, K. Katz, and M. Shepherd, 'The natural history of schizophrenia: a 5-year prospective follow-up of a representative sample of schizophrenics by means of a standardised clinical and social assessment', *Psychological Medicine,* 1983, 13: 663–70.

exhibited clinical symptomatology, compared with only 42 per cent of the women. The incidence rates are none the less equal in the two sexes. There is, therefore, the unusual profile of a condition with an identical cumulative sex incidence and a similar symptom picture, but dissimilar age of onset and outcome. Among the tentative explanations which have been advanced to account for these sex differences are stress, drug compliance, and the protective effects of natural oestrogens. None of these associations has been established, however, and all of them call for further investigation in the formulation of new research strategies.

Causation

Finally, a few words about causation. Here we can do no better than return once more to Griesinger, who recognized that the definition and classification of all mental illness must ultimately be based on causal factors but drew a fundamental distinction between aetiology and pathogeny. Of the former he wrote

> The conclusion, post hoc ergo propter hoc, depends...on a simple empirical (statistical) knowledge of the fact that these particular circumstances (for example, hereditary disposition) very frequently coincide

with, or precede, the commencement of the insanity...the province of *aetiology* in the narrow sense is only to enumerate empirically the known circumstances of causation.[21]

This is the province of what has been called clinical cartography or, more often, clinical epidemiology. By contrast, Griesinger states that it is the task of *pathogeny* to explain 'the physiological connection between cause and effect, to show the particular mechanical act by means of which insanity is induced through a given circumstance..., a task towards which we have hitherto done little more than prepare the way'. This is the province of biological science, and is conducted in or using the resources of the laboratory.

Traditionally the quest for pathogenic causes has been in terms of a single, pre-potent factor – a toxin, an infectious agent, a metabolic defect, a dietary deficiency. The evidence bearing on the genetic determinants of the schizophrenic syndrome, however, makes it necessary to consider a more complex multifactorial model, acknowledging that we may be confronted with either clinical diversity in genetic unity or genetic diversity in clinical unity. One of the most persuasive models of this type was advanced by Paul Meehl some years ago.[22] Meehl proposed what he termed a 'causal chain from gene through biochemical endophenotype (e.g. synaptic slippage) to behavioural dispositions to the ultimate learned behaviour' (see Figure 2.3).

Central to this notion is the postulate that 'clinical schizophrenia as such cannot be inherited because it has behavioural and phenomenal contents which are learned'. What is inherited is what he calls 'schizotaxia', a 'subtle neurointegrative defect' associated with a 'schizotypic' personality organization. It is this schizotaxia, according to Meehl, which represents the endophenotype which will eventually be identified in biochemical and neurophysiological terms. If environmental and interpersonal factors are favourable and there are also robust personality traits, the individual remains a well-compensated schizotype with no evidence of mental disease but with faint signs of what Meehl calls 'cognitive slippage and other minimal neurological aberrations'. This theoretical model has since received some support from empirical findings, including those of Kety and his co-workers on the Danish twin-study data.[23]

The causal chain is extended in Warner's model, to which I have already alluded.[24] Here 'predisposition' and 'vulnerability' make their appearance up to the outbreak of the schizophrenic episode and other factors bearing on outcome are identified. Much of the remainder of this symposium is devoted to the pathogenic and the aetiological links in this long, sequential chain. Future research will, I suggest, be concerned with the interaction between pathogeny and aetiology and, doubtless, among them and other, as yet unidentified factors. Meanwhile, I would emphasize that in the absence of an established biological marker for the clinical investigator, the significance

Figure 2.3 Meehl's causal chain

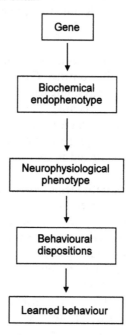

Source: P.E. Meehl, 'Schizotaxia, schizotypy, schizophrenia', *American Psychologist*, 1962, 17: 827–38.

of all such factors – whether they be life events or viruses, family communication, or season of birth – depends on the strength of an association and is therefore essentially epidemiological. Ideally, therefore, a representative population is needed within which it could be possible to study both these associations and the clinical features of the covert as well as the overt disorder.

In this task there is a key role for the clinician alongside the biological and epidemiological investigator, especially in the assessment of psychological dysfunction, still the elusive core of the schizophrenic syndrome. There, if anywhere, is where an operational definition of 'thought disorder', Meehl's 'cognitive slippage', has to be established. Psychological enquiry has already demonstrated that thought disorder is in part a form of perceptual aberration; that it is less specific than was formerly believed; that it is readily modifiable by operant techniques; and that most controlled experiments provide results that are unreliable and non-replicable. Recent work[25] suggests that neurological findings are less promising than studies of psychological constructs like the Thought Disorder Index,[26] but it is, I think, instructive to learn from Allen's recent report that while both sophisticated clinical and experimental tests failed to discriminate between the speech of non-speech-disordered schizophrenics and the speech of normal subjects, an experienced clinician was able to do so without being able to identify the factors contributing to his own success.[27] This would seem to indicate a need to examine clinical acumen still more carefully, in the light of the newer neuro-psychological techniques.

Finally, I would also mention another source of information for clinical enquiry, namely the patient, for whom the exclusion of the diagnosis of schizophrenia is as important as its confirmation. Let me conclude by citing a former patient of my own, one of the foremost living creative writers, who was originally admitted to a psychiatric institution in her teens with a diagnosis of schizophrenia. There she remained for three to four years, was treated with 200 ECTs and narrowly escaped prefrontal leucotomy. By chance we were able to see her some years later and eliminate the diagnosis on clinical grounds. Since then she has remained well and in her recently published autobiography she describes the impact of the clinical verdict:

I myself had suddenly been stripped of a garment I had worn for 12 or 13 years, my schizophrenia... I remembered how...I had accepted it, how in the midst of the agony and terror of the acceptance I found the unexpected warmth, comfort, protection: how I had longed to be rid of the opinion but was unwilling to part with it, and even when I did not wear it openly, I always had it by for an emergency, to put on quickly, for shelter from the cruel world. And now it was gone... banished officially by experts. I could never turn to it again for help.[28]

Her comment has, I would maintain, some relevance to the definition, outcome, and causation of schizophrenia and for any research strategy that may be adopted.

References

1 W. Griesinger, *Die Pathologie und Therapie der psychischen Krankheiten*, Stuttgart, Krabbe, 1845.
2 W. Janzarik, 'The crisis in psychopathology', *Nervenarzt*, 1976, 47: 73–80.
3 J.E. Myer, *Psychiatrie im XX. Jahrhundert: ein Rückblick*, Göttingen, Gotze, 1985.
4 M. Bleuler, 'Research and changes in concepts in the study of schizophrenia', *Bulletin of the Isaac Ray Medical Library*, 1955, 3, 1 and 2: 1–132.
5 N.C. Surya, 'Some remarks concerning an anthology of psychiatric definitions', in *Congress Report IV*, Second International Congress for Psychiatry, Zurich, Orell Fussli, 1959.
6 E. Stengel, 'Classification of mental disorders', *Bulletin of the World Health Organization*, 1959, 21: 601.
7 E. Kraepelin, 'Die Erscheinungsformen des Irreseins', *Zeitschrift für die gesamte Neurologie und Psychiatrie*, 1920, 62: 1–29.
8 M. Shepherd, E.M. Brooke, J.E. Cooper, and T.Y. Lin, 'An experimental approach to psychiatric diagnosis', *Acta Psychiatrica Scandinavica*, 1968, Supplement 210.

9   Report of a WHO Scientific Group, *Biological Research in Schizophrenia*, World Health Organization Technical Report Series no. 450, 1980.

10 J.J. Bartko and W.T. Carpenter, 'On the methods and theory of reliability', *Journal of Nervous and Mental Disease*, 1976, 163: 307–17.

11 W.T. Carpenter, D.W. Heinrichs, and A.M.I. Wagman, 'On the heterogeneity of schizophrenia', in M. Alpert (ed.) *Controversies in Schizophrenia*, New York, Guilford Press, 1985.

12 W. Griesinger, 'Herr Ringseis und die naturhistorische Schule', *Archiv für Physiologie und Heilkunde*, 1872, 1: 43–66.

13 R. Warner, *Recovery from Schizophrenia*, London, Routledge & Kegan Paul, 1985.

14 E. Bleuler, 'Die Prognose der Dementia praecox – Schizophreniegruppe', *Allgemeine Zeitschrift für Psychiatrie*, 1908, 65, 436–64.

15 O. Odegaard, 'Changes in the prognosis of functional psychoses since the days of Kraepelin', *British Journal of Psychiatry*, 1967, 113: 813–22.

16 E. Kraepelin, *Psychiatrie*, 5th edn, Leipzig, Barth, 1896.

17 C.A.H. Watts, 'A long-term follow-up of schizophrenic patients: 1946–1983', *Journal of Clinical Psychiatry*, 1985, 46, 6: 210–16.

18 D.C. Watt, K. Katz, and M. Shepherd, 'The natural history of schizophrenia: a 5-year prospective follow-up of a representative sample of schizophrenics by means of a standardised clinical and social assessment', *Psychological Medicine*, 1983, 13: 663–70.

19 E. Pulkinnen, 'Immunoglobins, psychopathology and prognosis in schizophrenia', *Acta Psychiatrica Scandinavica*, 1977, 56: 173–82.

20 A.W. Loranger, 'Sex difference in age on onset of schizophrenia', *Archives of General Psychiatry*, 1984, 41: 157–61.

21 Griesinger, *Die Pathologie und Therapie der psychischen Krankheiten*, op. cit.

22 P.E. Meehl, 'Schizotaxia, schizotypy, schizophrenia', *American Psychologist*, 1962, 17: 827–38.

23 S.S. Kety, 'Prospects for research in schizophrenia – an overview', *Neurosciences Research Program Bulletin*, 1972, 10, 4: 456–67.

24 Warner, op. cit.

25 J. Marcus, S.L. Hans, S.A. Mednick, F. Schulsinger, and F. Michelson, 'Neurological dysfunctioning in offspring of schizophrenics in Israel and Denmark', *Archives of General Psychiatry*, 1985, 42: 753–61.

26 C. Arboleda and P.S. Holzman, 'Thought disorder in children at risk of psychosis', *Archives of General Psychiatry*, 1986, 42: 104–12.

27 H.A. Allen, 'Can all schizophrenic speech be discriminated from normal speech?', *British Journal of Clinical Psychology*, 1985, 24: 209–10.

28 J. Frame, *The Envoy from Mirror City*, London, Women's Press.

Chapter three

Morbid jealousy: some clinical and social aspects of a psychiatric symptom

Introduction

Jealousy is more than a psychiatric symptom. Its language is universal: the conduct and feelings of the jealous man and woman have repeatedly drawn the attention of the great observers of human nature, the moralists and the philosophers as well as the poets and novelists. They have, on the whole, described the reaction more successfully than they have defined it. Even the most celebrated definitions – Descartes' 'kind of fear related to a desire to preserve a possession' or Spinoza's 'mixture of love and hate', for example – merely illustrate the complexity of a term whose many nuances of meaning can be detected in its roots. The English adjective 'jealous' and the noun 'jealousy' are derived respectively from the French *jaloux* and *jalousie*, both taken from the old Provençal *gilos*: *gilos* in turn may be traced back to the vulgar Latin adjective *zelosus* which comes from the late Latin *zelus* and so indirectly from the Greek ξηλος. In its transmission the word has thus been debased. It has ceased to denote 'zeal' or 'ardour'; the 'noble passion' which stood opposed to 'envy' for the Greeks has acquired a pejorative quality. In modern German the distinction is preserved verbally, *Eifersucht* having been formed from the original *Eifer* (zeal) and the suffix *-sucht*, which is cognate with *siech*, meaning 'sickly'. Amorous jealousy claims associations of its own. During the seventeenth century the French word *jalousie* acquired the meaning of 'blind' or 'shutter'; in this sense it entered the English language as a noun in the early nineteenth century; the transmutation is thought to have signified a jocular reference to the suspicious husband or lover who could watch unobserved behind the jalousie; the Italian word *gelosia* is used in this way as early as the middle of the sixteenth century. In the Scandinavian languages separate words designate amorous jealousy.[1] The Swedish *svartsjuk*, literally 'black sick', is taken from an old expression which identified jealousy with the wearing of black socks; the Danish *skinsyg*, 'afraid of getting skin (a rebuff)', harks back to an old link of

Originally published in *Journal of Mental Science*, 1961, 107: 687–753.

jealousy with skin which may in turn have been connected with hose or socks.[2] The origin of the colours which are traditionally employed to depict jealousy, especially black, yellow, and green, is obscure.

Though the belles-lettres of the world contain many observations of great clinical interest concerning behaviour and motivation, it was not until the emergence of psychology and psychiatry as branches of scientific enquiry during the nineteenth century that a number of states of mind and modes of behaviour associated with jealousy were studied systematically and classified as morbid phenomena. The older psychologists tended to treat the subject within the framework of their personal views on the psychology of emotion: their opinions, in consequence, frequently do no more than reflect their own theoretical constructs. Two examples will suffice. Wundt's tri-dimensional feeling-states, compounded of displeasure-pleasure, strain-relaxation, and excitement-calm, accounted for jealousy in terms of the elements of the first-named of all three diads; McDougall, on the other hand, regarded the reaction in hormic terms, though he did not accept jealousy as a sentiment so much as 'a complex play of painful, because conflicting emotions and tendencies'.[3]

Among psychologists the concept of jealousy as one of the human passions has been developed most fully in France, where, as Ernest Jones has pointed out, the features of the jealous state of mind have been described with particular subtlety and understanding.[4] The admixture of emotions, the affront to self-esteem, the yearning for total possession, the anger, the doubts, and the self-torment have all been analysed in themselves and in relationship to each other. To Ribot, the most prominent representative of the French school, *la vie sentimentale* consisted of the affective states, the emotions, and the passions proper.[5] He regarded the passions as the most complex of his three elements, calling them 'prolonged and intellectualized emotions'. Jealousy, for Ribot, was a complex state (*un mélange de sentiments*) made up of pleasure, anger, and chagrin, but he never quite succeeded in fitting it successfully into his elaborate system of affective categories.[6] Alongside amorous jealousy he recognized other varieties of jealousy associated with vanity, rivalry, and ambition, but he was in favour of confirming the application of the word to certain reactions of adult human beings; with animals and children, he maintained, the response aroused by the fear of dispossession should be classified differently. Other writers have been less circumspect. In his broad review of jealousy as a psychological concept Gesell ranged freely through the animal kingdom, the various phases of the human life cycle, and the fields of criminology, pedagogy, anthropology, sociology, and pathology. He attempted to avoid many semantic obstacles in his view of jealousy as a 'plastic complex which defies the circumscription of a definition'.[7] The plastic quality of this view finds its counterpart in the psychological definition of jealousy which has found widest clinical application: 'jealousy', according to Freud, 'is one of those affective states, like grief, that may be described as normal. If anyone appears to be without it, the inference is justified that it has undergone severe repression and consequently plays all the greater part in his unconscious mental life'.[8] The ramifications of this premiss will be examined later.

More recent attempts to classify human emotional states have not proved to be satisfactory, largely because of the dearth of experimental evidence.[9] In consequence clinical psychiatrists, unless they belong to a particular school of psychology, are likely to agree with Whitehorn's common-sense view that 'the "emotions" as we know of them empirically in the clinic and in ordinary life are the expression of sentiments in whose development there has been a large measure of cultural and conventional training'.[10] Among these emotions amorous jealousy is of particular clinical significance by virtue of its associations with mental illness. In accordance with general custom, discussion in this article will be confined to certain adult responses to real, suspected, or imagined sexual infidelity, but even within these limits a full review of the psychiatric aspects of morbid jealousy would demand an altogether larger canvas. Lagache has pointed out that 'there is no "problem of jealousy" which has given rise to an abundant literature and to controversy as there are problems of hysteria and hallucinations. The problem of morbid jealousy is scattered throughout the evolution of psychiatric thought.'[11] Some of the psychiatric themes which have been most closely related to morbid jealousy justify his verdict: they include the concept of 'monomania'; the psychopathology of chronic alcoholism; the theory and classification of the paranoid states and the psychoanalytical view of homosexuality; Mairet's delineation of emotional 'hyperaesthesia'; Jaspers's distinction between the 'delusion of jealousy' as 'process' and as 'personality development'; and the medico-legal problems raised by the crime of passion.

As a feature of mental illness morbid jealousy serves to illustrate Scott Buchanan's view that 'in diagnosis the single symptom is radically ambiguous; it belongs to many syndromes, and its only legitimate interpretation demands a thorough exploration of the possible syndromes to which it may belong'.[12] The standard textbooks devote little space to a symptom which may be encountered among patients suffering from functional psychoses, psychoneuroses, personality disorders, and organic, senile, or toxic states. Unfortunately much of the original work on the subject is scattered and not all of it is available in English. It has seemed therefore a useful task to colligate some of the available knowledge in order to outline the outstanding clinical features and to emphasize particularly the concomitant social problems. Illustrative case material is presented separately in the summarized case histories which have been selected from those of patients who have been encountered in the routine practice of one London teaching hospital and a nearby metropolitan observation unit. Many of the patients had been under the care of other physicians; the diagnoses given in the summaries are those of the individual physicians in charge of the patient. An effort to obtain follow-up information was made in every case, sometimes via the existing hospital facilities, sometimes by personal interviews, and sometimes by correspondence.

Clinical (general)

Clinical description has added little to the field which Mairet traversed fifty years ago.[13] Within his three broad subdivisions into hyperaesthetic jealousy, jealous monomania, and delusional jealousy he was able to find a place for most of the clinical phenomena. His elaborate and cumbersome system of classification, however, can be replaced profitably by Henri Ey's simple dichotomy into the so-called 'delusions of jealousy' and the 'small segment of emotionally jealous reactions which develop in the history of some abnormal personalities'.[14]

Jealousy is often encountered clinically in a delusional setting, though the term 'delusion of jealousy' (*Eifersuchtswahn*; *délire de jalousie*) is a misnomer: apart from an illogical conjunction of words it is the fidelity of the partner which is suspected and the delusions, when present, are of infidelity. In its florid form this mistaken belief is held with absolute conviction; in some cases or at some stages it may so dominate the clinical state as to constitute the outstanding indication of disorder. The clinical picture is usually extended further by the efforts of the patient to furnish evidence or proof of his accusations. His case is then supported by an accumulation of trivial incidents and experiences: everyday events and fluctuations of behaviour, chance encounters in the street, the untidiness of a room, blushing or slips of the tongue; such material is misinterpreted and invested with special meaning. But whereas it is the interpretation placed on such phenomena rather than the phenomena themselves which must be accounted abnormal, other experiences are patently morbid. Among the commonest of these are paranoid ideas associated especially with the belief that the suspected person has been giving the patient substances for the purpose of either poisoning him or of impairing his sexual potency; suspicions that the partner is suffering from venereal disease or has been indulging in sexual intercourse with a third person during the patient's sleep; the conviction that certain physical aspects of the sexual act itself, particularly a tell-tale moistness of the sexual organs, provide evidence of infidelity; and irrational doubts about the paternity of children. The content of the patient's morbid ideas may also be expressed in the form of imaginary visual scenes and in vivid dreams. Hypochondriacal preoccupations before or during the onset of symptoms are commonly present.

Some patients make strenuous efforts to corroborate their suspicions. They may approach lawyers, hire detectives, or take other measures appropriate to a justifiable suspicion of infidelity. They may also take extraordinary measures and search for evidence of seminal stains on clothing, bedlinen, chair covers, or wherever they believe adultery to have occurred; they may go through letters and find confirmation of their suspicions in innocent phrases; they may make excessive sexual demands in order to prove that the partner is sated or to ensure satiation and so prevent further indulgence. The desire to obtain proof of the offence is often overwhelmingly strong; it appears to be related to a need to resolve a tormenting doubt which in some cases leads to repeated attempts to extort a confession from the partner. Such patients declare this to be the only satisfaction which they demand, but the irrational nature of their request is strikingly demonstrated by the futility of the confession which is occasionally feigned by a blameless but desperate spouse. Attempts to obtain confession may lead to physical assaults; these also occur during the paroxysms of rage brought about by the supposed misdemeanours and they may result from the patient's belief in the need for vengeance. Aggressive conduct is often followed by periods of intense remorse which may in turn lead to suicidal action.

The clear recognition of these clinical features, only some of which can be expected in an individual case, is of practical importance. They make up abnormal patterns of symptoms and behaviour which render the morbid quality of the jealousy accompanying delusions of infidelity detectable on internal evidence; even when there is a factual basis for his suspicions the abnormality of the patient's reaction should become apparent. This point assumes special significance when the patient seeks legal or other non-medical advice and the more bizarre clinical features are absent.

It is evidence that many of these ideas and experiences may occur also in a non-delusional setting. If it be accepted further that some of these reactions – painful doubt, suspicious awareness of conduct previously regarded as innocent, attempts to obtain proof of guilt and even violence in certain circumstances – can be encountered among substantially healthy individuals who are confronted with reasonable evidence of infidelity on the part of a loved partner, then it is readily understandable why nosological problems arise in respect of the dividing line between 'normal' and 'abnormal' jealousy. Mairet's concept of hyperaesthetic jealousy as 'a readier and more intensive reaction than normal of jealous passion under the influence of doubt' is taken here to distinguish empirically between the two categories even though the boundary cannot always be demarcated easily. It follows that some of those people who are capable of a morbidly jealous reaction in the absence of delusional beliefs about their partner must be considered abnormal as much by virtue of the facility and intensity with which they react as by the abnormal quality of their reactions. While many of these individuals display other pathological personality traits there are some with nothing more overt than a seeming hyperirritability on a subject which tactful friends and marital partners learn to avoid. The borderline between such reactions and those of the 'normal', understandably jealous individual remains arbitrary in the present state of knowledge.

Between these extremes of a florid delusional state and a morbid readiness to react in a jealous fashion there must be inserted a universe of clinical variants. Though the individual's life-history moulds the content of each clinical picture a number of general factors enter into the phenomenology of every case. These factors include (1) the nature of associated clinical conditions; (2) the patient's personality-structure; (3) the age and sex of the patient; (4) the nature of the relationship which existed between the patient and partner before the onset of symptoms; (5) the tendency of the jealousy-reaction to be phasic and to be exacerbated by the physical proximity of the suspected person; (6) the speed of the development of symptoms. Reference to the more important clinical syndromes will illustrate the influence which these factors may exercise.

Clinical (special)

Morbid jealousy associated with toxic or organic cerebral disorders

Alcoholism constitutes the most widely recognized physical association of morbid jealousy. It was noted in the nineteenth century,[15] and given particular prominence by Krafft-Ebbing, whose view of morbid jealousy as a predominantly masculine reaction was derived in large measure from the much greater prevalence of alcoholism among men.[16] Many writers have described a classical picture which Lewis has condensed:

> chronic alcoholics may without passing through an acute hallucinosis, develop delusions of jealousy, which at first are only evident during intoxication but later pass, by way of constant suspicion and efforts to detect infidelity, into definite morbid beliefs, often very tenaciously held, which persist in the intervals when the patient is sober. He accuses his wife of adultery with neighbours or relations and attempts to extort a confession from her; he may treat her brutally, endangering her life. His diminishing potency, his sexual maladjustment, his bad conscience, and his wife's inevitable aversion from him when drunk may play a large part in the development of these delusions of jealousy.[17]

But, as this writer goes on to point out, the delusions can 'develop also in abstinent men during later life; alcohol and its effects cannot, therefore, be mainly blamed for the psychoses in all cases, even when there is a history of alcoholism'.

Attempts have been made to examine in more detail the states of morbid jealousy which are related to alcoholism. Lagache, for example, described eight separate types of reaction among his thirteen alcoholic patients, and Pohlisch has examined the association of morbid jealousy with the paranoid constitution of some alcoholics.[18] The most careful and satisfactory study, however, is that of Kolle who, following Schneider, distinguished clinically between three principal subgroups: (1) the reaction of the 'jealous drinker'; (2) the 'exogenous reaction' (with evidence of cerebral damage), and (3) the reaction of the 'delusional drinker'. A fourth category of 'organically provoked' cases included only three patients, all of whom were in the senium.[19] Only the patients in Kolle's third group exhibited a primary delusional process and these fell diagnostically into or near the schizophrenic category. The other two groups displayed less a delusional basis for their jealousy than a 'distrustful alertness' which attained conviction at times, especially in states of acute intoxication; the cerebral damage of those drinkers who displayed an 'exogenous' reaction modified the symptomatology.

The long and careful follow-up of his cases gives force to Kolle's views. Eleven of his thirteen 'jealous drinkers' were followed up for between fourteen and twenty-three years; they developed neither a spread of their ideas nor new psychotic symptoms and not one was readmitted to hospital; eight of the patients ceased to be addicted to alcohol, and it is of particular interest that six of these eight patients separated from their partners. The prognosis of the 'exogenous drinkers' (followed up for between five and nineteen years) was much worse and their mortality rate was high. The twelve 'delusional drinkers' followed up for between three and twenty-two years, also did badly; five of them died, one by his own hand and two after years of continuous stay in hospital; another five developed clear-cut schizophrenic illnesses. Kolle also examined the family pedigrees of these patients, their descendants as well as their ascendants. He concluded that the evidence, even though the numbers were small, was in favour of a genetic difference between the illnesses of his 'jealous drinkers' and those of 'delusional drinkers', and that the latter group bore a close relationship to schizophrenia.

A careful enquiry was made into the drinking history and habits of every patient in the present series of unselected psychiatric cases. In only a small minority was there evidence of excessive consumption of alcohol. Among the established alcoholics the most intimate association of morbid jealousy with bouts of heavy drinking was demonstrated by Case 1,[*] a patient who did not display jealous behaviour before she began drinking or between her bouts. Jealousy and suspicion had featured in the personality of other alcoholics (Cases 2, 3, and 4) but not more prominently than among patients with temperate habits. Case 5 is of particular interest in view of the emphasis which has been laid on the paranoid aspects of alcoholism: over many years of heavy drinking the patient had often entertained delusional ideas about his wife's infidelity, but not until they eventually separated did he come under medical care for the first time, in his fifties, with an episode of alcoholic hallucinosis.

---

[*] Cases referred to but not included in this edition (which contains numbers 1, 6, 11a, 20, 55, 75 from the total of 80) may be found in the original 1990 hardback edition.

Addiction to substances other than alcohol

Kraepelin regarded cocainism as one of the conditions most intimately associated with morbid jealousy.[20] Cocaine addiction is rare in England today; there were no cases among the patients examined for this study. Characteristically the delusional ideas supervene often, quickly, and with force, frequently leading to violence; they may remain in evidence for some time after the disappearance of other symptoms. Addiction to other drugs, e.g. morphine, probably leads to the development of morbid jealousy only when the patient is also taking either cocaine or alcohol, but in Case 6 the ideas of infidelity which presaged a paranoid illness did not appear until the patient, a grossly disturbed psychopath who had been an alcoholic for many years, became addicted to amphetamine.

Psychiatric disorders in the senium

Psychiatric patients in the older age group can display morbid jealousy as a prominently incongruous symptom. In 1901 Parant described the variety of its clinical associations,[21] which include organic and degenerative cerebral conditions, the late paranoid states, and the affective illnesses. In many instances the morbid ideas are accompanied by physical evidence of cerebral disease or by other psychological symptoms but they can open the clinical picture and raise diagnostic problems; morbid jealousy, according to Gruhle, can be most convincing as a seemingly isolated symptom in the senium.[22] Jealous traits are not necessarily apparent in the patient's pre-morbid personality. The patho-plastic effect of age on the delusional content probably contributes to the clinical picture, for jealousy is an understand-able reaction of the aged; the suggestion that the ideas of infidelity arise directly from the patient's awareness of his waning potency, however, is of specious simplicity (Case 7).

Other cerebral disorders

Morbid jealousy has been described among the symptoms of a number of cerebral pathological processes which include pre-senile dementia, cerebral arteriosclerosis, Huntington's chorea, Parkinson's disease, general paralysis of the insane, and cerebral tumour.[23] Among the patients of this series it was prominent in a case of secondary carcinoma (Case 8), of Alzheimer's disease (Case 9), of pan-hypopituitarism (Case 10), of disseminated sclerosis (Case 11), and of temporal lobe epilepsy as a post-ictal phenomenon (Case 11a).

Morbid jealousy in association with the functional psychoses

The schizophrenias and paranoid states

Morbid jealousy with delusions of marital infidelity constitutes a well-recognized symptom-complex in schizophrenic illnesses.[24] The ideas of infidelity may appear first and remain at the heart of the delusional process, however widespread its exfoliation (Case 12 and 13); alternatively they may become lost among other morbid ideas as the illness progresses (Case 14 and 15). In some cases delusions persist for many years with little obvious deterioration of the personality and with few associated symptoms in the absence of mental agitation (Cases 16 and 17). The mode of symptom development in these patients and its relationship to the pre-morbid personality served originally to illustrate Jaspers' distinction between delusions which develop understandably from the traits of a predisposed individual and the 'process' psychosis which attacks a relatively untainted personality.[25] The criteria on which this dichotomy was based are met by a sufficiently large number of cases to endow the distinction with some descriptive value but the categories overlap too often for unreserved application.

Within the congeries of the schizophrenic reactions morbid jealousy is most clearly related to the paranoid group. Examination of the case records of all 181 people attending the Maudsley Hospital as in-patients or out-patients during a three-year period and diagnosed as suffering from 'paranoia', 'paranoid illness', or 'paranoid schizophrenia' showed that 14 per cent included morbid jealousy among their presenting or most prominent symptoms. So many of the clinical phenomena associated with morbid jealousy are often of a frankly paranoid nature that Lagache has concluded that 'whatever the clinical setting the organization of the jealous experience is on a primitive level with paranoid patterns of projection and demand'. This view is supported by the cluster of symptoms demonstrated by several patients in the present series (Cases 18, 19, 20, 21, 22, 23): one man (Case 24), who was admitted to hospital with delusional ideas about his wife's infidelity, was discovered to have suffered eleven years before from a clear-cut paranoid psychosis with persecutory delusions unconnected with infidelity.

Affective psychoses

Disregarding Richard Burton's classical account of jealousy as a form of 'love-melancholy' most modern clinical observers of the depressive reaction have either paid it little attention or even argued against its inclusion among the phenomena of the syndrome.[26] Other authors[27, 28] have stressed an association which is clearly illustrated in this series by several patients who were morbidly jealous in the course of major depressive illnesses (Cases 25, 26, 27, 28, 29, 30). Diagnostic practice may account in some measure for disagreement on this issue, especially when there are coexistent paranoid symptoms. The case histories of the patients whose paranoid symptoms were manifested or exacerbated in the course of a depressive illness (Case 31 and 32) may be contrasted with other primarily paranoid illnesses which were complicated by depressive features (Cases 20 and 33); Case 20 is of particular interest in this regard as that of a man with a long-standing paranoid illness dominated by ideas of persecution whose delusions of infidelity appeared only when he became depressed and were dispelled by a course of electrical treatment which left his paranoid beliefs unaffected. The intimate association which can exist between paranoid and depressive symptoms is clearly illustrated by Cases 34 and 35.

Patients with less severe 'reactive' depression are more conveniently considered in the next section. The appearance of morbid jealousy in the course of affectively determined states of excitement is well recognized.[29] It has been explained in terms of the patient's interpretation of the sexual partner's failure to satisfy excessive physical demands and as part of the paranoid component of some manic reactions.

Morbid jealousy in association with neurotic and personality disorders

It is apparent from what has been said about morbid jealousy as a symptom of the major psychotic reactions that an abnormal pre-morbid personality is encountered in many cases. Even when the reaction can be related clearly to a particular precipitating event, whether this be physical or environmental, there is usually some evidence of unhealthy personality traits having antedated the illness. Clinical experience demonstrates also that many patients suffering from the large heterogeneous group of conditions which are loosely classified as the neurotic and personality disorders may become morbidly jealous in the course of their lives without evidence of clear-cut psychotic illnesses. The physical and biological events which Brousseau has emphasized as precipitants in such cases did not figure prominently in this series.[30] The clinical phenomena were more closely linked with interpersonal factors, especially the relationship between the patient and the sexual partner.

The diversity of these patients' reactions is covered inadequately by current systems of nosology. Perhaps the most clearly defined group of personality traits associated with morbid jealousy are those which have been taken to characterize the paranoid or hypoparanoid psychopath.[31] Such people display an irritable sensitivity and a wariness in their interpersonal relations which often go with a withdrawn, solitary existence (Case 36) but can also be compatible with a superficially gregarious and over-active mode of life (Case 37). Jealousy constitutes an indissoluble component of their attitude towards the sexual partner. It is readily exacerbated in times of stress and so tends to be episodic in intensity; at the height of the reaction the patients can hold to unshakable delusions of infidelity which usually recede rapidly after the passage of the crisis.

The majority of neurotics and personality deviants in this series were depressed at the time of examination. In Cases 38, 39, and 40 the depressive reaction was understandable in the light of incidents which had evoked suspicion and distress and in Cases 41, 42, and 43 sexual difficulties had played a major role. With most patients, however, the events leading up to the illness had their roots in the evolution of the marriage itself and in the part played by the patient towards its unsatisfactory development (Cases 44, 45, 46, and 47). Between jealous outbursts such patients were nearly all contrite, blaming themselves for having entertained groundless suspicions and for their past conduct. Case 48 demonstrates the appearance of jealousy as a transient phenomenon among other morbid traits. Overt anxiety and phobias were prominent in some instances (Cases 49, 50, and 51) while the insistent nature of admittedly irrational ideas assumed a compulsive character in Cases 52, 53, 54, and 55 in whom frankly obsessional features dominated the clinical picture. A retrospective variant of this reaction, in which the patient had become preoccupied with misconduct which he had previously condoned, is illustrated by Cases 56 and 57; this form of reaction was clearly described by Stefanowski in 1897.[32]

Psychopathology and social pathology

The foregoing observations demonstrate that morbid jealousy cannot be regarded as more than a convenient descriptive term which is applied to several forms of psychobiological reaction. Psychiatrists who have studied the psychopathology of these reactions have concentrated in the main on particular features of clinical interest. Kraepelin, for example, suggested that the morbid jealousy of alcoholics followed the inevitable estrangement between husband and wife and many clinicians relate the symptoms to the sexual impotence associated with chronic alcoholism. Bleuler paid attention to the affective accompaniments of morbid jealousy since, in his view, they constituted the complex which embodied the 'wish' in the delusional process.[33] Langfeldt has stressed the importance of the reaction among 'sensitive individuals with their tendency to suspiciousness, introspection and self-reference'.[34] Gruhle has pointed to the disturbance of thinking when obsessional features are prominent. Mairet's conclusions may be taken to exemplify the many attempts which have been made to provide an understandable interpretation of the links between morbid jealousy and paranoid states:

This association of ideas of persecutions and jealousy can be regarded as logical. Firstly, mistrust is at the basis of jealousy, as it is at the basis of the monomania of persecutions. Secondly, the individual who has the fixed idea that his spouse is deceiving him regards himself, naturally, as persecuted by her; it is not surprising therefore that he can extend to others his ideas of persecution. Thirdly, the jealous person with a fixed idea necessarily becomes a persecutor of his spouse, so that it is natural that he can become so for others, when he extends the number of his persecutors.

An extension of this reasoning would account for the development of either an overriding desire for revenge or an erotomania.

Clinicians holding to a theoretical framework for the classification of abnormal emotional response have advanced psychopathological formulations in terms of their particular systems. As a modern representative of the French school Borel, for example, recognizes the 'psychoses of passion' among which jealousy takes its place as an extreme form of a normally occurring emotion.[35] In Kretschmer's schema morbid jealousy is classified among his 'expansive' reactions, the patients displaying 'a spot in the core of their being, a hypersensitive nervous vulnerability, a buried focus, an old inferiority feeling'.[36] The psychoanalytical position was outlined by Freud in his essay on 'Certain neurotic mechanisms in jealousy, paranoia and homosexuality', where he described three 'layers or stages of jealousy': the first as competitive or normal, the second as projected, and the third as delusional. Freud asserted that even normal, competitive jealousy contained an element of homosexuality; projected jealousy, he maintained, sprang from ideas which the patient entertained about his own infidelity; while 'delusional jealousy represents an acidulated homosexuality, and rightly takes its place among the classical forms of paranoia'. The formula is epitomized in the memorable expression of the patient's conflict about his own feelings for the other man: 'I do not love him for she loves him'. Psychoanalysts have since added very little to Freud's original postulates. Fenichel, for example, refers to the frustration inherent in the Oedipus complex as being at 'the basis of all jealousy' and suggested that the jealous patient was striving to rid himself of impulses towards unfaithfulness and homosexuality by means of projection.[37] Melanie Klein has expressed views which are substantially similar, though they are coloured by her own theoretical standpoint.

> Jealousy is based on the suspicion of a rivalry with the father, who is accused of having taken away the mother's breast, and the mother. The rivalry marks the early stages of the direct and inverted Oedipus complex, which normally arises concurrently with the depressive position in the second quarter of the first year.[38]

Seidenberg has proposed a fourth category to be added to Freud's original three: emotional jealousy as 'a wish and gratification which the mechanism...itself fulfils',[39] and Schmeideberg has done no more than coin another complex, the 'Othello complex', which she suggests should be applied to some syndromes.[40]

The psychopathology of morbid jealousy has also been explored by the clinicians who have addressed themselves to the manner in which experience and perception are modified by the mental state of the jealous person. Some have employed psychoanalytical precepts but they have also drawn heavily on neo-phenomenological theory, with its focus on jealousy as 'a mode of being'.[41] Others have adopted a more eclectic position in their interpretation of the subjective changes and many different aspects of the jealous state of mind have been emphasized, ranging from 'the privacy of the experience'[42] to the insecurity of the 'wavering world'[43] in which the jealous person's emotion is expressed. Most of these workers represent morbid jealousy as a pathological reaction different in kind from the potential responses of a healthy person inasmuch as it constitutes a form of psychological regression and rests ultimately on a delusional basis. Against this view du Boeuff has argued on phenomenological grounds that a delusional structure does not underlie all pathological jealousy[44] and Minkowski makes allowance for a morbid *jalousie inauthentique* which he considers to be qualitatively different from the genuine *jalousie passionelle*.[45]

The patient efforts of investigators who have concentrated on the elucidation of mechanisms have yielded great insight into the mental processes of morbidly jealous people. But although individual patients in this series illustrate many of their observations, it would be difficult to generalize from them without reference to the environmental and interpersonal setting in which the reactions occurred; in no instance could these factors be neglected and in several cases they were of such importance as to justify Lund's view of jealousy as 'descriptive less of an emotional state than of a social situation'.[46] The influence of broad environmental factors is apparent in such phenomena as the rise in post-war crimes associated with jealousy among ex-servicemen in England or in the increased incidence of patients with delusional jealousy in Holland following periods of economic depression.[47] In general, however, the impact of social and cultural factors can be studied more intensively through the marriage contract or its equivalent. Widespread support can be found in many societies for Havelock Ellis's statement that 'the claims of jealousy fall within the claims of conjugal rights'.[48] Authority to enforce these obligations can claim scriptural precedent and modern anthropological investigations have illuminated many variants of the socially acceptable responses to real or threatened infidelity, especially when the female partner is taken to be the culprit.[49] The attitudes adopted in this situation are determined by emotions which in part reflect transmitted social values and expectations but the patterns of behaviour are so universal that Westermarck, after reviewing the evidence bearing on the customs and laws concerning adultery in several societies, concluded that masculine jealousy was a general human characteristic.[50] It is therefore to be expected that the social consequences of jealous behaviour will be felt most keenly in the domestic sphere. The quarrels, accusations, recriminations, suspicions, remorse, verbal abuse, and physical assaults are all detrimental to the well-being of the family group and Blacker has drawn attention to the prominent role of jealousy in broken marriage.[51]

When an individual displays morbid jealousy the repercussions become still more dramatic. The illnesses of two patients in this series were identified only after their spouses' admission to hospital following suicidal attempts which were directly related to the accusations of infidelity which had been made against them (Cases 58 and 59). A third patient entered hospital from prison to which he had been committed for a homicidal assault on his wife, who was subsequently discovered to be an old paranoid schizophrenic suffering from delusions of infidelity which had led her to torment her husband for many years (Case 60). The domestic discord may involve any or several or a number of social agents: the lawyer, the police officer, the probation officer, the private detective, the official of the citizens' advice bureau, or the marriage guidance counsellor played a part in the social histories of the majority of the patients in this series. Intervention of these non-medical intermediaries may not only determine referral to a physician; when effective it can dispense with the need for medical assistance or advice in an incalculable but probably large proportion of cases. A rounded view of the interpersonal difficulties posed by morbid jealousy is therefore difficult to obtain in any clinical sample. Experienced marriage guidance counsellors in particular are probably more familiar than the physician with the frequency of ruptured marital relations. They are also better placed to observe the different ways in which the reaction can become woven into the fabric of the marital relationship, a process which is enhanced by the reluctance of many spouses to interpret the symptoms as indices of mental disturbance. The tendency to regard the manifestations of jealousy as an aspect of the marital transaction constitutes an important determinant of the acceptance of even patently delusional ideas, especially when there has been little spread of symptoms and when a good relationship has previously existed.[52] On the basis of his experience at a marriage guidance clinic Revitch has used the term 'conjugal paranoia' to describe the difficult situation which arises when one spouse involves the other in a web of delusional ideas.[53] The most frequent responses to delusional ideas of infidelity among the partners of patients in this series were incredulity, resentment, fear of assault, depression, or remorse for previous misconduct. A realistic appraisal of the morbid nature of the patient's ideas was uncommon even when these were egregious (Cases 60, 61, 62, and 63).

The importance of interpersonal relations stands out even more clearly in the marriages of the neurotics in this series. Slater and Woodside have stressed the 'corrosive and ultimately destructive effect' of jealousy in such cases.[54] With only a minority of the patients could the reaction be related to past, current, or threatened extramural attachments on the part of the spouse; in most instances there had been a long history of an unhappy relationship in which unreasonable jealousy had played a large part. The patients were troubled principally by the thought of what had or might have occurred in the past or by the prospect of what might occur in the future. This uncertainty reflected not only a strong sense of inferiority *vis-à-vis* their marital partners but often a life-long insecurity of which some were explicitly aware (Cases 44, 45, 59, and 64). The role of overtly homosexual conflicts appeared to be relatively unimportant. Whatever the psychopathological basis of their sentiments, however, the patients' conduct was directed invariably towards the subjugation of the spouse and the gratification which they derived was linked closely to the eliciting of an appropriately submissive response (Case 65). The more compliant partners were humiliated by frequent displays of jealous behaviour which reduced their lives to a housebound, isolated routine and stifled their interest in extramural activities. The more robust partners resisted this pressure even when it was carried to the point of violence (Cases 66 and 67). Some exploited the situation by feigning indifference or by deliberate provocation (Cases 68, 69, and 70). The remorse which followed the jealous outburst served only to increase the patient's dependence. The interplay of both partners therefore entered into and modified the symptoms and the manifestations of behaviour to such a degree that the significance of the phenomena in an individual case could not be assessed without an understanding of the relationship between them.

Forensic

Jealousy is a notoriously dangerous passion and constitutes a well-recognized motive for crimes of violence, particularly of a gynocidal nature. While detailed statistics are difficult to obtain it has been established that the majority of murders in this country are committed by men and that their victims are mostly women.[55] In his examination of 200 'sane' murderers East found that forty-six had killed because of jealousy, an emotion which he put alongside 'anger, fear, love, lust, hate and the feeling of possession' as being most frequently associated with murder.[56] In a similar vein Brierly has reported that over a two-year period 54 out of 760 murders in Cook County, Illinois, were due to jealousy.[57] Morbid forms of the reaction have been recognized as important in the practice of forensic psychiatry since the nineteenth century; it is, for example, apparent even from the scanty clinical data which are included in Gray's study of 125 patients guilty of homicide and attempted homicide who were admitted to a criminal asylum in New York State between 1843 and 1873, that eight of these patients entertained florid delusions of marital infidelity.[58] Particular attention has been paid in the past to the part played by alcohol in such cases. Sullivan has gone so far as to claim that 'delusions of sexual jealousy are ... the characteristic disorder of thought in cases of alcoholic murder with conscious motive'.[59] The evidence of other workers, however, indicates that this extreme view is unjustified. Hopwood and Milner found 131 excessive drinkers among 1,000 male patients who were admitted consecutively to Broadmoor Asylum over a twenty-year period, but in fewer than half the cases did they consider alcohol to be of aetiological significance in the clinical history.[60] Eighty-one of their patients had been homicidal, fifty-one having murdered or tried to murder their wives, paramours, or sweethearts, but only thirty-three of these patients suffered from delusions of infidelity, conspiracy, or persecution concerning the victim. More recently Mowat has examined the records of the male and female patients admitted to Broadmoor during periods of twenty and fifteen years and has found morbid jealousy to have been a significant factor in 12 per cent and 15 per cent respectively; examining a sample of these cases he estimated that alcohol was an important aetiological factor in no more than a quarter.[61] East studied the place of alcohol as a precipitating factor among gynocidal murderers suffering from delusional states and concluded that 'perhaps the majority of delusions of this nature seen in the Criminal Courts are due to alcoholic insanity but clinical practice leaves little doubt that paranoid and other states of mental disorder may result in crime associated with delusions of this type'.[62] Homicidal behaviour associated with ideas of infidelity is illustrated in Cases 71, 72, and 73 in this series. The psychopathology of such patients has been explored by Myer, Apfelberger, and Sugar in their careful study of fourteen mentally ill men guilty of gynocide[63] and also by Karpman from a psychoanalytical standpoint.[64]

Crimes of violence committed by patients entertaining delusional ideas of infidelity raise the medico-legal problems implicit in the McNaughton Rules. The difficulty of assessing responsibility in individual patients was illustrated 100 years ago by the case of Victor George Townley, who confessed in 1863 to having murdered a young girl after learning of her intention to marry another man and raised a storm of conflicting opinions at his trial.[65] Former clinical fashion contributed to this legal dilemma, for morbidly jealous patients with little spread of their symptoms fell readily into one or other of the widely accepted groups of the monomas which Esquirol had introduced in his system of classification. The diagnosis of monomania was closely linked with the notion of partial insanity, a concept which met with the approval of such authorities as Hack Tuke who claimed that

> although it would be unsafe to employ it in a Court of Law, there are occasions on which a medical witness may truthfully contend for a partial insanity which allows of a patient exercising his judgment in some matters while admitting that there are others on which his opinion would be warped by his delusions.[66]

Despite his qualifications Tuke's argument leads inevitably to the legal correlate of partial responsibility and it was rejected by Maudsley who made his point with a telling and relevant example:

> if a so-called monomaniac has the delusion that his wife, whom he has hitherto loved and trusted entirely, is dishonouring or conspiring against him the existence of a delusion so foreign to the whole habit of his healthy thought and feeling marks a deeper and more general derangement of

mind, and it is impossible to foresee the extent of its possible influence upon his conduct.[67]

Maudsley's view has been upheld by subsequent medical and legal opinion. Partial responsibility is no longer acceptable as a medico-legal concept and Gruhle has developed Maudsley's argument to show why morbid jealousy cannot be taken to sustain it.

The assessment of responsibility for criminal behaviour motivated by abnormal emotional response which cannot be attributed to formal mental disease raises problems of a different order. Amorous jealousy constitutes a strong motive for the so-called crimes of passion so frequently that Claude assigned crimes of jealousy to a separate category in his classification of these offences.[68] The legal approach to such offences differs widely from country to country and in large measure reflects public attitudes towards sexual behaviour and codes of morality. Until recently English law has made few concessions to human frailty in this sphere. Even in the face of clear evidence of adultery a fatal act of vengeance on the part of the affronted cuckold was accounted murder unless it could be established that the defendant witnessed the legitimate spouse *in flagrante delicto* and took immediate action. In these circumstances, and in these circumstances only, provocation could be entered as a defence, and the crime reduced to manslaughter. This distinction becomes more comprehensible if it is viewed in the light of the canons of normal motivation and conduct which the lawyer applies to his own creation in the person of the 'reasonable man' of common law. On the evidence of collective legal opinion one jurist has attempted to define some of the pertinent qualities which characterize this model citizen:

> he is not impotent and he is not normally drunk. He does not lose his self-control on hearing a mere confession of adultery, but he becomes unbalanced at the sight of adultery, provided, of course, that he is married to the adulteress. Furthermore, he remains in control of his emotions, notwithstanding the vilest forms of oral provocation, and finally, even if he loses control he is expected to resort to no more than reasonable measures of retaliation.[69]

The boundaries of reasonable conduct have been redefined by the Homicide Act of 1957. Though English law refuses to recognize 'uncontrollable impulse' as a defence, the jury's deliberations on diminished responsibility must now be concerned with what the Act refers to explicitly as 'self-control'. The members of the jury are in effect being asked to consider whether the accused was unable to prevent himself from committing the act with which he is charged, a question which the Royal Commission on Capital Punishment recommended as an addendum to those which are demanded by the McNaughton Rules. By Part 1, Section 3 of the 1957 Act a case of murder in which the accused person has been provoked confronts the jury with the task of determining 'whether the provocation was sufficient to make a reasonable man do as he (the murderer) did' and for this purpose they must take into account 'everything both done and said according to the effect which in their opinion it would have on a reasonable man'. At the present time it is difficult to disagree with Lord Justice Devlin that the problems arising in association with self-control and provocation must be approached empirically.[70] In this context the trial of Ernest Fantle in 1958 is of great potential interest as the first reported case in which the defence of provocation was made under the 1957 Act. Gooderson has discussed the implications of the case, particularly as it may reflect 'a more liberal attitude to killers who have not unreasonably lost their self-control' though he has emphasized that public opinion and the law have yet to confirm this trend.[71]

But the limits of reasonable conduct have still be be defined for the aberrant individuals whose defects of personality impair their judgement and self-control rather than their reason. The clinical histories of several patients in this series (e.g. Cases 19 and 74) demonstrate numerous morbid traits which may accompany a 'hyperaesthetic' readiness to react in a jealous manner and lend force to de Greeff's statement that 'it is possible to explain all crimes of passion by jealousy and by vanity or by one of the major sins. The truth is that these sins only reach such proportions with psychopathic personalities.'[72] This association assumes some practical significance, for although modern legal opinion accepts the need for reform of the criminal law in respect of psychopathic behaviour and precedent exists for a plea of diminished responsibility, the Report of the Royal Commission on the Law relating to Mental Illness and Mental Deficiency has made it clear that medical knowledge is regarded as insufficiently secure to guide the lawyer in his management of individuals who cannot be classified as either mentally ill or mentally deficient. At the present time the heightened emotional reactions and correspondingly diminished self-control of the morbidly jealous neurotic or personality deviant remain legally dubious motives for criminal behaviour.

Legal advice may be sought by the spouse of a morbidly jealous patient who is considering marital dissolution because of domestic difficulties. The law, as it is embodied in the Matrimonial Causes Act, is straightforward when the afflicted partner is demonstrably insane; in Case 19, for example, the patient's wife was able to obtain a nullity decree after a few months of married life as she had been unaware of her husband's condition at the time of marriage. In other cases where the patient's sanity is not in question the spouse who seeks advice is likely to be advised to take proceedings on the grounds of cruelty. If the respondent accepts responsibility for his or her behaviour he has to rebut the charge of cruelty on factual evidence since 'motive' does not constitute an essential element of legal cruelty in English law;[73] Cases 12, 75, and 76 illustrate the background to successful actions of this type taken because of morbidly jealous behaviour. If the respondent alleges that he was in effect insane at the time his actions were committed it is of some theoretical and practical importance that by a ruling of Lord Chief Justice Goddard both limbs of the McNaughton Rules must apply to a criminal offence if a plea of insanity is to be sustained.[74] The concept of responsibility having been transferred from the criminal to the divorce courts in this way, the possibility of a respondent pleading diminished responsibility must be entertained in the future since the Homicide Act of 1957 has sanctioned this plea in criminal law.

(The Divorce Court has since ruled that the plea of diminished responsibility cannot be entertained in such cases.)

Management and outcome

A brief mention of these topics is justified by their clinical importance. In the opinion of one Victorian physician the most effective treatment of morbid jealousy was 'geographical rather than medical'.[75] Nowadays we can recognize that morbid jealousy accompanies several psychiatric states and that the value of symptomatic treatment depends partly on the nature of the associated illness, partly on the features of the individual case. The outcome and the indications for treatment depend therefore on a variety of factors and therapy cannot be limited to any single method. Where the symptoms constitute one component of an affective illness, for example, they may be expected to abate if the condition responds to electrical convulsive therapy. In a setting of chronic alcoholism the delusions of infidelity will usually recede when the patient's addictive habits are brought under control. Schizophrenics can lose their morbid suspicions if the illness remits spontaneously or is treated successfully. On the other hand, the prognosis of symptoms which appear for the first time to usher in a senile illness must be guarded.

As the one measure which has some place in the treatment of every case psychotherapy will demand particular consideration. Explanation, reassurance, support, and counselling are of particular benefit when the reaction is linked to a problematic life-situation and is not associated with a major disturbance of personality (Cases 77, 78, 79). Claims for successful psychotherapy can be sustained best by judicious selection from less severe cases of this type. The therapeutic value of the more radical methods of psychological treatment is dubious, however, especially when they are applied to the graver conditions, e.g. a ruminative or paranoid state.[76] A paradigm of the psychotherapeutic approach in such cases may be found in the detailed report of Brunswick;[77] whether the resolution of symptoms in this case can be ascribed to therapeutic intervention or to the natural course of the illness remains questionable in view of the marked fluctuations in duration and intensity of the symptoms. The same objection, which can be raised in most reports of this type, is reinforced by several cases in this series (e.g. Case 80).

The management of any case in which morbid jealousy is a prominent symptom imposes on the physician a double task. A medical opinion is clearly of most value when the interpersonal and social aspects of a case are as closely understood as the narrower issues of diagnosis and treatment. In particular, some understanding must be acquired of the character and likely reactions of the patient's marital partner who may also be in need of help and support. Without this knowledge the physician will be handicapped in the practical advice which he can provide about domiciliary management and, above all, about the desirability of a temporary or permanent separation which can so often bring about a subsidence of the turbulent emotions. These decisions can be ignored only at the risk of painful and even dangerous consequences and although effective treatment cannot always be instituted the mitigation of distress and suffering should be possible in most cases.

Case histories

Case 1

Mrs H.J.L., *aet.* 41, catering supervisor, was admitted to hospital on 5.4.55. She came from a middle-class French background. Her mother was an energetic woman, subject to mood swings, who had been a sporadically heavy drinker for many years. The patient was brought up in England from early childhood and was always regarded as a healthy, active person. Her work record in the catering business had been excellent and her sociable disposition made her very popular in the trade. She had had an uneventful heterosexual life and had been married three times. The failure of her first two marriages was principally attributable to her marital partners. Her third marriage had taken place at the age of 30 and was apparently happy; she had three healthy children. Neither the patient nor the husband had been unfaithful. Apart from tuberculosis of the left knee at the age of 13 her physical health had been good.

Shortly after her third marriage the patient assumed a responsible position in the catering trade which brought her into closer contact with alcohol. She soon began to indulge in heavy bouts of drinking; at first she drank in company but later she took to drinking spirits alone. In the course of these bouts she accused her husband of infidelity but otherwise she stated invariably that her accusations were groundless and that she knew him to be devoted to her. At no time did she search for evidence or make specific accusations about his conduct. Eventually she sought the help of her general practitioner and was referred to hospital.

On examination she was in good physical health except for an ankylosed left knee. She was friendly and co-operative and showed no overt signs of psychiatric abnormality. She attributed the suspicions of her husband to excessive indulgence in alcohol, stating that drink 'makes me have nasty thoughts'. She was treated with antabuse and supportive psychotherapy. She was discharged on 30.4.55, vowing not to drink again.

Diagnosis: Alcoholic addiction.

Follow up: The patient remained abstinent for a few months but then relapsed. She then made a more determined effort to overcome her dependence on alcohol and joined Alcoholics Anonymous. Three years after her discharge she was seen as an out-patient: she had remained teetotal for several months; she was working well and living a more settled married life. This improvement has since been maintained.

Case 6

Mr A.J.M., *aet.* 33, chef, was admitted to an observation unit on 17.7.56. He came from a working-class background, the youngest of five surviving siblings. One sister was unsettled and suffered from mood swings but there was no other family history of nervous or mental illness. The patient had exhibited numerous neurotic traits since childhood; his school record was adequate, however, and his culinary ability had always succeeded in stabilizing his work record. He was a reserved person, easily led, generous at times. He had indulged in bouts of very heavy drinking since his teens and had been sexually promiscuous with males and females since the age of 14. He married *aet.* 20 a tolerant woman who was fond of him despite his history; she had previously given birth to an illegitimate child by another man. She had remained faithful to the patient since the marriage although he had occasionally been unfaithful to her. Their sexual relationship had been satisfactory; there were three children *aet.* 16, 13, and 11 years. The patient had contracted tuberculosis in his 20s but he had been treated successfully.

From the age of 21 the patient had been admitted to various mental hospitals, observation units, and prison on at least twenty occasions. He was regarded as having become addicted to alcohol when he was *aet.* 21. From time to time he became depressed and made a number of suicidal attempts; he began to rely on barbiturates, paraldehyde, and benzedrine in addition to alcohol. At the time of each admission he usually expressed a determination to overcome his weakness; his mental state by the time of discharge was generally regarded as normal though on two occasions ideas of reference had been noted. The label of 'psychopathic personality' had been fixed to him since his early 20s. Two years before admission he had been hallucinating after taking large doses of benzedrine and there had been at least one episode of delirium tremens. Shortly after admission he had taken fifty tablets of benzedrine sulphate, twelve of sodium amytal and a quantity of promazine. He had been wandering about the streets for some hours; on his return home he complained about his being persecuted by strange men whom he said he saw in his house; he turned out cupboards to look for them.

On examination he stated that he suspected his wife of infidelity with the men in his house. He also had auditory hallucinations of his children's voices. His memory and other cognitive functions appeared intact. Within a few days he had come out of his psychotic state and it then emerged that his suspicions about his wife had begun during the previous year and coincided with his decision to rely on benzedrine sulphate as his principal stimulant. Close questioning failed to elicit evidence of his having been morbidly jealous while he had relied on alcohol. The patient admitted that in his morbid state he felt that men were going to his house for the purpose of having sexual relations with his wife, but he rarely accused her of this directly.

Diagnosis: Psychopathic personality with addiction to amephedrine.

Follow up: The patient was discharged home vowing to remain off drugs, but was soon re-admitted in a similar state to another hospital. Two years later he was seen in the same observation unit holding to a complex paranoid delusional system involving his wife and children. On this occasion his symptoms did not remit quickly in hospital and he was transferred to a mental hospital under certificate.

Case 11a

Mr J.D., *aet.* 52, stevedore, was admitted to an observation unit on 9.7.56. He came from a working-class background, the fifth of eight living siblings. There was no family history of nervous or mental illness. His early history was normal. He had been a hard-working, stable, energetic person, inclined to heavy social drinking. He was married happily at 29; there were six children ranging in age from 25 to 10, all of them healthy. Sexual relations had declined in the six months before admission but had previously been satisfactory. Though the patient had been occasionally unfaithful his wife had remained devoted to him.

At the age of 4 the patient was ill with chorea and shortly afterwards with a mastoiditis which was complicated by a suspected brain abscess. An EEG had revealed an abnormality in the right temporal lobe. He had suffered from epileptic attacks for at least ten years; these had consisted of grand mal fits preceded by an aura and easily precipitated by bouts of heavy drinking. After his fits he was frequently exhausted and at time disoriented; he had been admitted to a mental hospital on several occasions for this reason. During the post-ictal phases of the last three or four episodes the patient had expressed morbid ideas about his wife's misconduct though when he had emerged from this condition he had been apparently well and very contrite.

His admission to the observation unit had been necessitated by a violent outburst when he had destroyed the television set, stating that he saw his wife's lover as a vision on the screen. On admission he was very active and at times incoherent and irritable. He was excited and expressed some flight of ideas. He was fully orientated. His mood was depressed and he expressed a number of suspicions about his wife's behaviour, citing minor incidents which he had misinterpreted; he felt that his poor sexual performance might have been related to her misconduct. Two weeks later he had lost all his symptoms except for some irritability and was discharged home.

Diagnosis: Post-epileptic psychosis with temporal lobe epilepsy.

Follow up: The patient was known to have been admitted to hospital in a similar condition on at least three more occasions during the two years after discharge. His mental state improved after a few days in hospital on each occasion.

Case 20

Mr J.F.H., *aet.* 38, labourer, was admitted to hospital from an observation unit on 27.11.57. He was the younger of two siblings from a middle-class, comfortable background, with no family history of nervous or mental disease. He had always been a shy, serious person, dissatisfied with his milieu and disinterested in conventional society; there had been no overtly abnormal personality traits during childhood and adolescence. The patient did well at school and worked for a while in an insurance office and then as a surveyor's clerk. At the outbreak of war he registered as a conscientious objector and after having spent some time in prison he was released in order to undertake farm work. He then worked as a farm labourer for thirteen years in the West Country and never displayed any wish to improve his position despite his superior education. During the three years before admission he had been working in London in a menial capacity. The patient had been a heavy drinker for a few months when he was under considerable emotional strain some years before admission. He was married at the age of 20 and had five children, *aet.* 18, 14, 11, 8, and 6 months. His wife was a dreamy, dependent woman and suffered from poor sight which increased her dependence on the patient. During his stay in the country the patient had contracted a short-lived homosexual relationship with his landlord and there was some also experience of bestiality; the marriage on the whole was regarded as satisfactory by both partners despite these lapses. There was no history of serious physical or mental illness in the past.

In 1952 the patient had begun to feel that he was not longer acceptable to his friends and neighbours because of his sexual irregularities. Although he moved house he began to feel that he was surrounded by hostile observers and slowly he became convinced that they were spying on him and were obtaining information about him from hidden microphones in his house. He became unsettled and berated the family in order to get away from his persecutors. He then developed ideas that his children did not belong to him and that he had never been able to satisfy his wife's sexual demands. From this he reasoned that she must have been unfaithful to him; he became increasingly convinced of this belief, with which he confronted his wife frequently. Hitherto his wife had accepted his morbid ideas unquestioningly but she became very depressed at these accusations, especially as they continued after the birth of her fifth child. Eventually she threatened to commit suicide and she drew the attention of the mental health officer to her husband's mental state. Both marital partners were admitted to the observation unit at the same time and then transferred to a psychiatric hospital.

On examination the patient demonstrated no physical abnormalities. He was at first co-operative and friendly. The form of his talk was normal. He expressed systematized paranoid delusions with many ideas of reference and misinterpretations. There were no hallucinations; his memory and retention were normal and he was of high average intelligence. It was also apparent that he was depressed about his wife's supposed misconduct and after a few days in hospital he made a suicide attempt. After treatment with ECT his depression lifted and he began to hold less firmly to his belief in his wife's infidelity; he remained, however, convinced that he had been the victim of an organized plot as the only explanation of his morbid state of mind. Eventually he was discharged from hospital on 2.8.58, cheerful, but still entertaining morbid ideas about bodily dysfunction and ideas of reference.

Diagnosis: Paranoid schizophrenia.

Follow up: Two years after leaving hospital the patient was working well but had remained apart from his family. He had become convinced that his infirmities would impede a satisfactory reconciliation for some time.

Case 55

Mr L.J.P., *aet*. 30, film packer, was admitted to hospital from an outpatient department on 30.1.54. He had an unhappy working-class background; his father was a heavy drinker who had often behaved in a jealous manner towards his wife; his mother was blind, a possessive woman who drank heavily. There was no history of overt mental disease in the family. He had always been attached to his family and was regarded as an irritable, self-conscious person. His early work record had been irregular but his six years' service in the army were exemplary and he had boasted an excellent work record since demobilization. He drank alcohol rarely. Before his marriage the patient had had occasional heterosexual contact with prostitutes. He met his wife in 1952 and became unreasonably jealous almost immediately, accusing her of flirting with other men; he always recanted when she denied his accusations but he returned to them time after time. His wife had told him of her own premarital experiences, but he married her nevertheless in March 1953, eight months before admission. There was no previous history of significant illness.

From the time of his marriage the patient became more intensely jealous. He accused his wife of having had numerous affairs before marriage (this was untrue) and he made her leave her work as a telephonist because he feared her contact with other men; he tended to twist her conversation to show that she was faithless, and at the height of his paroxysms he would rake up old incidents and invent others. At no time, however, was he convinced that she was deceiving him and he admitted that he was aware of his tendency to fabricate when he became upset. After heated arguments with his wife he became contrite, apologetic, and very depressed. Their physical relations were satisfactory and he was never unfaithful. The marital difficulties eventually led the patient to consult his general practitioner who advised him to see a marriage guidance counsellor; the counsellor recognized the morbid nature of his difficulties and recommended psychiatric treatment.

In hospital he was at first anxious, tense, and also depressed, admitting that he had contemplated suicide in the previous weeks. There was no evidence of delusional thinking or of perceptual anomalies. He was treated with psychotherapy for six weeks. His feelings towards his wife fluctuated; at the time of his discharge on 30.3.54 he stated that he felt nothing but love for her.

Diagnosis: (1) Obsessional neurosis; (2) anxiety and depression.

Follow up: Three months after discharge the patient and his wife were known to be together though he remained moody and was jealous at times.

Case 75

Mrs C.P., *aet*. 37, housewife, was admitted to hospital on 12.3.55 following a domiciliary visit. She came from a middle-class family in Northern Ireland, the youngest of four sisters; there was no history of nervous or mental illness in the family. Though her mother died during her first year of life the patient was brought up capably by an aunt and her childhood was a very happy one. During her early years she had been an active, popular person, keen on games but disliking the academic side of school life. On leaving school at the age of 18 she led a pleasant, indolent life until her marriage and she never had to work for a living. She had never claimed more than a few friends, most of them women; she was subject to mood swings, very sensitive and shy but not suspicious. She drank alcohol only occasionally but was a heavy smoker. She had married *aet*. 27 and shortly afterwards came with her husband to England where she was at once unhappy. There was one child of the marriage, a girl aged 18. The marriage had been happy at first; neither the patient nor her husband had been unfaithful. There was no history of serious physical illness.

In March 1951 the patient had been referred for a psychiatric opinion and was seen once in the out-patient department of a general hospital. At the time she was complaining of feelings of depression and an inability to cope with her domestic responsibilities. She was regarded as suffering from a mild reactive depressive illness and the connection between her reaction and her nostalgia for her home was noted. She also admitted at the time that although she wanted another baby the thought of pregnancy so frightened her that she was considering the adoption of another child. In March 1955 she was seen on a domiciliary visit by the same psychiatrist who had seen her four years earlier. At this time she was expressing ideas about her husband's infidelity and admitted to a fantastic series of morbid beliefs on the subject. A diagnosis of paranoia was made and admission to hospital was advised. It appeared that she had been suspicious of her husband's fidelity at intervals throughout their married life but during the past year she had become certain of his guilt. She had followed him in the streets and had been through his clothes on many occasions; she had on occasion hidden herself in the boot of his car and claimed that she had heard him making love to another woman; she had maintained that her husband's clothes were stained with seminal fluid and that there was lipstick on his handkerchiefs. She also stated that her husband's attitude had changed towards her and that he had admitted his guilt. The relationship between them had deteriorated in consequence of her changed attitude.

On examination in hospital she was found to be poorly nourished with a rachitic deformation of the chest. There was no other evidence of physical disease. She was listless and fidgety and nodded her head frequently when talking. She appeared to be depressed for much of the time and was wholly taken up with her ideas about her husband's conduct. She admitted that some of her accusations might have been unfounded. She was treated with ECT, modified insulin, and supportive psychotherapy without any change in her condition becoming manifest. While she was in hospital she stated that her physical feelings for her husband increased in intensity. It was suggested that many of her ideas about her husband's infidelity represented a projection of her own feelings in the same direction. She was discharged from hospital on 28.5.55 without any substantial change in her mental state.

Diagnosis: Hysterical psychoneurosis with paranoid features.

Follow up: The patient was seen at regular intervals in the out-patient department and it gradually became clear that her delusions were becoming more firmly held and were proliferating. She stated that her husband was having an affair with a fictitious person and she maintained that she had discovered seminal stains on his socks, shoes, and raincoat. She hired a private detective to have her husband followed. She attacked an innocent woman on one occasion and was fined. Quarrels between the two marital partners began to increase in frequency. In 1958 the husband applied for a divorce but even after their physical separation the patient continued to accuse her husband of misconduct and also of homosexual activities. Divorce proceedings were commenced in October 1959; the application was eventually granted on the grounds of cruelty alone with a cross-petition by the patient on the same grounds. The following extracts of the legal proceedings were reported in 1960:

A charge that the wife had committed adultery with the co-respondent...was rejected, the co-respondent having been dismissed from the suit at the close of the evidence on the part of the husband, under section 5 of the Matrimonial Cases Act, 1950. The husband was ordered to pay the costs of the wife and of the co-respondent.

The essence of the husband's case of cruelty against the wife was that, from about September 1954 onwards, she falsely accused him of carrying on with other women. She made these accusations incessantly, for hours at a time. She checked and kept a record of the daily mileage of the husband's car; she kept a list of phone numbers, and invented names of women with whom she said the husband was associating. On one occasion she told the husband she had been concealed in the boot of his car while he had been making love to a woman in the car. On another occasion she said that she had received a letter saying that one of the women the husband was carrying on with had a venereal disease. When the husband asked to see the letter, she was unable to produce it.

In the spring of 1955 the wife was seen by a consultant psychiatrist.... His diagnosis was that she was paranoid and suffered from delusions. She sincerely believed, contrary to the fact, that her husband was carrying on with other women. She knew, when she made these accusations, the nature and quality of her acts, in that she knew she was accusing her husband of having affairs with other women, but she did not know that she was doing wrong. She did not make the accusations in order to be cruel to her husband, but because she felt herself wronged by his unfaithfulness...

After the wife's discharge from hospital, she soon renewed her accusations against her husband, suggesting that he had been carrying on with women while she was in hospital. Later the wife recanted, and admitted that her accusations were untrue, saying that some of them had been made to trick her husband. There was a legal presumption that a person was sane, so as to be responsible for his or her acts. The burden was on the wife to prove that she was in such a state of mind that either she did not know what she was doing or that she did not know that what she did was wrong. It was quite possible that in the autumn of 1954, and until her discharge from hospital in May 1955, she did not know that in making these accusations against her husband she was doing what was wrong. After she had recanted, however, it was impossible to hold that she was not legally responsible for her actions. The husband's case of cruelty had accordingly been established.

The wife's case against the husband which consisted essentially in the complaint that from 1955 onwards he had treated her with contempt and indifference, had also been made out.

References

1   E. Hellquist, *Svensk Etymologisk Ordbok*, Gleerup, Lund, 1920.
2   S. Stenberg, 'Beitrag zur Kasuistik des Eifersuchtswahnes', *Acta Scandinavica Neurologica et Psychiatrica*, 1943, 18: 59.
3   W. McDougall, *The Energies of Men*, London, Methuen, 1948.
4   E. Jones, 'La jalousie', *Revue française de Psychanalyse*, 1929, 3: 228.
5   T. Ribot, *Essai sur les Passions*, Paris, Alcan, 1910, p. 90.
6   A.F. Shand, 'M. Ribot's theory of the passions', *Mind*, 1907, 16: 477.
7   A. Gesell, 'Jealousy', *American Journal of Psychology*, Worcester, 1906, 17: 437.
8   S. Freud, 'Certain neurotic mechanisms in jealousy, paranoia and homosexuality', *Collected Papers*, vol. II., London, Hogarth Press, 1924, p. 232.
9   C.A. Ruckmick, 'The classification of emotions', in J.F. Dashiel (ed.) *The Psychology of Feeling and Emotion*, McGraw-Hill, 1936, p. 111.
10 J.C. Whitehorn, 'Physiological changes in emotional states', *Research Publications of the Association for Research in Nervous and Mental Disease*, 1939, 19: 256.
11 D. Lagache, *La Jalousie amoureuse*, 3 vols, Paris, Presses Universitaires de France, 1947.
12 S. Buchanan, *The Doctrine of Signatures*, London, Kegan Paul, 1938.
13 A. Mairet, *La Jalousie: Étude Psycho-physiologique, Clinique et Médicolégale*, Montpellier, 1908.
14 H. Ey, 'Jalousie morbide', in *Études Psychiatriques*, vol. II, Paris, Desclée de Brouwer et Cie, 1950, p. 483.
15 J. Escombe, *La Jalousie Morbide des alcooliques*, Paris, 1899.
16 R. Krafft-Ebing, 'Uber Eifersuchtswahn beim Manne', *Jahrbuch für Psychiatrie*, 1891, 10: 221.
17 A.J. Lewis, 'Alcoholic psychoses', *British Encyclopaedia of Medical Practice*, 1938, 8: 332.
18 K. Pohlisch, 'Die Persönlichkeit und das Milieu Delirium-tremens-Kranker der Charité aus den Jahren 1912 bis 1925', *Monatsschrift für Psychiatrie und Neurologie*, 1927, 63: 82.
19 K. Kolle, 'Uber Eifersucht und Eifersuchtswahn bei Trinkern', ibid., 1932, 83: 128.
20 E. Kraepelin, *Psychiatrie*, 7th edn, vol. II, Leipzig, Verlag von Johann Ambrosius Barth, p. 158.
21 V. Parant, quoted by R. Semelaigne, 'Delusions resulting from jealousy', *Journal of Mental Science*, 1902, 48: 131.
22 H.W. Gruhle, 'Partielle Geschäftsunfähigkeit, partielle Zurechnungsfähigkeit (Eifersucht)', *Nervenarzt*, 1940, 13: 544.
23 E. Redlich, 'Die Psychosen bei Gehirnerkrankungen', in A. Aschaffenburg (ed.) *Handbuch der Psychiatrie*, Leipzig, G. Deuticke, 1912.

24 P. Abély and C. Feuillet, 'Les idées délirantes de jalousie dans la démence précoce', *Annales Médico-Psychologiques*, 1941, 99, 2: 75.

25 K. Jaspers, 'Eifersuchtswahn', *Zeitschrift für Neurologie.*, 1910, 1: 567.

26 . D. Lagache, Discussion, in *L'Évolution Psychiatrique*, 1955, p. 64.

27 J.D. Campbell, *Manic-Depressive Disease*, Philadelphia, J.B. Lippincott, 1952.

28 B. Alapin, 'Zazdrose Zwykla, Charakteropatyczna I Urojeniawa (Etiologia, patogeneza', klinika)', *Neurologia, Neurochirurgia i Psychiatria Polska*, 1958, 8: 441.

29 J. Lange, 'Die endogenen und reaktiven Gemütserkrankungen und die manisch-depressive Konstitution', in O. Bumke (ed.) *Handbuch der Geisteskrankheiten* (Special), Berlin, Springer, 1928, vol. II, p. 91.

30 A. Brousseau, 'Variétés de la personnalité des jaloux au regard de la clinique', *L'Évolution Psychiatrique* 1955, p. 33.

31 F. Kehrer, 'Paranoische Zustände' in O. Bumke (ed.) *Handbuch der Geisteskrankheiten* (Special), Berlin, Springer, 1928, vol. II, pp. 245 and 260.

32 D. Stefanowski, 'Morbid jealousy', *Alienist and Neurologist*, St Louis, 1893, 14: 375.

33 E. Bleuler, *Dementia Praecox*, New York, International Universities Press, 1911 (trans. 1950), p. 399.

34 G. Langfeldt, 'The hypersensitive mind', *Acta Psychiatrica et Neurologica Scandinavica*, 1951, Supplement 73, p. 53.

35 J. Borel, *Les Psychoses Passionnelles*, Paris, Expansion Scientifique Française, 1952.

36 E. Kretschmer, *A Textbook of Medical Psychology*, London, Hogarth Press, 1952, p. 268.

37 O. Fenichel, *The Psychoanalytic Theory of Neurosis*, New York, W.W. Norton, 1945, p. 512.

38 M. Klein, *Envy and Gratitude*, London, Tavistock, 1957, p. 32.

39 R. Seidenberg, 'Jealousy: the wish', *Psychoanalytic Review*, 1952, 39: 345.

40 M. Schmeideberg, 'Some aspects of jealousy and of feeling hurt', *Psychoanalytic Review*, 1953, 1: 1.

41 J. Tiggelaar, 'Pathological jealousy and jealous delusions', *Fol. Psychiatr. Nederl.*, 1956, 59: 552.

42 Lagache, op. cit.

43 Ey, op. cit.

44 C.W. du Boeuff, *Over Jaloerschheidswan*, Zutphen, Ruys, 1938.

45 E. Minkowski, 'Jalousie pathologique sur un fond d'automatisme mental', *Annales Médico-Psychologiques*, 1929, 87, pt 2: 24.

46 F.H. Lund, *Emotions*, New York, Ronald Press, 1947, p. 228.

47 H. Rumke, in *Transcript of Comments and Discussion of the Work Conference on Problems in Field Studies in the Mental Disorders*, American Psychopathological Association, 1959 (unpublished), p. 370.

48 H. Ellis, 'Studies in the psychology of sex', vol. VI, *Sex in Relation to Society*, Philadelphia, F.A. Davis, 1928, p. 569.

49 K. Davis, 'Jealousy and sexual property', *Social Forces*, 1936, 14: 395.

50 E. Westermarck, *A Short History of Human Marriage*, London, Macmillan, 1908.

51 C.P. Blacker, 'Disruption of marriage', *Lancet*, 1958, i: 578.

52 J.F. Lovel Barnes, 'Marriage, paranoia and paranoid states', *Medical Press*, 1954: 232.

53 E. Revitch, 'The problem of conjugal paranoia', *Diseases of the Nervous System*, 1954, 15: 271.

54 E.T.O. Slater and M. Woodside, *Patterns of Marriage*, London, Cassell, 1951, p. 156.

55 J. Macdonell, in *Report of the Royal Commission on Capital Punishment* (1949–1953), London, HMSO, p. 330.

56 W.N. East, *Medical Aspects of Crime*, London, J.A. Churchill, 1936, p. 364.

57 H.C. Brierley, *Homicide in the United States*, Chapel Hill, NC, 1932.

58 J.P. Gray, 'Responsibility of the insane: homicide in insanity', *American Journal of Insanity*, 1875, 32: 1 and 153.

59 W.C. Sullivan, 'The relation of alcoholism to insanity and crime', *Proceedings of the Royal Society of Medicine*, 1924, 17: 37.

60 J.S. Hopwood and K. Milner, 'Alcoholism and criminal insanity', *British Journal of Inebriety*, 1940, 38, 51.

61 R.R. Mowat, 'Incidence of morbid jealousy in murderers', Dissertation for the University of London Diploma of Psychological Medicine, 1956 (unpublished).

62 W.N. East, *Forensic Psychiatry*, London, J.A. Churchill, 1927, p. 198.

63 A.F. Myer, B. Apfelberger, and C. Sugar, 'Men who kill women', *Journal of Clinical Psychopathology*, 1947, 8, 3: 481.

64 B. Karpman, *Case Studies in the Psychopathology of Crime*, vol. III, Washington, DC, Medical Science Press.

65 *Journal of Mental Science*, 1864, 9: 591; 1865, 10: 21; 1865, 11: 66.

66 D.H. Tuke, 'Monomania', in *Dictionary of Psychological Medicine*, London, J.A. Churchill, 1892, p. 82.

67 H. Maudsley, *Responsibility in Mental Disease*, New York, Appleton & Co., 1897, p. 213.

68 H. Claude, *Psychiatrie Médico-Légale*, Paris, G. Doin et Cie, 1932, p. 135.

69 J.W.J. Edwards, 'Provocation and the reasonable man: another view', *Criminal Law Review*, London, Sweet & Maxwell, 1954, p. 898.

70 P. Devlin, 'Criminal responsibility and punishment: functions of judge and jury', *Criminal Law Review*, London, Sweet & Maxwell, 1954, p. 661.

71 R.N. Gooderson, 'The charge was murder', *The Listener*, 1959, 61: 549.

72 E. de Greeff, *Introduction à la Criminologie*, vol. I, Brussels, Joseph Vandenplas, 1946, p. 366.

73 *Report of the Royal Commission on Marriage and Divorce*, London, HMSO, 1956, p. 39.

74 The Law Reports (Probate), Palmer *v.* Palmer, 1955, p. 4.

75 W. O'Neill, 'A case of jealousy', *Lancet*, 1898, *i*: 223.

76 C.F. Wendt, 'Die "Eifersuchtsparanoia" im psychotherapeutischen Aspekt', *Archiv für Psychiatrie und Nervenkrankheiten*, 1951, 186: 496.

77 R. Brunswick, 'A case of paranoia (delusions of jealousy)', *Journal of Nervous and Mental Disease*, 1929, 70: 1 and 155.

Chapter four

Changing disciplines in psychiatry

One of Virginia Woolf's late essays bears the interrogative title, 'Why?'.[1] In it she questions many widely accepted precepts and practices, and singles out the lecture for particular attention. 'Why lecture?' she asks, 'Why be lectured?'

> In the old days, [she continues] when newspapers were scarce and carefully lent about from hall to rectory, such laboured methods of rubbing up minds and imparting ideas were no doubt essential. But now, when every day of the week scatters our tables with articles and pamphlets in which every shade of opinion is expressed, far more tersely than by word of mouth, why continue an obsolete custom which not merely wastes time and temper, but incites the most debased of human passions – vanity, ostentation, self-assertion, and the desire to convert?

By way of illustration she goes on to give a memorable description of the prototypical lecture:

> The chairs in the room were occupied intermittently, as if they shunned each other's company, by people of both sexes; some had note-books, others had none and gazed with the vacancy and placidity of bull frogs at the ceiling.
>
> A large clock displayed its cheerless face, and when the hour struck in strode a harried-looking man, a man from whose face nervousness, vanity, or perhaps the depressing and impossible nature of his task had removed all traces of ordinary humanity. There was a momentary stir. He had written a book, and for a moment it is interesting to see people who have written books. Everybody gazed at him. He was not bald and not hairy; had a mouth and a chin; in short he was a man like any other, although he had written a book. He cleared his throat: the lecture began. . . . But why – oh,

Maudsley lecture to the Royal College of Psychiatrists, 1987. Originally published in *British Journal of Psychiatry*, 1988, 153: 493–504.

why – since printing presses have been invented these many centuries, should he not have distributed his printed lecture instead of speaking it?

One of the few satisfactory answers to this question was provided by Mrs Woolf's friend, E.M. Forster, in the encomium on her work which he delivered shortly after her death in the form of an eponymous lecture.[2] Here he touched on the ceremonial function of the lecture as ritual, conferring public honour on speaker, sponsoring body, and subject alike. And despite her stated views, he surmises slyly that Mrs Woolf herself would not have been displeased by the occasion.

Since its inception in 1919 the Maudsley Lecture has come to assume a ceremonial function in the programme of this College, and it would seem incumbent on anyone who is honoured by an invitation to deliver it to familiarize himself with the preceding lectures of the series. For me the task has been unexpectedly instructive. The list of lecturers is impressive by virtue of not only their eminence, but also the heterogeneity and range of their selected topics. Taken as a group, the lectures emerge as a line of beacons which illuminate the direction, if not always the advances, of psychological medicine over the past three generations.

In the pre-war period this variety reflected in some measure the original nature of the bequest, according to which two categories of lecture were to be delivered in alternate years, the one 'scientific' and devoted to original work, the other 'popular' and concerned with any subject connected with the hygiene of the mind.[3] The scientific category included such topics as Sir Frederick Mott's 'Further researches on dementia praecox',[4] Edwin Goodall's 'Dealing with some of the work done to elucidate the pathology of disease failing to be considered under the rubric "insanity"',[5] and C.E. Spearman's 'The psychiatric use of the methods and results of experimental psychology'.[6] To the popular category were allocated more general themes: Sir Farquahar Buzzard's 'Education in medicine',[7] Lord Macmillan's 'The professional mind',[8] and Mr Justice McCarthy's 'Truth'.[9]

In the post-war years this system of alternation appears to have given way to a more uniform pattern. As Erwin Stengel pointed out, every lecture has tended to focus on a large issue, drawn either from the field of clinical psychiatry or from one of the many areas of basic or applied studies in which psychiatrists are interested.[10] In most instances the lecturer has chosen to speak on some topic within his or her sphere of expertise, and the spectrum has proved broad enough to incorporate themes ranging from Sir Frederick Bartlett's 'Intelligence as a social problem',[11] to Grey Walter's 'The function of electrical rhythms in the brain',[12] and John Ryle's 'Nosophobia',[13] the first Maudsley Lecture that I attended and the one that is indirectly linked most closely with my own.

To maintain the tradition I have deemed it appropriate to relate my contribution to some of the work with which I have been associated, but the content prompted less difficulty than the form in which it might be presented. The occasion is clearly no longer appropriate for popular lectures, now that the mass media have taken over the field to such an extent as to have given rise to Henry Miller's diatribe on the psychiatrist as magician, prepared to 'misuse his jargon to confuse any and every topical issue in an incessant series of television appearances'.[14] But nor, I think, should it provide no more than a platform for the specialized presentation of clinical or scientific material, some of which might otherwise qualify for publication in the 'Journal of Irreproducible Results'. I felt there was something to be said for a broader framework than has sometimes been evident and I was glad to find a guiding precedent in Adolf Meyer's Maudsley Lecture, which was constructed in what he called a 'semi-historical and semi-personal' format.[15]

The historical element opens the door to mention of Henry Maudsley. His work and influence on British psychiatry have constituted the subject of two previous lectures,[16] and most lecturers have endorsed Sir David Henderson's vignette of 'a sensitive, solitary man, a keen student, a brilliant and independent thinker, with something of the quality of genius'.[17] More recently some medical historians have called for a reevaluation.[18] My own concern, however, is more with the roots and soil of Maudsley's outlook than with its flowering, for the familiar portrait of the white-bearded patriarch who died in 1918 tends to obscure the fact that his formative years were passed in the high noon of the nineteenth century. His first paper, 'The correlation of mental and physical forces',[19] was published at the age of 24 in 1859, the year when Landseer's lions appeared in Trafalgar Square, when Gladstone became Chancellor of the Exchequer, and the Franco-Austrian war commenced; the year that also saw the appearance of Mill's *Essay on Liberty*, Samuel Smiles's *Self-Help*, Dickens's *Tale of Two Cities* and, most significantly, Darwin's *Origin of Species*. To that most perceptive of historians, G.M. Young, 1859 ushered in the 'years of division' between early and late Victorian England, separating what he called the 'statistical' from the 'historical' age:

We are passing from the statistical to the historical age, where the ground and explanation of ideas, as of institutions, is looked for in their origins: their future calculated by observation of the historic curve. As early Victorian thought is regulated by the conception of progress, so the late Victorian mind is overshadowed by the doctrine of evolution. But the idea of progress – achieved by experiment, consolidated by laws or custom, registered by statutes – had, without much straining of logic or consequence, been made to engage with the dominant Protestant faith, and thus, equally in both its modes: in the individualism of the soul working out its own salvation, in the charity which sought above all things the welfare of others.... Religion, conceived as a central system of ideas, aspirations, and practices to be imposed on society, was losing its place in the English World.[20]

Not only the English world, it might be added. The drift away from religion was part of a wider process, one which Owen Chadwick has aptly termed the 'secularisation of the European mind'.[21]

Maudsley's period of maturation, then, coincided with a crucial period in the history of ideas. Unlike most physicians, as Sir John Macpherson pointed out in his Maudsley Lecture, he was 'a man in advance of his time – one of the galaxy of intellectuals which adorned the mid-Victorian period',[22] and as such he was well aware of the impact of evolutionary theory and scientific materialism on what Harold Nicolson described as 'that intricate weaving and unweaving of taste and distaste, that kaleidoscopic and continuous reshaping of intellect and indifference, of surprise and expectation, which we call, somewhat indolently, "the spirit of the age" '.[23] Writing in the 1890s, Bernard Shaw could look back in pleasure:

> Let any man of middle age . . . consider what has happened within a single generation to the articles of faith his father regarded as eternal, nay, to the very scepticisms and blasphemies of his youth . . . and he will begin to realize how much of our barbarous Theology the man of the future will do without.[24]

But Shaw, secure in his socialist faith, was in a minority. For a majority of late Victorian thinkers the strain was overwhelming, so much so that Gertrude Himmelfarb has concluded that:

> Victorian intellectuals dwelled, for the most part, upon the plains of madness – that deceptively peaceful countryside where philosophers paraded as journalists and writers showed off their Rugby Blues more proudly than their Oxford Firsts. Here lived those scientists and rationalists (Darwin, Huxley, Spencer) who suffered from lifelong illnesses which defied medical diagnosis and cure; novelists of domestic manners and morals (Bulwer Lytton, Thackeray, Meredith, Dickens) whose marriages were tragically unhappy; religious libertarians (Harrison, Stephen, Morley) who were zealous puritans; successful and wealthy writers (Macaulay, Dickens, Darwin) who were obsessed with the fear of bankruptcy; moral critics (Carlyle, Eliot, Mill, Ruskin) who lived in the shadow of sexual aberrations and improprieties; and in general an intellectual community suffering a larger proportion of nervous breakdowns, it would seem, than almost any other.[25]

With his adherence to notions of 'degeneration' and his sceptical views on treatment, what Maudsley had to offer his troubled contemporaries must have been cold comfort. From the beginning his writings are deeply imbued with an analytical, agnostic, ultimately pessimistic approach to the major philosophical questions associated with religious belief, moral conduct, and the mind-body problem. That first paper contains a credo which underpins many of his subsequent expositions:

> Man, indeed, only progresses in knowledge in so far as he progresses in physical science; it is in this mainly that the progress of civilisation has consisted ... it is so far true, that no change has taken place of late in the principles of morality; but it seems impossible to deny that there has been an extension of the application of those principles – an increase in practical morality; and this, not as the result of any supposed exacerbation of moral principle, but as the simple and inevitable result of the progress of science. The abstract moral truth, that man 'should do unto others as he would have others do unto him' though for ages preached, and for ages recognized as true, would not avail to induce the rich man to improve his poor neighbour's pig-sty habitation. And the poor man being left, morality notwithstanding, to live like a pig, acted also in some measure like a pig but modern science has taught us that a filthy habitation, and a foul atmosphere and unwholesome food, are directly destructive to human life; and cholera and fever have done what religion and morality had attempted and failed to do; and now, as a result, is appearing the dawn of a social science.[26]

When Maudsley here speaks of progress he does so in the spirit of G.M. Young's 'historical age'. There is nothing endaemonical in his use of a word which to Herbert Spencer was 'not an accident, but a necessity. Surely must evil and immorality disappear; surely must men become perfect.'[27] And Maudsley's final sentence suggests that for him Young's 'statistical age' had been superseded rather than merely succeeded by the burgeoning of the natural sciences, for he ignores altogether the large claims to the scientific study of society on a statistical basis which had been lodged thirty years earlier. Melioristic and overtly political in outlook, and drawing on Benthamite utilitarianism and on philosophical radicalism for their ideas, the advocates of the statistical movement participated in a widespread reaction to industrialization in a society which was rapidly changing its values and looking for a way of rationalizing political economy and formulating social 'laws'.[28] The term 'social statistics' was coined to cover moral as well as vital statistics. The former were concerned mainly with education, crime, and intemperance, the latter with the collection of data on birth and mortality. And from these collections of facts and figures there emerged the study of 'sanitary statistics', conceived as the numerical relationship between the hygienic conditions of living and the risks to health and life, especially in urban conditions, which constituted the basis of the concept of public health in Britain during this epoch in the work of men like Owen Chadwick, William Farr, Thomas Southwood Smith, and John Snow. On the European mainland there developed a slightly different but parallel trend that was to lead to Neumann's challenging assertion that medicine is intrinsically and essentially a social science.[29]

Much of this early work was focused on epidemics of infectious disease, correlating death rates with the hygiene of the living conditions of the population at large. Paradoxically its impetus was impaired by the emergence of bacteriology in the 1870s when the microscope of the laboratory worker came into its own and the emphasis was placed on the biological causation of disease. The statisticians diversified their activities and loosened their political links, some to concentrate on what was to become empirical sociology, some to develop the field of biometrics, and others to apply medical statistics to the study of morbidity and mortality. By the beginning of this century Alfred Grotjahn was able to construct a framework of social hygiene,[30] and in his autobiography he put the matter plainly:

> I was, from the beginning, convinced that medical statistics must be regarded as the basis of socio-pathological and social-hygienic study and therefore needed the most careful cultivation. At that time the victorious march of bacteriology had relegated medical statistics to the background. ... It was not necessary to rob bacteriology of a single leaf of her garland in order to insist that this view was erroneous and that a quantitative study of the theory of epidemics was as indispensable as before the bacteriological era.[31]

Grotjahn's words cast a long shadow. The debate over these two approaches to medicine was to extend far beyond the infectious diseases and continues to the present day. Reviewing the characteristics of these two complementary forms of clinical science, Sir James Spence referred to the one as clinical cartography, aiming chiefly to map the contours and terrain of disease; the other he called clinical phenomenology, an experimental discipline that 'studies the isolated phenomena of disease or of disordered function and its aim is to explain their mechanisms and their clinical significance'.[32] For a while the spectacular achievements of experimental medicine appeared to hold out boundless prospects, founded on Lewis Thomas's claim of fifty years ago that 'medicine was changing into a technology based on genuine science'.[33] By 'genuine' he meant biological. Since then a period of disillusionment has set in and no less an authority than Macfarlane Burnet has gone so far as to assert that 'the contribution of laboratory science to medicine has virtually come to an end'.[34] Colin Dollery has spelt out the reasons for a more sober verdict in his monograph explicitly entitled, 'The end of the era of optimism'.[35]

Perhaps the most far-sighted overview of this dichotomy, however, was provided by John Ryle, the first Professor of Social Medicine in this country.

Unlike most earlier representatives of this viewpoint Ryle was an eminent clinician, a former physician at Guy's Hospital, and Regius Professor of Physic at Cambridge.[36] Towards the end of his career, in 1948, he summarized his standpoint in a volume of essays which he entitled *Changing Disciplines*:

> Looking back, it has seemed to me that while Medicine – through scientific and technical advances – has greatly gained in potentiality during the past quarter of a century, it has in the process become less surely attuned to some fundamental human needs – to the broader social needs of the group or community. . . . In the midst of great social changes we have not succeeded in registering and explaining the accompanying changes in the quantity and quality of many of our main diseases some of which I shall later refer to as our 'modern endemics'. . . . We no longer believe that medical truths are only or chiefly to be discovered under the microscope, by means of the test-tube and the animal experiment, or by clinical examination and increasingly elaborate pathological studies at the bedside. Psychological and sociological studies have an important part to play. Even so, it is not yet appreciated how intimately disease and social circumstances are inter-related. The whole natural history of disease in human communities, as well as in individuals, is ripe for a fuller and more exhaustive study.[37]

It was on this basis that Ryle constructed his own concept of social medicine, drawing on the 'changing disciplines' of his – and my – title. These included demography, biostatistics, history, sociology, some branches of psychology, and above all, epidemiology, especially the epidemiology of non-infectious disease, a notion that was then still controversial. Ryle himself spoke of 'endemics' and in many ways, as Erik Strömgren has argued, the word endemiology would have been more appropriate.[38] None the less the term 'epidemiology' has stuck because of its historical associations and has come increasingly to be the term of choice for the mass aspects of disease. It is a word, incidentally, which – as far as I can determine – has received explicit mention, and that in passing, by only two previous Maudsley lecturers.

How did these 'changing disciplines' impinge on the study of psychological medicine? The nineteenth century witnessed numerous debates on such topics as moral treatment, the increase and the prevention of insanity, and the putative nexus between civilization and mental disease. Most of them were conducted in very general terms, though a few individuals appreciated the potential significance of employing the numerical approach to mental disease under institutional care exemplified by Black as early as 1811.[39] By and large, however, this was not the use to which the statistics of insanity were widely put. The professional world of most nineteenth-century psychiatrists was limited by the asylum walls where, as Gerald Grob has pointed out, psychiatry developed as 'a managerial and administrative speciality'.[40] In consequence, the statistics of mental disorder were collected and published primarily to canvass public support and to establish the legitimacy of public mental hospitals. For the purposes of scientific enquiry, the data were gravely handicapped by the inadequacy of psychiatric diagnosis, and most psychiatrists were largely unaware of the importance of classification which William Farr, the first Registrar General, had early recognized as 'another name for generalisation', adding that 'successive generalisations constitute the laws of the natural sciences'.[41]

The isolation of mental hospital practice further retarded the interest of psychiatrists in the mainstream of general medicine as well as public health. This separation was reinforced by the seeming irrelevance of the bacteriological revolution to the aetiology of most mental disorders. The tenacious beliefs held by a few clinicians in the causal importance of micro-organisms for many mental illnesses may have represented their tribute to the successful public-health campaigns against infectious diseases but by and large, as the published deliberations of the Medico-Psychological Association demonstrate, most psychiatrists seem to have taken little account of these developments.

By the early years of this century a change of opinion can be detected, stimulated in part by the progressive policy adopted in Germany. Like Henry Maudsley, R.G. Rows, Assistant Medical Officer and Pathologist to the Lancaster County Asylum, was much impressed by the organization and work of the German university psychiatric clinics, but he drew quite different conclusions from his observations. Maudsley himself, as J.R. Rees pointed out in his Maudsley Lecture, was unable to see much future for the public-health movement in the field of mental illness,[42] but in 1912, in a paper entitled 'The development of psychiatric science as a branch of public health', Rows commented adversely on the British asylum service, and concluded that

> the causes of insanity resemble the causes of the diseases to combat which our service of Public Health has been instituted; and that in order to achieve as good results in the treatment of mental disorder, the work must be undertaken by a service of men of high scientific training and keen enthusiasm.[43]

The First World War temporarily interrupted this trend, but it reappears shortly afterwards in the report of the Royal Commission on Lunacy and Mental Disorder (the Macmillan Commission), which emphasized that mental disorder was 'essentially a public health problem, to be dealt with on public health lines'.[44] In that same year, 1926, a Royal Charter was granted to the Medico-Psychological Association, and Lt-Col. J.R. Lord delivered his presidential address on the topic of 'The clinical study of mental disorders'. Seventy-nine pages long, it was printed as a special number of the *Journal of Mental Science* (presumably only a portion was delivered verbally!) and contains a strongly worded critique of the isolationism of the mental hospital and a plea for a broader view of the discipline. 'Mental anthropology', he stated, 'would not be an inapt synonym for modern psychiatry' and, he went on, 'The Royal Medico-Psychological Association is concerned with the practice of psychiatry in the broadest sense. Psychiatry and mental hygiene are to be regarded as part of the large problem of public health.'[45] Emphasizing the need for research, Lord drew particular attention to the inadequacies of diagnosis and classification for statistical analysis, commenting bluntly that 'the terms used, with a few exceptions, are confusing and meaningless'.

The same trend is discernible among the early Maudsley Lectures. In 1924 John Carswell devoted his address to 'Some sociological considerations bearing upon the occurrence, prevention and treatment of mental disorders', drawing on some dubious statistics from the Glasgow area.[46] Two years later George M. Robertson chose as his theme 'The prevention of insanity: a preliminary survey of the problem'.[47] On the basis of data derived from the Twenty-First Annual Report of the Commission in Lunacy of the State of New York, he generalized, none too convincingly, on prevention, eugenics, mental hygiene, temperance, education, early treatment, and the putative increase of insanity, concluding with an exhortation to the psychiatrist of his day:

> Far too long has he sulked in his tent: now he must come out into the market-place. He must co-operate with the general practitioner, and get into touch with the outer world, the out-patient department and the social service worker.

Fine words, but how little force they carried was evident from the Maudsley Lecture delivered twenty years later by Sir Laurence Brock, a Chairman of the Board of Control, on 'Psychiatry and the public health service'.[48] For Brock the cream in the professional bottle apparently consisted in what he called the Olympians of Harley Street. As for the milk, his views on training reflect his own outlook and that, presumably, of officialdom:

> The new entrant should be treated as a cadet – i.e. someone having the status of an officer but still needing instruction and supervision ... it is difficult if not impossible to determine whether a young doctor is worth postgraduate training until he has lived in mental hospital long enough to decide whether he likes the life or not.

In the face of such an outlook it is less surprising that although the application of epidemiological principles to the cause and treatment of pellagra had already provided a convincing demonstration of the public-health approach to mental illness, during the inter-war years the concept of mental hygiene carried more meaning for public-health workers than for psychiatrists. Since its inception in the USA, the mental hygiene movement had been primarily concerned with psychiatric issues in the community at large – the school, the home, and the courts – and so became involved with a broad spectrum of social problems. In Britain much of the ground was broken by the voluntary organizations, as exemplified by the pre-war activities of the Mental After-Care Association, the Child Guidance Council, the Central Association for Mental Welfare, and the National Council for Mental Hygiene.

The full impact of these currents of opinion on psychiatry in this country, however, had to await the Second World War, when the potential psychological ill-effects of bombing and of internal migration on the civilian population were recognized as potential public-health problems.[49] In the army the need to evaluate and treat psychiatric morbidity was soon appreciated, and selection procedures and rehabilitation programmes were introduced. In the RAF a number of far-reaching medico-statistical studies were carried out on the classification, distribution, and causation of psychological disorders among flying personnel. Outstanding among these were the epidemiological enquiries on pilot stress conducted by Donald Reid,[50] and Austin Bradford Hill's little-known work on the reliability of psychiatric diagnosis,[51] which anticipated much research in this sphere.

During the war, furthermore, a remarkable series of planning activities was initiated, including the 1944 Education Act, the Beveridge Report, and the preparation of the foundations of the National Health Service. Medicine itself underwent a penetrating self-examination by the Goodenough Committee on Medical Education,[52] which emphasized both the need for recognition of the importance of psychiatry and its affiliation with social medicine. The Royal College of Physicians' broad view of psychiatry as the study of human behaviour in a social setting led naturally to its conclusion that psychiatry and social medicine be regarded as 'the inside and outside of the same glove'.[53]

The early 1940s, then, constituted a historical turning-point in the confluence of factors bringing psychiatry into the new field of force generated by social medicine and the changing disciplines associated with it. And at this juncture the historical becomes the personal, though at the time I was barely aware of the process, thereby exemplifying G.M. Trevelyan's observation that people who are present at a turning-point in history are usually unaware that history is turning. For me the pre-potent factor was the exposition of these ideas by several outstanding teachers, foremost among them John Ryle himself during my undergraduate years. One of the consequences of their teaching was an awareness that for the systematic investigation of mental disorder there were many advantages attaching to a clearly defined catchment area. Some years later chance, possibly favouring the prepared mind, brought me into contact with the Buckinghamshire County Mental Hospital, St John's Hospital at Stone, near Aylesbury. There I was given free access to the institutional records, which enabled me to mount a study of the whole population of an area hospital. Since this investigation and its sequelae bear directly on my theme, I propose to summarize them briefly. All the work to which I shall be referring was conducted in Buckinghamshire and could not have been undertaken without the support of several local colleagues, especially Dr David Watt, with whom I have worked closely on several studies.

Some years before I began my first study, Sir Aubrey Lewis had observed that

So far as psychiatry is conceived as a branch of social medicine and public health, it must rely for its advancement upon methods which require accurate statistics such as it is the business of official intelligence to supply, as well as upon the individual and perhaps more original methods which are in keeping with its main tradition.[54]

A major obstacle to investigations of this type, however, had been the disparity between the basic demographic and clinical data and the outdated and uninformative diagnostic categories recorded in the case notes, a point made explicitly by Lord sixty years ago. Commenting on the need for 'the collection, registration and classification of clinical data for the purposes of psychiatry generally and research work in particular', he went on:

I have never written up a good case in the records of a mental hospital without finding that it was a pure waste of time. The sex, age, occupation, civil state, diagnosis and result would appear in statistical form, but otherwise the rest of my labour would be hidden, perhaps for centuries, between heavy brass-mounted boards and that would be the end of it. Why should such labour in large measure be lost to the common good and the advancement of psychiatry?[55]

Why indeed? It seemed to me worth exploring the possibility of combining the carefully recorded accurate statistics of a county mental hospital with a clinical analysis of the case notes based on the study of all recorded sources, including follow-up information. The task proved unexpectedly rewarding, and with these data it became possible to undertake a trend analysis by comparing intramural events in two separate time-periods.[56] The initial triennium, 1931–3, covered the final phase of the custodial era, symbolized by the Mental Treatment Act of 1930. This preceded a more active phase of administration that was to be exploited by the appointment in 1934 of a forward-looking physician-superintendent who was wedded to the concept 'of a Mental Health Service rather than one of mere Mental Hospital administration – a policy of co-operation rather than custody'.[57] His vigorous reforms resulted in a sharp increase in medical personnel, the creation of out-patient clinics, the introduction of domiciliary consultations, and the provision of beds in a local general hospital, all aiming to render the mental hospital, in his words: 'more a centre of active medical treatment and less a place of care and custody for the chronic harmless case'.

By the mid-1940s the fruits of this policy were apparent in the form of a local system of community care which had been established long before the notion became fashionable. Over this period the outcome of patients with functional psychoses admitted during the second triennium 1945–7 had become significantly superior to that of the initial cohort in terms of discharge rates, length of stay in hospital, remissions, re-admissions, and mortality. An investigation of the related circumstances identified three possible reasons for this amelioration: namely the new administrative policy, the admission of less severe cases, and the arrival of new forms of somatic treatments such as continuous narcosis, ECT, sedatives, deep insulin coma therapy, and pre-frontal leucotomy. A closer analysis made it clear that the physical measures were of least importance and that the changes were largely attributable to what Cheney and Drewry had referred to twenty years earlier as the 'non-specific effects of treatment'.[58] By this term they indicated not only the impact of environmental and interpersonal factors but also, by implication, the need to demonstrate the superiority of any new treatment over the intensive application of good hospital care and management. 'Non-specific' in this context was largely synonomous with 'non-biological' and constituted the standard by which any supposedly 'specific' treatments would be assessed.

The role of these non-specific, psychosocial factors seemed to me to carry wider significance. Behind the discussion of the seemingly remote question of the interpretation of mental hospital statistics there lay, and still lies, a profound difference of opinion concerning not only the place of somatic treatments but also the causation of the illnesses themselves. In large measure the specific–non-specific dichotomy reflects the divide between the biological and the psychosocial approaches to the aetiology and treatment of mental disorder.[59]

The practical aspects of this issue soon became apparent when the psychotropic drugs entered the scene in the mid-1950s. The action of these drugs was supposedly 'biological' or 'specific' and their impact, it was claimed, overshadowed any 'non-specific' or 'psychosocial' effects which were dismissed as supposedly placebogenic. The consequences of this contention were highlighted when the claims for the efficacy of these compounds were employed in support of the national policy of running down the mental hospitals. The so-called 'pharmaceutical' era was seen as spearheading a major shift in policy, and the terms 'deinstitutionalization' and 'community care' began to attract widespread support.

In the subsequent debate, as several commentators made clear, a closer examination of the facts, or rather the figures, showed that the official view represented a gross over-simplification of a complex phenomenon. Essentially the policy was based on national statistics that took no account of local variation. How relevant this could be became apparent from our extension of the original trend analysis at St John's Hospital to cover the four-year period, 1954-7, that is from the year before the introduction of psychotropic drugs to the year in which they were prescribed on a large scale. The findings showed that very little change had occurred during this time.[60] The major movement of the hospital population, defined in terms of a higher discharge rate and a shorter hospital stay, had in fact taken place ten years earlier, largely as a result of the setting up of the active mental health service in the area. A very similar pattern was reported from Norway by Ødegaard, who drew the seemingly paradoxical conclusion that

in hospitals with a favourable situation the psychotropic drugs brought little or no improvement or even a decrease in the rate of discharges. In hospitals with a low pre-drug discharge rate, on the other hand, the improvement was considerable.[61]

This factor had, of course, long been recognized by clinical observers, particularly with regard to the schizophrenias. As long ago as 1908 Eugen Bleuler commented on the difference in outcome and prognosis of two groups of schizophrenic patients who were under his care.

In New-Rheinau the patients with 'favourable' outcome were more severely ill than those allocated to the same category in Burghölzli or in Alt-Rheinau. As I had known most of the patients personally for years, it seemed unlikely that this was due to an error. The observation was confirmed by the physicians in Alt-Rheinau. The explanation for this fact, I concluded, was that New-Rhineau was run in accordance with new ideas and, from the start, had been organised so as to be filled by patients from every quarter of the globe. Here it was possible to create a new spirit which allowed the transformation of a number of severe and chronic catatonics into good workers. This difference between different parts of the same psychiatric service is very striking.[62]

The introduction of long-acting drugs administered by injection as 'maintenance' or 'continuation' treatment of schizophrenics in the late 1960s enabled us to apply similar methods to a more focused issue. The putative advantages attaching to continuation therapy were dominantly social, in that it was claimed (1) to facilitate the return of patients to the community, (2) to reduce the burden on the family, and (3) to render rehabilitation easier and more economical. Several reports conformed well to what had become the expectations of the day, though the hard evidence delineating the relative efficacy of short- and long-acting neuroleptic continuation treatment was negligible. None the less in Britain, as elsewhere, the climate of clinical opinion came to favour the view that a diagnosis of schizophrenia in hospital should lead to pharmacotherapy by the parenteral route in a majority of cases.

Accordingly we carried out a retrospective study of the outcome of two cohorts of all schizophrenics discharged from St John's Hospital during 1967–8 and 1970–1 respectively.[63] The first period preceded the establishment of special clinics for the administration of long-acting drugs, the second followed their introduction. By comparing the numbers of patients readmitted and their length of stay in hospital we were able to obtain an index of the impact of the drug on the movement of the schizophrenic population. The result of this analysis showed clearly that while fewer discharged schizophrenics were readmitted to hospital when on long-acting medication, this finding characterized only those patients who enjoyed a more favourable prognosis regardless of treatment.

Such findings underlined the importance of examining more closely the natural history of the disorder, on which a rational approach to treatment ultimately depends. Within the National Health Service it is probable that most schizophrenics make contact with hospital facilities which can therefore be employed as a method of case identification. For the study of outcome, however, the limitations of any enquiry based on hospital statistics had clearly been reached and prospective enquiries became indispensable.

Ideally any such study should be based on the four criteria needed for the establishment of reliable data. These are (1) a representative population; (2) a standardized method of diagnosis; (3) a prospective enquiry over at least five years; and (4) the recording of independent clinical and social criteria. No investigation has so far met all four specified criteria but it proved possible to construct and follow up a reasonably representative cohort of patients diagnosed as schizophrenic by standardized criteria of known reliability so as to ascertain the clinical and social outcome independently over the subsequent quinquennium.[64] This proved to be much better than most earlier workers had maintained, most strikingly among women.

While some of this improvement may be attributable to drugs it is apparent that even if a particular form of treatment can be shown to facilitate discharge from hospital and maintain an extramural existence, its importance cannot be adequately assessed without reference to the subsequent quality of life in the community. Earlier studies had emphasized the point by suggesting that 'the mental hospital atmosphere had merely been transferred to the home'. A direct examination of this issue demands an assessment of the impact of treatment on both the patients' clinical status and social capacity within the framework of a controlled therapeutic trial.

My own involvement in such investigations dated back some years, one of the first having been carried out at St John's Hospital as early as 1956.[65] Subsequently my work on the MRC Clinical Trials Committee, which had been set up for the evaluation of treatment modalities in psychiatry, brought me into close collaboration with Sir Austin Bradford Hill who helped demonstrate for the first time that the basic principles of the multi-centred clinical trial could be applied to mental disorder.[66]

Under the auspices of the MRC Clinical Trials Committee we were able to organize a comparative double-blind clinical trial of two drugs at St John's Hospital. Its aim was to assess the relative efficacy of the two compounds in the continuation therapy of patients returning to the community following hospitalization for an acute schizophrenic episode. For the purpose standardized clinical and social assessments were made independently over a period of twelve months.[67]

With regard to the results of this complex experiment I would emphasize here only the two most relevant. First, in terms of the clinical criteria employed there was nothing to choose between the two drug regimes. Second, and quite unexpectedly, one of the drugs – originally introduced as no more than a control for the other – proved to be superior on the various measures of social functioning. Other workers have made it clear that an adequate explanation of these findings involves more than drug action and the authors of a comparable American study have concluded: 'The development of successful treatment programmes may hinge on our learning more about the nature of this social dysfunction'.[68] If this could prove to be the case, the psychosocial factors in treatment could, paradoxically, be regarded as 'specific' as the postulated biological factors.

So much for hospital-based enquiries which, as I have tried to demonstrate, carry some meaning for major mental illness. However, their scope is clearly limited and must be complemented by examination of psychiatric morbidity in the community at large. The term 'community psychiatry' has been widely misapplied by restricting it to the fate of patients discharged from hospital. In a public-health context, it should refer to the general population. Only then is it possible to examine the distribution of illness in its early and less severe forms and to approach the vexed question of what Ryle called 'The meaning of normal and measurement of health',[69] an objective particularly important for mental disorders characterized by 'dimensional' rather than 'categorical' phenomena.

Buckinghamshire provided an early example of such work in the records of the seventeenth-century practitioner, Richard Napier, whose material has been carefully evaluated by Michael MacDonald.[70] The primary care health services for adults in the county in the twentieth century, however, proved too scattered for investigation and it was more feasible to concentrate on the population of children via the county schools and the child-guidance services which provide a reliable statistical framework.[71]

The basic information was derived from specially constructed questionnaires (6,300 in all) dealing with health, behaviour, and family background, which were sent to the parents of a one-in-ten random sample of all children aged between 5 and 15 years attending local authority schools in the county. The items of conduct in the questionnaire covered most of the common behavioural problems characterizing the schoolchild population attending child guidance clinics. At the same time separate questionnaires were prepared for despatch to the children's schools, where they were completed by the class teachers.

The availability of quantitative and qualitative data obtained independently from school and home made it possible to examine the areas of concordance and discordance between the reported behavioural disorders in the two settings. It emerged that while difficulties at home were significantly associated with poor academic performance and also with behaviour 'problems' at school, some children exhibited disorders of behaviour only at home or only at school. Furthermore, many of the recorded items of supposedly disturbed behaviour could not in themselves be taken as indices of abnormality: several items were reported as occurring very rarely, others so frequently as to characterize a majority of the population.

To take account of these factors, operational criteria of 'deviant' behaviour were constructed to provide a quantitative index of behaviour typical of the child's age and sex. As many as four-fifths of the sample of children attending the county child guidance clinics were characterized by a deviant total score; there was a significant association between the reported occurrence of deviant conduct at home and the reporting of behavioural problems in school. This concept of deviance, however, has nothing to say about duration, which is closely bound up with the notion of morbidity, since disturbed behaviour in childhood can represent no more than a developmental phase or a transient reaction to short-lived stresses. For this reason a follow-up study was carried out on two matched groups of 400 children, one of which was originally characterized as deviant and the other not. An analysis of associated factors showed the former group of children and their families to be less healthy, less successful, and more exposed to stress at home and at school, than were the control group. None the less, two and a half years later approximately three-quarters of the deviant group were reported as exhibiting a reduced number of deviant items, and about half were said to exhibit no evidence of such behaviour. The notion of morbidity attaching to an item of conduct therefore must incorporate frequency, intensity, behavioural associations, and duration before it transcends the boundaries of 'normality'.

So much for a brief summary of a body of work which has extended over thirty years. In relation to the historical background that I have attempted to sketch I would stress, first, its dependence on close collaboration with colleagues whose professional skills lie in 'changing disciplines' outside the biomedical orbit – in particular, epidemiology, statistics, sociology, and social psychology.

Second, in retrospect it is now apparent that such work exemplifies a movement in psychiatric research which has come into its own during the post-war period. This has been characterized by the plethora of studies on diagnosis and classification; on measurement, and especially on what Alvan Feinstein calls 'clinimetrics', the design and application of 'instruments' for the assessment of psychopathology;[72] on the evaluation of treatments and of health services; and on environmental studies. In themselves none of these topics is new. The novelty consists in the increased frequency and intensity with which they are being applied to the study of mental disorder. All of them incorporate the criteria implicit in Michael Oakeshott's definition of science as the study of quantitative generalizations,[73] and in a medical context they share an adherence to the epidemiological method.

I am not, of course, suggesting that these methods and techniques constitute the only form of relevant scientific enquiry. The post-war period has also witnessed a fresh influx of experimental studies of mental disorder and dysfunction and a welcome quickening of interest among laboratory-based neuroscientists in the somatic substrata of mental illness: much of what is now designated 'biological psychiatry' has resulted from their efforts. Nor am I disregarding the traditionally idiographic approach of clinical psychiatry, with its emphasis on the description and interpretation of general psychopathology. If I have chosen to highlight the third leg of the tripod it is because it is still relatively less familiar and has been more widely misunderstood. It significance may be summarized by a brief mention of the research objectives associated with the six principles enunciated by Alfred Grotjahn in his *Social Pathology*: namely, prevalence, clinical phenomena, outcome, treatment, aetiology, and prevention.[74]

An appreciation of the extent of mental illness is probably the best-established result of the work so far, underlining Grotjahn's verdict: 'the significance of illness from a social point of view is primarily determined by its frequency'. One major finding has been the identification of a large volume of conspicuous psychiatric morbidity at the level of primary care which falls outside the purview of the mental health services, and about which the specialist psychiatrist knows all too little.[75] In addition, the search for inconspicuous morbidity in the community at large has renewed interest in the vexed issue of case definition and the boundaries of mental ill-health. *Pari passu* there has been a quickening of interest in clinical phenomena in their own right: first, with the aim of quantification; second, to complete the clinical picture of syndromes derived from hospital studies; and third, to delineate more accurately the so-called 'minor' forms of mental disorder. All this assumes increasing practical importance as epidemiological enquiries become recognized as the basis of rational health policy.[76]

The study of these various syndromes further incorporates a temporal dimension, since all too often their natural history, especially of the non-psychotic conditions, remains to be firmly established. In this task it becomes necessary to examine clinical and social criteria independently since disorders of function figure prominently in the presenting picture. The evaluation of therapeutic intervention also demands an acknowledgement of this distinction, especially since the adoption of the clinical trial as a standard method of assessment has exposed the role of non-specific factors and the need to examine the much underestimated placebo effect.

With regard to aetiology, it is relevant to recall that not unitl 1951 were the statistics of morbidity as distinct from mortality made the subject of a Registrar General's report which stated squarely that if 'the search for specific (aetiological) agents halted the progress of social medicine, then the role of nutrition, psychological medicine, stress and other trends have reawakened interest in "broader domains of aetiology"'.[77] These 'broader domains' imply the concept of multiple causation, whose counterpart in mental illness is the notion of 'multidimensionality' which has come to underlie several systems of classification. The search for aetiological factors within this framework is, in Griesinger's terminology, that of causal association rather than causal mechanisms,[78] leading to the realms of predisposition, and to precipitating, pathoplastic, and preformative factors rather than to the exogenous, pathogenic link in the aetiological chain which, when identified, lends itself more readily to preventive action. Such noxae which have so far been identified in relatively few mental disorders, are, by contrast, closely linked to genetic predisposition and to patterns of living or lifestyle which are less susceptible to modification.[79] The scope for prophylactic intervention is correspondingly limited.

From all these considerations the message is clear. 'Medicine', as the sociologist Robert Merton once observed, 'is at heart a polygamist becoming wedded to as many of the sciences and practical arts as prove their worth.'[80] His comment applies *a fortiori* to psychological medicine, but it is now apparent that in these liberated times the new wives are already showing signs of independence not only from the older females but also from the polygamous male, viewing themselves not so much as help-mates as partners, even senior partners, in a joint enterprise.[81] The emergence of 'behavioural medicine' in the USA indicates which way the wind is blowing and psychiatrists have now to familiarize themselves with unfamiliar viewpoints and techniques if their role is not to be diminished.

Finally, I would emphasize the significance of this trend for members of this College. Much of the work, as I have tried to illustrate, can be carried out in area hospitals or centres as well as university clinics or specialized laboratories. Accordingly it provides ample opportunity for psychiatric physicians, with or without academic affiliations, to conduct research on their own patients in their own setting, drawing on their knowledge of the ecological matrix in which mental illness is embedded. Here the College can and should play a crucial role. Many of us deplored the low priority given to research at its foundation and have applauded the recent moves to remedy that deficiency. They will surely help regain something of that 'breadth of vision' which, according to a recent Maudsley lecturer,[82] the profession has lost in the past few years. Fortunately we need no longer argue the case for changing the disciplines required for the task. They have already been changed.

References

1   V. Woolf, 'Why?', in *The Death of the Moth*, London, Hogarth Press, 1942.
2   E.M. Forster, *Virginia Woolf*, Cambridge, Cambridge University Press, 1942.
3   J. Crichton-Browne, 'The first Maudsley lecture', *Journal of Mental Science*, 1920, 66: 199–25.
4   F. Mott, 'The second Maudsley lecture: Further researches on dementia praecox', *Journal of Mental Science*, 1921, 67: 319–39.
5   E. Goodall, 'Dealing with some of the work done to elucidate the pathology of disease failing to be considered under the rubric "insanity" ', *Journal of Mental Science*, 1927, 73: 361–90.
6   C.E. Spearman, 'The psychiatric use of the methods and results of experimental psychology', *Journal of Mental Science*, 1929, 75: 357–70.
7   E.F. Buzzard, 'Education in medicine', *Journal of Mental Science*, 1933, 79: 4–17.
8   Lord Macmillan, 'The professional mind', *Journal of Mental Science*, 1934, 80: 469–81.
9   Mr Justice McCarthy, 'Truth', *Journal of Mental Science*, 1931, 77: 4–21.
10 E. Stengel, 'Pain and the psychiatrist', *Journal of Mental Science*, 1965, 111: 795–802.
11 F. Bartlett, 'Intelligence as a social problem', *Journal of Mental Science*, 1946, 93: 1–8.
12 W.G. Walter, 'The functions of electrical rhythms in the brain', *Journal of Mental Science*, 1950, 96: 1–31.
13 J.A. Ryle, 'Nosophobia', *Journal of Mental Science*, 1948, 94: 1–17.
14 H.G. Miller, 'Psychiatry – medicine or magic?', *World Medicine*, 1969, 5: 44.
15 A. Meyer, 'British influences in psychiatry and mental hygiene', *Journal of Mental Science*, 1933, 79: 435–63.
16 H. Bond, *Henry Maudsley* (unpublished), 1931; A. Lewis, 'Henry Maudsley: his work and influence', *Journal of Mental Science*, 1951, 97: 259–77.
17 D. Henderson, 'A re-evaluation of psychiatry', *Journal of Mental Science*, 1939, 85: 1–21.
18 T. Turner, 'Henry Maudsley – psychiatrist, philosopher and entrepreneur', *Psychological Medicine*, 1988, 18. M.J. Clark, 'Late Victorian psychiatry', D.Phil. dissertation, University of Oxford, 1982; and E. Showalter, *The Female Malady*, London, Virago, 1987.
19 H. Maudsley, 'The correlation of mental and physical forces; or, man a part of nature', *Journal of Mental Science*, 1859, 6: 50–78.
20 G.M. Young, *Victorian England: Portrait of an Age*, London, Oxford University Press, 1936.
21 O. Chadwick, *The Secularization of the European Mind in the Nineteenth Century*, Cambridge, Cambridge University Press, 1975.

22 J. MacPherson, 'The new psychiatry and the influences which are forming it', *Journal of Mental Science*, 1928, 74: 386–99.

23 H. Nicolson, *The Development of English Biography*, London, Hogarth Press, 1968, p. 134.

24 G.B. Shaw, *Shaw's Music*, ed. D.H. Laurence, vol. III, London, Bodley Head, 1891, p. 446.

25 G. Himmelfarb, *Victorian Minds*, London, Weidenfeld & Nicolson, 1968, p. 218.

26 Maudsley, op. cit.

27 H. Spencer, *Social Statics*, New York, D. Appleton, 1892, p. 32.

28 M.J. Cullen, *The Statistical Movement in Early Victorian Britain*, Hassocks, Harvester Press, 1975; K.H. Metz, 'Social thought and social statistics in the early nineteenth century', *International Reviews of Social History*, 1984, 29: 254–73.

29 S. Neumann, *Die öffentliche Gesundheitspflege und das Eigentum. Kritisches und Positives mit Bezug auf die preussische Medizinalverfassungsfrage*, Berlin, Adolph Reiss, 1847, p. 64.

30 A. Grotjahn, *Soziale Pathologie*, 2nd edn, Berlin, August Hirschwald, 1911.

31 A. Grotjahn, *Erletztes und Erstrebtes*, Berlin, Heibig, 1932.

32 J. Spence, 'The methodology of clinical science', in *Lectures on the Scientific Basis of Medicine*, vol. 2, London, Athlone Press, 1954, pp. 1–12.

33 L. Thomas, *The Youngest Science*, Oxford, Oxford University Press, 1984, p. 32.

34 F.M. Burnet, *Genes, Dreams and Realities*, Lancaster, Medical and Technical Publishing Co., 1971.

35 C. Dollery, *The End of an Age of Optimism*, London, Nuffield Provincial Hospitals Trust, 1978.

36 G. Rosen, 'Approaches to a concept of social medicine: a historical survey', *Milbank Memorial Fund*, 1948, 26: 7–21; and C. Webster, 'The origins of social medicine in Britain', *Bulletin of the Society for the Social History of Medicine*, 1986, 38: 52–5.

37 J.A. Ryle, *Changing Disciplines*, London, Oxford University Press, 1948.

38 E. Strömgren, 'Introduction', in *Contributions to Psychiatric Epidemiology and Genetics*, Acta Jutlandica, x: 4, Medical Series, Copenhagen, Munksgaard, 1968, p. 9.

39 W. Black, *A Dissertation on Insanity: Illustrated with Tables, and Extracted from between Two and Three Thousand Cases in Bedlam*, 2nd edn, London, G. Smeeton, 1811.

40 G.N. Grob, 'The origins of American psychiatric epidemiology', *American Journal of Public Health*, 1985, 75: 229–36.

41 W. Farr, cited in M.J. Cullen, op. cit., p. 34.

42 J.R. Rees, 'Psychiatry and public health', *Journal of Mental Science*, 1957, 103: 314–25.

43 R.G. Rows, 'The development of psychiatric science as a branch of public health', *Journal of Mental Science*, 1912, 58: 25–39.

44 Report of the Royal Commission on Lunacy and Mental Disorder (Macmillan Report), Cmd. 2700, London, HMSO, 1926.

45 J.R. Lord, 'A clinical study of mental disorders', *Journal of Mental Science*, 1926, 72, special number.

46 J. Carswell, 'Some sociological considerations bearing upon the occurrence, prevention and treatment of mental disorders', *Journal of Mental Science*, 1924, 70: 347–62.

47 G.M. Robertson, 'The prevention of insanity: a preliminary survey of the problem', *Journal of Mental Science*, 1926, 72: 454–91.

48 L. Brock, 'Psychiatry and the public health service', *Journal of Mental Science*, 1946, 92: 387–404.
49 J.M. Mackintosh, *The War and Mental Health in England*, New York, The Commonwealth Fund, 1944.
50 D.D. Reid, 'Some measures of the effect of operational stress on bomber crews', FPRC Report 605, in *Psychological Disorders in Flying Personnel of the Royal Air Force (1939–1945)*, Air Publication 3139, pp. 245–58, Air Ministry, London, HMSO, 1947.
51 A.B. Hill and D.J. Williams, 'Reliability of psychiatric opinion in the Royal Air Force', FPRC Report 601, in *Psychological Disorders in Flying Personnel of the Royal Air Force (1939–1945)*, Air Publication 3139, pp. 308–20, Air Ministry, London, HMSO, 1947.
52 Report of the Inter-Departmental Committee on Medical Schools (Goodenough Report) London, HMSO, 1944.
53 Interim Report on Undergraduate Education in Psychiatry: Committee on Psychological Medicine, London, Royal College of Physicians, 1943, p. 4.
54 A. Lewis, 'Letter from Britain', *American Journal of Psychiatry*, 1945, 101: 486–93.
55 Lord, op. cit.
56 M. Shepherd, *A Study of the Major Psychoses in an English County*, London, Oxford University Press, 1957.
57 J.S.I. Skottowe, 'Medical Superintendent's Report for the Year 1941', in *Fifty-Second Annual Report of the Visiting Committee Elected by the County Council on the Bucks County Medical Hospital*, 1941, p. 15.
58 C.O. Cheney and P.H. Drewry, 'Results of non-specific treatment', *American Journal of Psychiatry*, 1938, 95: 203–17.
59 M. Shepherd and N. Sartorius (eds) *Non-Specific Aspects of Treatment*, Bern, Huber, 1989.
60 M. Shepherd, N. Goodman, and D.C. Watt, 'The application of hospital statistics in the evaluation of pharmacotherapy in a psychiatric population', *Comprehensive Psychiatry*, 1961, 2: 11–19.
61 Ø. Ødegaard, 'Pattern of discharge from Norwegian psychiatric hospitals before and after the introduction of psychotropic drugs', *American Journal of Psychiatry*, 1964, 120: 772–8.
62 E. Bleuler, 'Die Prognose der Dementia Praecox – Schizophreniegruppe', *Allgemeine Zeitschrift für Psychiatrie*, 1908, 65: 436–64.
63 M. Shepherd and D.C. Watt, 'Impact of long-term neuroleptics on the community: advantages and disadvantages', in J.R. Boissier, H. Hippius, and P. Pichot (eds) *Neuropsychopharmacology*, New York, Excerpta Medica, 1975.
64 D.C. Watt, K. Katz, and M. Shepherd, 'The natural history of schizophrenia: a prospective 5-year follow-up of a representative sample of schizophrenics by means of a standardized clinical and social assessment', *Psychological Medicine*, 1983, 13: 663–70.
65 M. Shepherd and D.C. Watt, 'Chlorpromazine and reserpine in chronic schizophrenia: a controlled clinical study', *Journal of Neurology, Neurosurgery and Psychiatry*, 1956, 19: 232–5.
66 Medical Research Council, Report by its Clinical Trials Committee, 'Clinical trial of the treatment of depressive illness', *British Medical Journal*, 1965, i: 881–4.
67 I. Falloon, D.C. Watt, and M. Shepherd, 'A comparative controlled clinical trial of pimozide and fluphenazine decanoate in the continuation therapy of schizophrenia', *Psychological Medicine*, 1978, 8: 59–70; I. Falloon, D.C. Watt, and

M. Shepherd, 'The social outcome of patients in a trial of long-term continuation therapy in schizophrenia: pimozide vs. fluphenazine', *Psychological Medicine*, 1978, 8: 265–74.

68 C. Schooler and H.E. Spohn, 'Social dysfunction and treatment failure in schizophrenia', *Schizophrenia Bulletin*, 1982, 8: 85–98.

69 J.A. Ryle, *Changing Disciplines*, op. cit.

70 M. MacDonald, *Mystical Bedlam*, Cambridge, Cambridge University Press, 1981.

71 M. Shepherd, A.N. Oppenheim, and S. Mitchell, *Childhood Behaviour and Mental Health*, London, London University Press, 1971.

72 A.R. Feinstein, *Clinimetrics*, New Haven, Conn., Yale University Press, 1987.

73 M. Oakeshott, *Experience and its Modes*, Cambridge, Cambridge University Press, 1985, p. 221.

74 Grotjahn, *Soziale Pathologie*, op. cit.

75 Shepherd *et al.*, 1966, op. cit.

76 S. Levine and A. Lilienfeld, *Epidemiology and Health Policy*, London, Tavistock, 1987.

77 D. McKay, *Hospital Morbidity Statistics: Studies on Medicine and Population Subjects, No. 4*, London, General Register Office, 1951.

78 W. Griesinger, *Mental Pathology and Therapeutics*, trans. C.L. Robertson and V. Rutherford, London, The New Sydenham Society, 1867, pp. 127–8.

79 Report of the WHO Scientific Working Group, *Stress, Lifestyle and the Prevention of Disease*, Geneva, World Health Organization, 1982.

80 R.K. Merton, 'Some preliminaries to a sociology of medical education', in R.K. Merton, G.G. Reader, and P. Kendall (eds) *The Student Physician*, Cambridge, Mass., Harvard University Press, 1957.

81 M. Shepherd, 'Who should treat mental disorders?', *Lancet*, 1982, i: 1, 173–5.

82 K. Jones, 'Society looks at the psychiatrist', *British Journal of Psychiatry*, 1978, 132: 321–32.

Chapter five

Psychological medicine *redivivus*: concept and communication

Introduction

Although the term 'psychological medicine' is widely used in Britain to label academic titles, hospital departments, textbooks, and examination diplomas, it does not appear in most dictionaries and is rarely defined. The ambiguity can be traced to its origins. From the time of its inception the term would appear to have carried two distinct meanings. One of these was well enough established by the middle of the nineteenth century to have been employed by Sir John Bucknill and Daniel Tuke to designate their influential *Manual of Psychological Medicine*[1], which incorporated 'the lunacy laws, the nosology, aetiology, statistics, description, diagnosis, pathology and treatment of INSANITY'. A fitting title too, one might think, for the official organ of the Association of Medical Officers of Asylums and Hospitals for the Insane, which had appeared five years earlier and of which Bucknill was the founder editor. In the event, however, this was called the *Asylum Journal of Mental Sciences* and Bucknill gave his reasons for this choice:

> Our journal does not contain a single article which can be truly called *psychological*. Its character is strictly *psychiatric*, and the matters discussed in its pages are restricted to such as have immediate reference to the pathology and therapeutics of insanity, to the construction and management of asylums and to the diseases, accidents and difficulties likely to arise therein. We aim not at the discussion of those higher branches of metaphysical science, the able and learned treatment of which has so long distinguished the pages of our contemporary. Our desire is to be collectors of facts, the active practical pioneers in the march of mental science.[2]

Here Bucknill is being disingenuous, knowing as he did that the 'pages of our contemporary' to which he refers were those of the *Journal of*

Presidential address to Section of Psychiatry, Royal Society of Medicine, 10 October 1985. Originally published in *Journal of the Royal Society of Medicine*, 1986, 79: 639–45.

Psychological Medicine and Mental Pathology, the first British journal to be concerned exclusively with mental illness, which had appeared in 1848. The stated purpose of the *Journal of Psychological Medicine* was much broader than that of the *Asylum Journal of Mental Science*. It aimed to examine theories as well as facts, not to focus on insanity but, in the words of its founder, 'to establish a periodical devoted to the discussion of questions in relation to the Human Mind in its abnormal condition'.[3]

Winslow

The driving force behind this publication was a remarkable and strangely neglected figure, Forbes Benignus Winslow (1810–74) (Figure 5.1), who first conceived of the journal in the 1820s and then put up £1,000 of his own money to launch it. For the first ten years of the journal's life Winslow acted as proprietor, editor, and sub-editor, revising papers and proofs, writing many of the articles and reviews himself, and superintending the mechanical side of the printing.

Who was Winslow? He was the ninth son of a military father and a religious mother, a lineal descendant of the Pilgrim Fathers who left England in the *Mayflower*. Having supported the Royalists in the American War of Independence, the family returned to England in straitened circumstances and Winslow had to battle hard to obtain the medical education that he had passionately desired from an early age. His energy was prodigious. It was said of him by an obituarist that, as a student:

> he would work all day at the hospital, and then as a reporter for the Times go in the evening to the Gallery in the House of Commons, so paying for the expenses of his own education.... It was no uncommon thing for him to leave the Times' office at seven or eight in the morning, take a hasty breakfast and be ready to receive patients by 10 o'clock. He managed to steal two or three hours sleep in the course of the day, but was always ready, and apparently fresh, to take his turn in the Gallery when he was required...he was made of the right stuff for work, and possessed a cheerfulness of spirit, a hopefulness and self-reliance, which carried him through.[4]

Winslow was also the proprietor of two private establishments where humane methods of treatment were *de rigueur*, and he had an extensive private practice with a particular bias towards medico-legal work. He was a key witness in the McNaughton case and wrote extensively on forensic matters. He was also a public-spirited man, who refused parliamentary seats on four occasions. He received an honorary DCL from Oxford, and was appointed President of the Medical Society of London and of the Psychological Association. 'No wonder', says his biographer, 'he could

Figure 5.1 Forbes Winslow

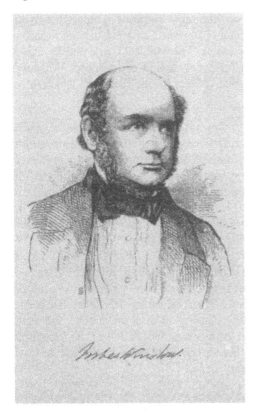

Source: From a photograph by John Watkins.

claim for 10 years he had never dined at home or spent an evening away from his patients.'[5]

From the age of 18 Winslow described himself as having 'lived out of an inkstand'. His voluminous writings included not only many articles but also several books on a variety of topics, including *Physic and Physicians* (1839), *The Anatomy of Suicide* (1840), *On Preservation of the Health of Body and Mind* (1842), *On Softening of the Brain from Anxiety* (1859), *Light: its Influence on Life and Health* (1867), *On Uncontrollable Drunkenness, Considered as a form of Mental Disorder* (1867), and the volume in which he took greatest pride, *On the Obscure Diseases of the Brain, Disorders of the Mind*, first published in 1860 and running to four editions over the next eight years. Here he discusses at length the importance of ascertaining the symptomatology of early mental disorder, and adumbrates the need to develop methods of so doing by means of developing clinical interview techniques, psycho-diagnostic testing, and what he called 'chemico-cerebral pathology'.

Journal of Psychological Medicine

Of all these achievements, however, the most enduring is undoubtedly his journal, which ran to thirteen volumes under its original title and then, in 1861, continued for three more issues as 'The Medical Critic and Psychological Journal', to indicate a still further widening of its scope. Winslow's style and character beam out of his 'Address to our Readers'[6] which introduces volume 3:

> With the present number of our Journal we enter upon the *third* year of our eventful existence. We have outlived a most unfavourable prognosis. Dismal were the forebodings with which our entrance into life was greeted. Persons who wished us a happy and prosperous voyage, speculated (as kind friends often do) either upon our gradual decay or premature dissolution. Thank God, we still breathe, we can throw ourselves into the editorial chair, and with philosophical benignity, look back with pleasure upon the PAST, and with glowing anticipation towards the FUTURE. We do not wish our kind friends to misunderstand us. We have not for the last two years been reposing upon a bed of down. Our editorial life has not been one of ease and quiet. Our path has not been across flowery meads, and by the side of purling streams. The road we have travelled has been a rugged and circuitous one, often full of great discouragement, and as we have paused on our journey we have occasionally allowed the thought to glance through our mind, whether we should even reach the goal towards which we were bending our weary steps.

The goal proved to be inseparable from the man, for the journal ceased publication following the editor's serious illness. In 1875 it reappeared as 'a new series' under its original title and edited by Winslow's son, only to expire after three years.

The title of Winslow's journal was highly significant, pointing as it did to the emphasis on psychology and philosophical enquiry in relation to mental disorder. Its generic content included original commentaries, analytical reviews, translations, notes on medical jurisprudence, a correspondence column, and monograph/supplements. To illustrate the spectrum of material, some of the early articles were devoted to epidemic insanity, religious mania, the statistics and pathology of insanity, the transmission of mental qualities, hallucinations, puerperal insanity, the aesthetics of suicide, literary fools, and the significance of Cartesian philosophy.

Concept of psychological medicine

For Winslow, it should be noted, the term 'psychology' was synonymous with 'all that relates to the soul or mind of man in contradistinction to his material nature'; the word, he claimed, had come to denote 'all that relates to the department of science which takes cognizance of irregularities and aberrations and diseases of the mind (hence "psychological physician")... mental pathology would be a far more exact but also a more cumbrous term'. Here, as throughout his mature work, Winslow was reflecting the impact of Ernst von Feuchtersleben's seminal book, *The Principles of Medical Psychology*,[7] which was published in 1844, and translated into English in 1847. This course of lectures for medical students was designed for

> not only... the psychiatric practitioners in lunatic asylums but... physicians in general, every one of whom ought to have a clear view of the relations of the body to the mind... an exposition of all the relations under which mental operations may be represented to medical observations and medical treatment.

Feuchtersleben speaks explicitly of a 'psychological medicine' which broadens the framework of the discipline to incorporate history, phenomenology, nosography, the natural history of psychosis and of therapeutics. To represent psychological medicine he sketches the character of the 'psychological physician', a man not only with 'quick apprehension and correct judgement... a refined perspicacity and a philosophically cultivated understanding', but one who possesses a high moral character and undergoes a 'second education... to obtain influence over the minds of other men... a gift that Nature often refuses to the most distinguished men, and yet without which, mental disease however thoroughly understood, cannot be successfully treated'.

Winslow endorsed and elaborated on this notion in one of his Lettsomian Lectures of 1851–2, which he devoted to the 'Psychological Physician',[8] and he made his position explicit when reviewing a volume called *The Elements of Psychological Medicine*, a book which he dismissed as a 'flimsy elementary treatise upon insanity... instead of being an introduction to the Study of Medical Psychology – or Psychological Medicine (we are indifferent as to how the words are played upon)'.[9]

Essentially, therefore, this concept of psychological medicine overlaps with, but is larger than, its more restricted identification with what was to be termed 'psychiatry'. Its orbit was to include not only mental disorders in *sensu strictu*, but also the study of abnormal behaviour from the medical standpoint. This was the core of Winslow's outlook. In the words of a contemporary medical historian, he 'did more than anyone else... to popularise the term and concept of psychological medicine with all the implications of a recognised speciality'.[10] And the instrument by which he did so was 'the first non-partisan psychological journal to be published in this country, uncommitted... to particular causes'.[11]

An adequate account of the subsequent fate of the notion of psychological medicine would demand nothing less than the development of the specialty in this country and has still to be written. My primary concern here, however, is with nothing so ambitious. It is limited to some reflections on the communication of the concept, deriving partly from its subsequent evolution, and partly from my own experiences as a participant observer of the process.

Medico-scientific journals

In historical perspective the *Journal of Psychological Medicine* can be seen not only as a periodical in its own right but also as an early specimen of the medical scientific journal, a vehicle for the spread of information which was becoming indispensable to nineteenth-century medicine as it began to lay claim to scientific status. Up to the mid-seventeenth century the basic means of communication among scientists had been letters and books, of which there were a great number. 'One of the diseases of this age', wrote Barnaby Rich in 1613, 'is the multiplicity of books; they doth so overcharge the world that it is not able to digest the abundance of idle matter that is every day hatched and brought forth into the world.'

Partly from this sense of dissatisfaction and partly from the growing need for contact among scientists, there emerged the scientific journal, whose purpose has been defined as 'to facilitate communication among scientists . . . whose . . . goal . . . is the discovery of scientific knowledge and the verification of such discovery'.[12] The first scholarly scientific journal, *Le Journal des Sçavans*, appeared in 1665, followed shortly afterwards by the *Philosophical Transactions of the Royal Society*. At the heart of the scientific journal was the scientific paper, which has been described by a historian of science as 'a major achievement of our civilisation', one whose form 'has changed less in nearly 300 years than any other class of literature except the bedroom farce'.[13] The conjunction is not fortuitous. Both bedroom farce and scientific papers are concerned with the public presentation of private activities.

And in the wake of the scientific journals there emerged the scientific editor to join the ranks of the larger editorial tribe. One of the greatest of these, Denis Diderot, defined the editorial function in the *Encylopédie* as follows:

The term editor is applied to a man of letters who takes the trouble to publish the works of other people. Such a person should have two essential qualities: first, he should understand the language in which the work is written, and secondly, he should have a working knowledge of the author's material.

Matters have become more complicated since the eighteenth century. At first the roles of editor and publisher were closely intertwined, and Sir Leslie Stephen – in outlining the history of the subject – remarks that

The normal process of the evolution of editors ... is the gradual delegation of powers by the printer or bookseller who had first employed some inhabitant of Grub St as a drudge, and when the work became too complex and delicate, had handed over the duties to men of special literary training.[14]

By contrast, editors of the early scientific and medical journals were not men of letters. They were characterized more by a professional training, a feeling for words, and, often, a strong personality and a determination to impose their points of view on their peers and their readers. This was especially true of those men who edited journals that were independent of professional associations. Thomas Wakly of *The Lancet* was one such man, and Forbes Winslow was another.

In the second half of the nineteenth century, medical and scientific journals began to proliferate in such numbers as to provide historians of various disciplines with a rich source of information, nowhere more so that in the field of psychiatry. As Helen Marshall has pointed out:

the general psychiatric journals reflect the history and nature of the subject. Their changes in title, like those of their parent societies, indicate changing concepts of and attitudes towards mental illness ... Some of its [psychiatry] branches are esoteric, semantically confusing and often subtle, as journal titles sometimes show.[15]

By way of example, mention may be made of the metamorphosis of the *Asylum Journal of Mental Science* (1855) into the *Journal of Mental Science* (1859) and eventually into the *British Journal of Psychiatry* (1963), reflecting as it does the corresponding titular and functional evolution of the Association of Medical Officers of Asylums and Hospitals for the Insane to the Medical-Psychological Association to the Royal College of Psychiatrists.

Psychiatric journals

Where, amid what was to become a confusing welter of journals, was the successor to Winslow's *Journal of Psychological Medicine*? The short answer is: nowhere. While the term survived in Britain and for a time was probably best represented by the philosophical and psychological writings of Henry Maudsley, the adjective and the noun moved in different directions. With the emergence of psychology as an independent and verbose discipline in the last quarter of the nineteenth century, the adjective 'psychological' was purloined by a flood of journals on psychology with so many shades of meaning – normal, abnormal, general, clinical, physiological, philosophical – as to call for the talents of a W.S. Gilbert to do them justice. In the twentieth century the term 'medical psychology' took on a colouring that would have surprised von Feuchtersleben, especially in its psychodynamic reincarnation, and, more recently, there has been a proliferation of specialist interdisciplinary journals (e.g. *Psychophysiology, Neuropsychologia, Biological Psychology*) which exhibit further adulterations of the psychological sciences.

The noun 'medicine', on the other hand, drifted towards the evolving specialty of neurology. The six volumes of the *Reports of the West Riding Asylum*, published between 1871 and 1876, were edited by the superintendent, Sir James Crichton-Browne, who attracted the interest of such eminent neurologists as Charles Ferrier and John Hughlings Jackson. The *Reports* preceded the appearance of the journal *Brain* in 1878, edited originally by two psychiatrists (Crichton-Browne and Bucknill) and two neurologists (Ferrier and Jackson), but eight years later this was taken over by the Neurological Society of London and became increasingly an organ of clinical neurology and neurophysiology.

This cannibalistic tendency was to be repeated as neurologists began to make their reputations out of organic disease and their income out of mental disorder. To many of them, as Adolf Meyer pointed out fifty years ago, psychiatry became a 'mere subordinated appendix, useful for diplomatic reasons'.[16] In 1903 there appeared the *Review of Neurology and Psychiatry*, in which the case for combining the two disciplines was explicitly presented in the first issue:

> The British Medical Schools are surely to be congratulated on the production of a journal in which the subjects of Neurology and Psychiatry are to be dealt with in combination. During the 19th century, and especially during the last 50 years, the students of scientific medicine, and also the practical clinician have recognised with steadily increasing conviction of the importance, the essential unity of the two subjects.[17]

As it turned out, this journal was to be dominated by neurologists, whose interests were reflected in its contents. In 1926 it was taken over by the British Medical Association and renamed the *Journal of Neurology and Psychopathology*, again with a neurologist as editor and relatively little psychiatric representation. This was nominally one of the three major British inter-war journals of psychiatry, the others being the *Journal of Mental Science* and the *Archives of Neurology and Psychiatry*. The latter was founded in 1902 to present the work of the Pathological Laboratory of the London County Asylums and was first entitled *Archives of Neurology*. Later it came to consist of a collection of reprints of the published papers of staff members of the Central Pathological Laboratory, the London County Hospitals for Nervous and Mental Diseases, and the Maudsley Hospital and the associated Institute of Psychiatry, until its demise in the immediate post-war period.

In 1938 the *Journal of Neurology and Psychopathology* was re-named *Journal of Neurology and Psychiatry*, once more with a neurologist as editor and a bare quorum of psychiatrists on the editorial board. In 1944 it incorporated neurosurgery to become the *Journal of Neurology, Neurosurgery and Psychiatry*. By the time I joined its editorial board in the early 1960s, the proportion of psychiatric papers per annum was under 1 per cent and after discussion with the editor of the *British Medical Journal* I suggested that the journal should cease to include psychiatry in either its title or its subject matter, and that the British Medical Association create a new specialist journal devoted to psychological medicine in the original, larger sense of the term.

The first of these proposals received warm support until it was learnt that the great majority of subscribers were North American psychiatrists who would be unlikely to continue their subscription if the recommendation were adopted. This information resulted in a sharp U-turn of opinion, supported by references to tradition and the importance of preserving an image, and the proposal was in consequence rejected. None the less, a decision to proceed with a new journal was endorsed, and for five years the BMA was responsible for the publication of two titular psychiatric journals. A glance at the *Journal of Neurology, Neurosurgery and Psychiatry* today demonstrates that not much has changed, though elsewhere psychiatry and neurology have gone their separate ways, and journals like *Archives of Neurology and Psychiatry* and *Acta Neurologica et Psychiatrica Scandinavica* have long since split into two separate publications.

Psychological Medicine

The new journal was launched in 1969 with the help of a distinguished editorial board and an international advisory committee. Our initial task was to tackle three questions: namely the colour of the dust-jacket, an agreement on objectives, and a title. The first was easily resolved: since nothing in psychiatry is black or white, grey was evidently the colour of choice. With regard to objectives, we had thought originally of aiming at the education of professors in psychiatry, but their halo of omniscience appeared to be impenetrable, so we settled for the goal of indispensability by determining to concentrate on original, high-quality work across the wide spectrum of both psychiatry and its allied disciplines. In so doing we were virtually compelled to resurrect Winslow's title.

Psychological Medicine has now been in existence for about as long as its predecessor, and during this period I, like Winslow, have been its sole editor, responsible for the appearance of a journal which has so far carried some 2,000 articles and many million words. In the process I have come to appreciate that to most readers a journal is little more than an object which appears on desks or through letter-boxes at regular intervals and may or may not be scrutinized, according to inclination. Very few readers of journals have assumed editorial responsibility, though some may have served on editorial boards or refereed manuscripts. And their professional contact with editors largely comes about in their capacity as potential authors, one of whom has indicated the emotion latent in the relationship by defining an editor as a person with a mission to suppress rising genius. Many people who have submitted a paper can understand why he did so: the preparation of a manuscript is all too often invested with strong feelings, spiced with the wish for priority, professional ambition, and a high degree of self-regard. And since, as Stephen Lock has pointed out,[18] the survival of editors of a scientific journal depends on the acceptance of good articles, they must get to grips with their authors in full awareness of the personal aspects of the situation. It has been said that one person can understand another individual well only if they have been together in bed or in a submarine. I would add a third, less intimate but comparably revealing site, namely the editor's desk. Some aspects of the view from this desk merit comment in their own right.

Medical editors

In one respect the situation is now very different from Winslow's day. The meadows may still contain flowery meads and purling streams, but modern editors no longer have the field to themselves and confront a very different situation. In the first place, the number of medical journals, including those devoted to psychiatry, has greatly increased. When *Psychological Medicine* was founded in 1969, there were in existence more than 250 listed journals and they have continued to proliferate, being devoted not only to subdisciplines like mental subnormality and psychogeriatrics but also to individual conditions, such as schizophrenia, affective illness, and eating disorders. The expansion of these journals, moreover, must be viewed in the context of a much larger phenomenon, the explosion of information in medicine and science which has transformed the editorial role and function. It has recently been estimated that the number of scientific journals is increasing by 6–7 per cent annually, doubling every ten to fifteen years and increasing tenfold every thirty-five to fifty years. At the turn of the century there were a thousand journals in biomedicine alone; this number had risen to four thousand by the early 1950s and to more than twenty thousand by 1983.[19] A former editor of the *Lancet* has put it more graphically: 'If we held a world jamboree for medical journals, the procession of chief editors, marching three abreast at three miles an hour, would take three-quarters of an hour to pass the saluting-base.'[20]

The editors of these journals have become the epicentres of a network of forces generated by the information explosion. Within this area they constitute one group of what Menzel has termed the 'scientific troubadours',[21] those men and women who spread the word or disseminate information in the modern era of medical science, whether by sitting on committees, awarding fellowships, reviewing research grants, or organizing formal and informal seminars and conferences. Here we find the so-called 'invisible colleges' of communication. The scientific journal, however, remains at the heart of this process and as such has been subjected to detailed analysis by historians and philosophers of science and by students of information science. Three of their preoccupations carry particular significance for my theme.

Scientific journals

First, there is the central fact that science has become public knowledge, dependent on the storage as well as the retrieval of information.[22] It has been estimated that most scientists read no more than four to five hours weekly, and Price has shown how little routine use is made of most journals.[23] None the less, as repositories of observations, experimental data, and speculations, journals subserve an essential function, one which is embodied in Ludwig Fleck's[24] distinction between journal science, essentially personal and provisional, and science in its vademecum (or handbook) form, which requires a critical synopsis in an organized system. Fleck summarizes the relationship between journal science and vademecum science by means of a telling metaphor:

It [scientific knowledge] resembles a column of troops on the march. Every discipline, in fact almost every problem, has its own *vanguard*, the group of research scientists working practically on a given problem. This is followed by the *main body*, the official community. Then come the somewhat disorganised stragglers. This structure becomes the more conspicuous the greater the progress in the field of investigation. Journal science, which comprises the latest work, becomes more or less removed from vademecum science, which always lags behind. The vanguard does not occupy a fixed position. It changes its quarters from day to day and even from hour to hour. The main body advances more slowly, changing its stand – often spasmodically – only after years or even decades.

On the basis of my experience as editor of a handbook as well as a journal of psychiatry, I can testify to the truth of this comment.

Second, I would refer to Bradford's law of scatter, enunciated in the late 1940s by the librarian of the Science Museum in London. By ranking all the journals related to a particular subject in terms of their productivity, Bradford[25] found there to be a constant ratio of productive to peripheral to marginal journals in a progression of $1:5:5^2$. Bradford himself regarded his law as conforming to the mathematician's criterion of being of no practical use whatsoever. In fact, it has been extended by Zipf[26] to the field of linguistics and to other areas of human behaviour, showing that people operate according to a law of obtaining maximal results from a small amount of work, i.e. the principle of least effort or least average rate of probable work. For medical journals in general, and psychiatric journals in particular, the application of Bradford's law leads to the notion of a 'nuclear' group of journals which computerization now relates to the citation and impact indices. Some years ago, for example, the librarian of the Institute of Psychiatry examined the *Index Medicus* over a period of 17 months to see which journals had published papers on schizophrenia, the psychoses, and the neuroses.[27] She found that 427 articles came from 6 journals, the next 402 references from 29 journals, and the next 387 from 169 journals. Among the six 'nuclear' journals, incidentally, was the *Proceedings of the Royal Society of Medicine*.

Third, there is the vexed matter of peer review. Faced with a proliferation of new methods of enquiry and whole new subdisciplines, the task of modern editors is much more complex than that of their predecessors. For this reason alone, submitted manuscripts cannot be assessed by any one individual and most editors now make extensive use of peer review by external referees.[28] In *Psychological Medicine*, for example, a minimum of three (and often more) referees is employed for most articles. The refereeing system, which has been described as 'the lynchpin around which the whole business of Science is pivoted',[29] is, by its very nature, confidential but it has been subjected to considerable discussion and to several significant empirical studies, some of which carry wider implications.

Peer review

Gordon has investigated the way in which referees are used in a sample of thirty-two British research journals by interviewing their editors and obtaining basic information about such objective data as the annual number of submitted papers and their rejection rates.[30] Table 5.1 indicates the pattern which confirms the conclusions reached by Zuckerman and Merton in their earlier study of eighty-three American journals, namely: 'the more humanistically orientated the journal, the higher the rate of rejecting manuscripts for publication; the more experimentally and observationally orientated, with emphasis on rigour of observation and analysis, the lower the rate of rejection'.[31]

In addition to this distinction between 'hard' and 'soft' areas of research, there were differences in editorial practices between medical and non-medical journals. Not only did medical editors tend to select referees by virtue of their scientific expertise, but also, when compared with the editors of natural science journals, they gave more weight to the social status and seniority of the referee in the formal academic hierarchy, thereby reinforcing a conservatism in the choice of papers. Furthermore, the editors of three wide-ranging medical journals, including the *British Journal of Psychiatry*,

Table 5.1 Institutional characteristics and editorial preferences of the sample of journals investigated

Journal	Rejection rate (%)	Submissions per year (no.)	Circulation	Editors (no.)	No. of critical readers per paper (modal) Internal	No. of critical readers per paper (modal) External	Are more critical readers required for acceptance or rejection	Which is the greater error A or B
Mineralogical Magazine	10–15	70–80	2,000	6	1	1	Rej	B
Journal of the Institute of Physics	18–30	300–450 each	–	1+1	0	2	Rej	B
British Journal of Psychiatry	40–60	500	9,250	1+4	up	1,2,3	=	B
Nature	65	7,000	20,000	3	1	1	Acc	B
British Journal of Sociology	80	132	3,500	2	2	1	=	A
Philosophy	92	300	3,000	1	1	0	=	=

Source: M. Gordon, A Study of the Evaluation of Research Papers by Primary Journals in the UK, Leicester, Primary Communications Centre, 1978

admitted to having to bear in mind their heterogeneous readership in order to maintain a high circulation, so that 'somewhat journalistic criteria entered into the selection of manuscripts'. Such criteria, of course, play a greater role in the case of 'medical newspapers', directed primarily at clinical practice, than in the case of 'medical readers', directed at the advancement of knowledge.[32]

But perhaps the most intriguing of Gordon's findings was that a substantial degree of disagreement was displayed by the expert biomedical referees, making it necessary for the editor to make many of the decisions himself. This shadow on the surface of peer review has been deepened by the notorious investigations of Peters and Ceci, who selected twelve papers by well-known American psychologists, each already published in a prestigious journal with a high rejection rate and a well-developed refereeing system. They then submitted fictitious names and institutions for the originals and resubmitted the same articles to the journals in which they had originally appeared 18–32 months earlier. Only three out of thirty-eight editors and reviewers detected their activities; nine out of the twelve papers were sent out to referees again, and eight of these nine were rejected.[33]

Though to the best of my knowledge this study has not been repeated in psychiatry, I would not hold out hope for a different result if it were. It illustrates what Mahoney[34] has dubbed the 'filtration-processes' by which editors play a necessary part in influencing the information to which readers have access. Advocates of a more objective, supposedly more efficient system have not been lacking since the demise of medical journals was predicted fifty years ago by J.D. Bernal,[35] who argued for a more rational, more impersonal procedure. Instead of scattering pollen in the wind, he maintained, we might advance at least to the more selective stage of insect-borne pollination, where more pollen gets to the right flowers.

The editorial function

Modern computer techniques have rendered this notion both more feasible and potentially attractive. None the less, scientific, medical, and psychiatric journals continue to multiply along with their editors, who are far removed from James Thurber's description of Harold Ross's self-image of 'an infallible omniscience...a dehumanised figure, disguised as a man'. Their function and their fallibility were pungently summarized by Adlai Stevenson, who defined them as people who separate the wheat from the chaff and print the chaff; but a more charitable and more accurate view was expressed by one of Walt Disney's colleagues, who said of him: 'Walt was no good at music, drawing or animation. He was just a good editor, a guy who knew a good thing when he saw it.' Maeve O'Connor refers to this quality as 'an indefinable and elusive talent owing as much to intuition as to a deep knowledge of the subject'.[36]

Most medical editors are untrained, unpaid, solitary figures. Why do they do it? One of the best of them, Morris Fishbein, was in no doubt: 'an editor does not edit for the benefit of the owners. He does not edit for the benefit of the advertisers. And he certainly does not edit for the benefit of the politicians. He edits a medical journal for the readers, and the readers are the only ones who have a right to his basic consideration.'[37]

I would go further and claim that the editorial obligation also resides in representing and, if necessary, helping to create standards which unify a professional group. In this sense it is an active role, one which demands a point of view. No computer has a point of view. A good journal both reflects current trends and points constantly towards the future. It also functions by laying down criteria which act as guidelines and incentives to younger recruits in the field. In Ziman's words: 'the hallmark of a new discipline is the establishment of a specialised journal catering to the scholarly needs of its exponent. It constitutes an act of solidarity and sodality, and polarizes the subject around it.'[38]

Psychological medicine, as I have endeavoured to show, is not a new discipline but until recently its elements have been widely scattered. My colleagues and I have been associated with a journal which attempts to draw together these elements and cement the discipline by virtue of the impact made on the thought collective of its professional membership. Such, at least, has been and still is the objective. How far it is realized depends on the response of the readership as well as the content of the journal. At the very least, however, I can say that to participate in so important a process is both a privilege and a responsibility. And I feel sure that Forbes Winslow would have agreed.

References

1   J.C. Bucknill and D. Tuke, *A Manual of Psychological Medicine*, London, Churchill, 1858.
2   J.C. Bucknill, 'Editorial', *Asylum Journal of Mental Science*, 1855: 11.
3   F.B. Winslow, 'Preface', *Journal of Psychological Medicine*, 1845, 1: iii.
4   F.B. Winslow, 'In Memoriam: Forbes Benignus Winslow', *Journal of Psychological Medicine*, 1875, NSI: x–xvi.
5   Anonymous, 'Biographical Notice: Forbes Winslow', *The Medical Circular and General Medical Advertiser*, 1853, II: 209–11.
6   F.B. Winslow, 'Address to our Readers', *Journal of Psychological Medicine*, 1850, 3: iii–iv.
7   E. von Feuchtersleben, *The Principles of Medical Psychology*, trans. H. Evans Lloyd, London, Sydenham Society, 1847.
8   F.B. Winslow, 'The psychological vocation of the physician (Lettsomian Lecture, No. 1)', *Journal of Psychological Medicine*, 1854, 7: 106–50.
9   F.B. Winslow, '*Elements of Psychological Medicine*: review', *Journal of Psychological Medicine* 1854, 7: 24–35.
10 R. Hunter and I. Macalpine (eds) 'Forbes Benignus Winslow', in *Three Hundred Years of Psychiatry*, London, Oxford University Press, 1963.

11 L.S. Hearnshaw, *A Short History of British Psychology: 1840–1940*, London, Methuen, 1964, p. 25.
12 L. DeBakey, *The Scientific Journal*, St Louis, Mosby, 1976, p. 1.
13 J.M. Ziman, *Public Knowledge*, London, Cambridge University Press, 1976.
14 L. Stephen, 'The evolution of editors', in *Studies of a Biographer*, vol. 1, London, Duckworth, 1898.
15 H.M. Marshall, 'Psychiatry', in L.T. Morton (ed.) *Use of Medical Literature*, Edinburgh, Butterworth, 1975.
16 A. Meyer, 'The psychological point of view', in M. Bentley and E.V. Cowdry (eds) *The Problem of Mental Disorder*, New York, McGraw-Hill, 1934.
17 J. Sibbold, 'Psychiatry in general hospitals', *Review of Neurology and Psychiatry*, 1903, 1: 4–12.
18 S. Lock, 'How editors survive', *British Medical Journal*, 1985, 11: 1, 118–19.
19 S. Lock, 'Futurology and medical journals', *Journal of the Royal College of Physicians*, London, 1983, 17: 92.
20 T. Fox, *Crisis in Communication*, London, Athlone Press, 1965.
21 H. Menzel, 'Physician for tomorrow', in D. McCord (ed.) *Bibliotheca medica*, Cambridge, Mass., Harvard Medical School, 1966, p. 112.
22 Ziman, op. cit.
23 D.J. de Salla Price, *Little Science, Big Science*, New York, Columbia University Press, 1963.
24 L. Fleck, *Genesis and Development of a Scientific Fact*, Chicago, Ill., University of Chicago Press, 1979.
25 S.C. Bradford, *Documentation*, London, Crosby Lockwood, 1948.
26 G.R. Zipf, *Human Behaviour and the Principle of Least Effort*, Cambridge, Addison-Wesley Press, 1949.
27 H. Marshall, 'The mental hospital's medical library', in D. Watt and B. Barraclough (eds) *Clinical Tutors in Psychiatry*, Royal Medico-Psychological Association, 1971, pp. 39–47.
28 S. Lock, *A Difficult Balance*, London, Nuffield Provincial Hospitals Trust, 1985.
29 Ziman, op. cit.
30 M. Gordon, *A Study of the Evaluation of Research Papers by Primary Journals in the UK*, Leicester, Primary Communications Research Centre, 1978.
31 H. Zuckerman and R.K. Merton, 'Patterns of evaluation in science: institutionalisation, structure and functions of the refereeing system', *Minerva*, 1971, 9: 66–100.
32 Fox, op. cit.
33 D.P. Peters and S.J. Ceci, 'Peer-review practices of psychological journals: the fate of published articles, submitted again', *Behavioural and Brain Sciences*, 1982, 5: 187–255.
34 M.J. Mahoney, 'Publication, politics, and scientific progress', *Behavioural and Brain Sciences*, 1982, 5: 220–1.
35 J.D. Bernal, *The Social Function of Science*, London, Routledge & Kegan Paul, 1939.
36 M. O'Connor, *Editing Scientific Books and Journals*, Tunbridge Wells, Pitman Medical, 1978.
37 W.B. Bean, 'My sampler of editors', *New England Journal of Medicine*, 1980, 303: 229–33.
38 Ziman, op. cit.

Chapter six

The sciences and general psychopathology

The subject-matter of this volume develops the map charted by Karl Jaspers in his *General Psychopathology*, which remains the clearest and most convincing outline of the whole field.[1] Jaspers nowhere provides a clear-cut definition of psychopathology, and points out that its 'essence . . . as a study can only emerge from a composite framework'. Inveighing against the futility of 'endlessness', the attempt to establish absolute knowledge through the application of any one scientific discipline, he urges the psychiatrist to 'acquire some of the viewpoints and methods that belong to the world of the Humanities and Social Studies . . . since the methods of almost all the Arts and Sciences converge on psychopathology'. With this ambiguous phrase Jaspers indicates the complex nature of a discipline which, in his view, extended the notion of scientific enquiry as it is usually understood.

Jaspers refers to science in relation to psychopathology repeatedly but disconnectedly throughout the several sections of his text. While claiming scientific status for psychopathology he also asserts that

> Science is wrongly identified with Natural Science . . . natural science is indeed the groundwork of psychopathology and an essential element in it but the humanities are equally so and, with this, psychopathology does not become in any way less scientific but scientific in another way.

According to Jaspers there are no fewer than four modes of scientific thought which are relevant to psychopathology: descriptive phenomenology, causal explanation, genetic understanding (the psychology of meaningful connections), and the construction of complex unities.

The phenomenological approach to psychopathology, involving as it does the careful analysis of the phenomena of mental disorders, constitutes a basic contribution to clinical knowledge. The careful and systematic delineation of abnormal forms of experience and behaviour provides the descriptive

Originally published in M. Shepherd and O.L. Zangwill (eds), *Handbook of Psychiatry*, vol. I, Cambridge, Cambridge University Press, 1983, pp. 1–8.

groundwork of the subject but even though such material can be given quantitative expression, its heavily subjective nature has led some observers to distinguish it from scientific enquiry proper. According to Zubin, for example, 'Science deals with public events while phenomenology deals with the still private events.'[2] To Jaspers, on the other hand, phenomenology remained not only a form of scientific enquiry but also one which, by its very nature, separated itself from the study of all infra-human organisms, lacking as they do capacity for comparable self-expression. 'In psychopathology', he maintains, 'the human being has himself become the object of scientific study and thus observations on animals do not contribute anything essential'. Further, he speaks pointedly of 'physical findings that have or may have some relation to psychic events but they do not portray them nor reveal them in any sense which we can understand'.

From this point it is a short step to his distinction between 'explanatory' and 'understandable' processes in the sphere of psychopathology, a dichotomy borrowed from Dilthey and Weber, who applied it originally to philosophy and the social sciences. For Jaspers the establishment of 'explanatory connections in psychopathology belongs to the sphere of natural science, leading to the formulation of rules and eventually to mathematical laws'. Here he comes close to a generally held opinion, summarized by Oakeshott, for whom 'The explicit character of scientific experience is a world of absolutely stable and communicable experience: the explicit purpose in science is to conceive the world under the category of quantity.'[3] In psychopathology, by contrast, Jaspers asserts that particular causal connections and some general laws are attainable but that the discovery of more specific, immutable laws 'would presuppose a complete quantification of the events observed and since these are psychic events which by their very nature have to remain qualitative, such quantification would as a matter of principle remain impossible without losing the actual object of the enquiry'.

In Jaspers's schema natural science is equated with biology. 'It is an absolute necessity', he says, 'for the psychopathologist to *see life* the way biologists do.' Inasmuch as this statement implies the subordination of the physical sciences his meaning is clear enough:

> The concrete phenomenon is part of a living whole and it never permits the isolation of a simple fact, a simple cause which operates like a cannoning billiard-ball; it can be conceived only as a *complex event* taking place among a host of conditioning factors.

This distinction between inanimate mechanisms and a living biological causality, however, runs counter to the outlook of many practising biologists. To Mainz, for example, biology 'has developed special methods and special subdivision, but these are nevertheless not different in principle from those of other natural sciences'.[4] And for Monod: 'Science rests upon a strictly *objective* approach to the analysis and interpretation of the universe, including Man himself and human societies. Science ignores, and must ignore, value judgements.'[5] Jaspers, on the other hand, rejects the need to suspend value judgements except when attempting causal explanations and regards this view of science as insufficient:

> Psychopathological phenomena may also be reinterpreted as *biological events* against a general ground of biological theory, e.g. genetics, where human existence and mental illness can be studied from this point of view. Only when the biological aspects have been clearly distinguished can we proceed to discuss what essentially belongs to man. Whenever the object studied is Man and not man as a species of animal, we find that psychopathology comes to be not only a kind of biology but also one of the Humanities.

It is on this proposition that Jaspers bases his argument for the need of a science of 'understanding', as opposed to 'explanation', in which meaningful psychic connections can be established because 'psychic events "emerge" out of each other in a way which we understand'. This form of 'genetic' or 'psychological' understanding underpins the empathic, interpersonal components of Jaspers's schema:

> The scientific attitude suspends all value-judgement in order to arrive at knowledge. But though this is possible when attempting causal explanation it is not possible with empathic understanding, at least not exactly in the same sense. We can, however, make an analogous claim to impartiality when we have shown an understanding that is fair, many-sided, open and critically conscious of its limitations. Love and hate bring values which are indeed the pacemakers of understanding but their suspension brings us a clarity of understanding that amounts to knowledge.

The application of psychological understanding, however, extends only to the field of 'empirical experiment and free existential achievement'. Beyond this, knowledge is derived only from 'metaphysical' understanding which is attainable by philosophy rather than by any form of scientific enquiry.
According to Jaspers,

> Metaphysical understanding (as distinct from psychological understanding) reaches after a meaning into which all the other limited meanings can be taken up and absorbed. Metaphysical understanding interprets the empirical facts and the free achievement as the language of unconditioned Being. This interpretation is not a mere device of reason, something futile, but the illumination of fundamental experiences with the help of symbol

and idea. As we look at the inanimate world, the cosmos, the landscape, we experience something we call 'soul' or 'psyche'.

And what is 'psyche'?

1 Psyche means *consciousness*, but just as much and, from certain points of view it can even, in particular, mean 'the unconscious'.
2 Psyche is not to be regarded as an object with given qualities but as 'being in one's own world', the integrating of an inner and outer world.
3 Psyche is a becoming, an unfolding and a differentiating, it is nothing final nor is it ever fully accomplished.

The concept of psyche, therefore, is the gateway to an existentialist universe: 'There is no valid theory of the psyche, only a philosophy of human existence.'

Here is the language of Kierkegaard and Nietzsche, a transcendentalism which Jaspers was later to develop at length in his philosophical writings but which is also central to his outline of psychopathology:

> The sciences through knowledge provide a springboard for thought which transcends. It is only where scientific knowledge is at its fullest that we first have the experience of *really not knowing* and in this not knowing we transcend the situation with the help of specific, philosophic methods. But the sciences also tend to *obscure Being itself* by the knowable facts and keep us tied to preliminaries without end. They tend to make absolutes of our limited insights and convert them into a supposed knowledge of Being itself.

Again: 'Human beings . . . constantly transcend their own empirical human self which is the only self that scientific research can recognise and grasp.' Within this context Jaspers also develops his notion of 'wholes' in relation to science, the 'whole' being 'the proper theme for philosophy whereas science is only concerned with particular aspects of the whole'. He argues that 'science, if it is to be productive, will vacillate constantly between the elements and the whole' and goes on to conclude:

> Some exact experiment in biological research may often make us feel that we have grasped life in its original wholeness and that we have at last penetrated it through and through and yet in the end we find it is still only a widening of the mechanistic insight. . . . In the end we have comprehended only elements and the problem of the whole appears again in new form.

As for the scientific method with its reliance on hypothesis formation: 'Where our theories may seem to have some kinship with the natural sciences it is in the forming of tentative hypotheses, which we make for limited research ends only and which have no application to the psyche as a whole.'

In sum, then, Jaspers enlarges the field of general psychopathology to extend from the natural sciences, and in particular biological science, via descriptive phenomenology to existentialist philosophy. The psychopathologist employs the scientific method and the scientific attitude even when dealing with phenomena like subjective experience or meaningful connection, but his own position is ultimately non-reductionist and transcendental. In the preface to the seventh edition of his book, written in 1959, Jaspers acknowledged that after sixty-five years his methodological principles had remained largely unchanged but that there was room for modification in the light of recent research. The hypsography and the contours of his map have both been modified by the evolution of new areas of scientific enquiry, many of which have emerged since the completion of the final revision of his text. Some of these have developed as a result of new techniques of investigation, and the intensive study of the central nervous system and its functions has led to the recognition that many traditional areas of psychopathology involve a variety of disciplines not traditionally associated with psychopathological enquiry. The investigation of memory, to take one example, now involves the microbiologist, the physiologist, the anatomist, and the pharmacologist, as well as the clinician.[6] In consequence, psychopathology has been subject to a series of shifting 'paradigms' which, as Kuhn has so convincingly argued, indicate the turmoil of a science on the move.[7] The boundaries between the older scientific disciplines have been redrawn to generate the emergence of new, compound sciences whose nature is tellingly indicated by a multiplicity of prefixes – 'neuropsychopharmacology', 'neuropsychoendocrinology', 'psychobiology', 'sociobiology'.

The bearing of these scientific methods and disciplines on general psychopathology has already been profound. This overview gives a brief general account of their impact on the clinical and basic sciences.

Clinical sciences

Jaspers's outline of the clinical conditions calling for psychopathological investigation corresponds to most of the widely accepted classifications. He grouped the conditions into three broad categories:

Group I. Known somatic illness with psychic disturbances
   Cerebral illnesses
   Systemic diseases with symptomatic psychoses
   Poisons
Group II. Major psychoses
   Genuine epilepsy

Schizophrenia
Manic-depressive illness
Group III. Personality disorders
Isolated abnormal reactions that do not arise on the basis of illnesses
belonging to Groups I and II
Neuroses and neurotic syndromes
Abnormal personalities and their developments

It may be noted that this scheme is hierarchical, that precise diagnosis is feasible only in Group I, and that classification in Group III is least satisfactory. The somatic basis of the diagnoses in Group I brings these conditions most intimately into the orbit of conventional scientific enquiry, where advances in the spheres of physical investigation and treatment have proved to be most fruitful. At the same time, however, these advances have underlined the need to re-categorize the major 'functional psychoses' in Group II. In the case of epilepsy, for example, while Jaspers originally stated that the diagnosis is psychological, 'made on the basis of convulsive attack linked with a psychological diagnosis', the introduction of electroencephalography has provided a physical substrate for the disorder in the form of cerebral dysrhythmia.[8] Similarly the work of Gjessing demonstrated the importance of metabolic disorders in the genesis of periodic catatonia, thereby rekindling interest in the physiobiology of the schizophrenias.[9]

New knowledge has stimulated an increasing awareness of the need to establish the principles of psychiatric diagnosis and classification which in general follow conventional lines. An exception, however, has been provided by the claims of psychoanalysis which, because of their radical nature, calls for separate mention.[10] The complicated system derived from psychoanalytical theory and practice does not lend itself to a detailed summary.[11] Essentially, however, it is a reductionist schema which, to Freud, was 'a dynamic conception which reduces mental life to an interplay of reciprocally urging and checking forces'. These forces are conceived in terms of schema of 'libidinal' energy which ultimately determines the basic attributes of the individual and is dependent on a variety of postulated 'mechanisms', such as sublimation, repression, and fixation. One of the suggested contributions to general psychopathology has been the hypothesis that some of these 'mechanisms' are causally related to particular phenomena of mental disease, e.g. the links between hostility and depression. Another major implication of psychodynamic theorizing for general psychopathology has been the proposed nexus between early childhood experience and mental disturbance in later life, e.g. maternal attachment and adult homosexuality.

Jaspers was one of the first to point out the fundamentally unscientific nature of 'psychodynamic' theory, to which he allocated the limited role of establishing meaningful connections by way of genetic understanding. This view has been vigorously contested by Hartmann who, while accepting the value of the phenomenological method, asserted that psychoanalysis 'has come to see the most essential processes of the human mind from the causal point of view'.[12] The goal of psychoanalysis, according to Hartmann, is not the understanding of the mental, but rather the explanation of its causal relationships, for psychoanalysis is

a science which proceeds inductively and is rooted in biology... a natural science not only in its manner of conceptualization... but also in the scientific goals it sets itself – namely the knowledge of laws and regularities, ... an inductive science of the connections between complex mental structure.

Closer examination, however, has shown that these constructs are metaphors rather than models and are not susceptible to operational definitions so that they cannot be subjected to scientific enquiry. The protean theoretical system has none the less led to a vast amount of experimental work, only a small proportion of which has supported the operationally derived hypotheses,[13] even when the work can overcome the twin methodological problems of poor inter-observer agreement and the confusion between 'interpretation' and observation. A great deal of ingenuity has been expended in an effort to render these studies scientific, and the psychodynamic model has probably been of most value as a stimulus to provoking such work rather than as an accurate picture of human behaviour.

Perhaps the impact of 'psychodynamic' theorizing would have been greater if its therapeutic claims had been substantiated.[14] In the event, the efficacy of psychotherapy has been rendered questionable by the application of techniques of evaluation to new forms of treatment which have themselves exercised a major impact on psychiatry and psychopathology as a clinical science.[15] For Jaspers, physical treatment occupied a tiny section of his discussion and was confined to a brief mention of anticonvulsants, opiates, diet, and the shock therapies. He was unable to take account of recent advances in the pharmacological therapy of the functional psychoses which were introduced in the early 1950s[16] and whose implications for psychopathology have been twofold. First, by modifying the outcome of many forms of these disorders medication has provided another axis of classification in an area where prognosis is a central issue: the postulate, for example, of a 'drug-responsive' or 'non-responsive' depression[17] has been to introduce a novel dichotomy far removed from the traditional, clinically based endogenous – exogenous or neurotic-psychotic type of categorization. Second, and still more important, the apparent response of the functional psychoses to substances acting on the central nervous system has raised the possibility of identifying a physico-chemical basis for these disorders via the mode of drug action. The older idea of psychosis resulting from a 'metabolic disorder' or a 'biochemical lesion' has been superseded by the modern concept of disorders of neuro-transmitters[18] in which the functional psychoses take their place alongside neurological and other medical conditions. The 'dopamine hypothesis' of schizophrenia[19] and the 'catecholamine hypothesis' of the affective disorders[20] exemplify this mode of thinking (see below).

The other large area of clinical science which receives inadequate consideration in Jaspers's schema is epidemiology, the study of the nature and distribution of disease in populations, whose methods and techniques have been applied increasingly to non-infectious as well as infectious conditions.[21] Jaspers's account of the need to establish the demographic and social associations of disease and his searching discussion of the methods of correlation are close to the core of the epidemiological method. What is lacking, however, is an explicit awareness of the role which can be played by epidemiology in establishing causal connections, as in the cases of pellagra,[22] or twin research in schizophrenia,[23] as well as in extending the scope of descriptive enquiry. The central part played by epidemiology in the development of the controlled clinical trial is also missing, understandably, from a text which pays so little regard to treatment.

Yet though Jaspers nowhere uses the term, an epidemiological perspective is apparent in his chapter on heredity (devoted largely to population genetics), on eidology, on the social and historical status of the individual, and on diagnosis and classification. Indeed, he explicitly extends the boundaries of general psychopathology to cover the population at large:

> our science starts in the field of the 'normal' and with the study of personality. Once psychiatry began to designate personalities as 'sick' it became simply a practical matter where to draw the line in regard to all the individual variations.

He goes on to say that 'the personality disorders (the psychopathies and neuroses) and the psychoses are veritable sources of human possibilities, not only deviations from a health norm'. Within this framework the socio-cultural contributions to psychopathology fall naturally into place.[24]

Basic sciences

Alongside the advances in the clinical study of psychopathology which have been made in recent years must be placed the contributions from the so-called basic sciences, each elaborating on its concepts and techniques to demarcate an area of relevance. In general, the representatives of these disciplines proceed not so much by tackling clinical phenomena directly as by constructing 'models'. Jaspers, while referring to the significance of 'analogy' in the study of biological processes, does not discuss the value of scientific models which are susceptible to experimental manipulation. As

Alinstein has pointed out,[25] such models possess four attributes: (1) a set of assumptions about the subject under investigation; (2) the derivation of properties of hypotheses derived from these assumptions which can be tested; (3) the view that the model employed is an approximation to the 'true' model which excludes other theories; and (4) the analogical nature of the model employed. Having constructed the model the scientist has to establish its reliability and validity by appropriate examination and then to test its applicability, being prepared to discard or modify it when the limits of its relevance have been determined.

The broad objective of experimental science in using its models is to investigate the mechanisms of disease by the controlled manipulation of relevant variables and then to test these directly on the human subject. The mechanisms in question may be neurobiological or behavioural, according to the methods and standpoint adopted. The use of infra-human species plays a large part in such work and the question of the degree to which the animal model can be regarded as a homologue for the study of human psychopathology has constantly to be considered.

The neurobiological sciences

The recent explosion of research in the neurosciences has impinged on psychopathology in a number of ways. First in order of significance is the impact of psychopharmacology following the introduction of a variety of new drugs in the 1950s. The scientific significance of these compounds has extended beyond their use in clinical practice to involve their mode of action and, by implication, the biological mechanisms assumed to underlie the conditions for which they are used therapeutically. The case of schizophrenia may be taken to illustrate the issues:

> In so far as schizophrenia is not a purely linguistic disorder, but involves abnormalities in more elementary perceptual, attentional, and cognitive processes, such paradigms can be used to investigate the anatomical, physiological, and neurochemical mechanisms underlying the disease.[26]

Translating this view into testable hypotheses, Matthysse and Haber lay down four minimum and essential requirements for a model of schizophrenia:[27] (1) that aberrant animal behaviour should be restored to normal, at least in part, by drugs which are therapeutically effective in schizophrenia; (2) that substances which are chemically similar to anti-psychotic drugs but are therapeutically ineffective in schizophrenic psychoses should fail to normalize aberrant behaviour in the model animal; (3) that drug tolerance, which does not develop to anti-psychotic drugs, should not develop in the animals; (4) that the effect of drugs on abnormal animal behaviour should not be counteracted by anticholinergic agents. The underlying assumption in such reasoning is that schizophrenia results from a defect of neuro-transmission, as exemplified by the 'dopamine hypothesis'.[28]

Clearly, however, the gap between a basically neurochemical disorder and the complex symptoms associated with schizophrenia is difficult to close conceptually without the postulation of mediating mechanisms, such as elementary psychological processes which may be studied in terms of either experimental biology or the phenomena of the disease itself. Thus from the biological standpoint it has been suggested that relevant dopamine-related behaviour includes stereotypy and motor disinhibition,[29] corresponding to perserveration of thought and distractibility respectively; the clinical features of the psychosis have, in turn, been related to the psychology of attention and its disturbances,[30] especially since the identification of 'focal attention' neurons in the parietal lobe.[31] Whatever their detailed nature, such psychological mechanisms could thus be associated with anatomico-physiological systems utilizing neurotransmitters or even constitute predisposing factors to overt disease in a manner akin to the inherited 'risk factors' in some physical diseases.

A model of this type, which has been applied to other forms of functional psychoses and to the neurotic disorders, refurbishes the old notion of mental disorder as dependent on cerebral dysfunction. The concept of the 'lesion', however, has become more complex, reflecting a multi-factorial framework which incorporates neurochemical, endocrinological, genetic, psychological, and even environmental factors. A major emphasis here is on the elucidation of physical mechanisms which have been extended to traditionally psychological domains. In the field of memory, for example, animal experiments have been carried out to examine the hypothesis that nucleic acids or protein molecules synthesized in the learning process may constitute a chemical basis for memory.[32] Anisomycin and cyclohexicide, both of which suppress cerebral protein synthesis, have been used for this purpose in the study of discrimination tasks and habituation; the results have then been compared with the retrograde amnesia which follows the administration of ECT to human subjects to construct a model for short-term memory in terms of synaptic conductance.

The behavioural sciences

For the advocates of a behavioural approach to psychopathology the subject has been defined, significantly, as 'the scientific study of disordered behaviour'.[33] Without minimizing the importance of biological disorders, these workers concentrate on the overt behavioural disturbances which characterize many forms of psychopathology, and attempt to reproduce them in the laboratory with animal or human subjects by experimental means. Perhaps the most fundamental examples of the behavioural approach have come from the field of genetics. While the study of population genetics has successfully demonstrated through pedigree analyses and twin studies the hereditary basis for much human variation, including several forms of mental disorder, geneticists have also turned their attention to behavioural syndromes. Recognizing that such syndromes are multifactorial in aetiology, they have attempted to identify controlling factors by taking advantage of the fact that some genetic polymorphisms can be used as linkage markers; the use of these in conjunction with the familial distribution of a syndrome renders it possible to construct a genetic taxonomy within the syndromal spectrum. Several different psychopathological areas have already been explored along these lines. Animal models for epilepsy, for example, have been developed through the study of mice which carry a gene for susceptibility to audiogenic seizures.[34] Again, the genetic selection of aggressive animals has received an impetus from the suggested association of the extra Y-chromosome with aggression in human males, while breeding experiments and the cross-fostering of mice indicate that certain Y-chromosomes are associated with a propensity for aggressive behaviour in combination with certain autosomal genes, possibly by regulating the testosterone level of puberty.[35]

So far, though, perhaps the most promising application of behavioural genetics relating to mental disease has been in the area of drug response to a drug as a phenotypic property, the resultant of a genotype modified by a change in the internal milieu induced by drugs.[36] The marked individual variation in response to drugs and in the exhibition of their adverse effects has drawn attention to differences in pharmacokinetics, susceptibility of cell-receptors, and the physiopathology of psychiatric syndromes. The well-established tendency for alcoholism to occur in families, for example, has been matched by the breeding of mouse strains which vary in their ability to metabolize ethanol, to exhibit preference for alcohol, and to exhibit widely differing behavioural responses to low doses of alcohol.[37] Again, the biochemical effects of morphine on inbred strains of mice have shown that analgesia and locomotor activity can be genetically differentiated, suggesting that striatal dopaminergic systems are involved in the latter, and cholinergic neurones in the former, syndrome.[38] In the field of mental disorder attention has been drawn to the inactivation of isoniazed and related drugs by the liver by an acetylating enzyme because of the use of monoamine oxidase inhibitors in the treatment of depression. 'Slow' acetylation, a trait determined by a simple gene and attributable to less enzymic activity, has been reported to be associated with greater therapeutic effectiveness of phenelzine in the treatment of neurotic depression among patients carrying the genetic predisposition to acetylate slowly.[39] Another example is minimal brain dysfunction, a condition which is known to respond unpredictably but strikingly to stimulants like amphetamine and methylphenidate. Attempts to reproduce the syndrome have been made by breeding hyperactive beagle hybrids whose responses to large doses of amphetamine have been used as analogous to the human condition.[40]

Other significant behavioural approaches to clinical conditions have been via the conflict paradigms of 'experimental' neurosis[41] and the various uses made of the conditioned reflex in relation to schizophrenia[42] and phobias.[43] In addition, attempts at behaviour modification by means of psychological techniques derived from learning theory have introduced new notions about the genesis and outcome of such disorders as the phobias and the obsessional states.[44]

By way of a more detailed example depression stands out with particular clarity. Though the response to ECT and to certain psychotropic drugs has pointed to a biological substrate in some forms of depression, the phenomena of the disorder also lend themselves to behavioural analysis by meeting 'the assumption that the variables controlling normal behaviour also control deviant behaviour'.[45] This outlook represents the application of principles developed from the laboratory study of normal behaviour in terms of learning, motivation, and perception as developed in the laboratory. For depression the model becomes most telling when the behavioural analogues can be most closely approximated to the conditions under study, as is the case with two currently productive concepts, namely 'learned helplessness' and 'separation'.

'Learned helplessness' and depression

The experimental observations here are based on the defective escape-avoidance behaviour of infra-human organisms after receiving inescapable traumata, e.g. electric shocks. Those animals which make no attempt to escape from the traumatic situation, passively accept the noxae, and learn the effectiveness of response with difficulty are said to exhibit 'learned helplessness'.[46] They also exhibit other deficits in adaptive behaviour, e.g. food-seeking, appetite, and aggression, and depletion of norepinephrine has also been established. A comparable state induced in human subjects exposed to inescapable high noise or electric shocks exhibits several parallel features characterizing morbid depression – inertia, passivity, retardation, slowness, and negative attitudes. The suggested links between depression and a diminution of norepinephrine at receptor sites in the brain have also been adduced as a further feature of similarity. On the other hand, the associations of intense anxiety and of peptic ulceration with 'learned helplessness' in the laboratory animal do not find a counterpart in depression, and the treatment measures which prove effective in clinical practice cannot be fitted readily to the model.

'Separation' and depression

Most of the work on separation has centred on the so-called anaclitic or dependency depression which can occur in some very young children as a consequence of prolonged separation from the mother.[47] Clinicians have described a sequence of 'protest' leading to 'despair' and eventually to a state of 'detachment', characteristically responding to maternal reunion. Since this constitutes a model in pre-verbal subjects it can be established in purely behavioural terms with a causal factor, a natural history, and a response to 'treatment'. Such a situation suggests the possibility of creating laboratory models with subhuman primates and this objective has been pursued by animal ethologists.[48] The complexities and limitations of employing monkey analogues of depression have been carefully summarized by Suomi and Harlow, who conclude that despite certain defects the model can be defended.[49]

Conclusion

The foregoing outline may serve as a ground plan of the current status of general psychopathology. It remains to be emphasized that the area between the formal methods of science and those areas of psychopathology which Jaspers regarded as the province of philosophical enquiry has become an area of study in its own right.[50] Against the various reductionist theories of physicalism and behaviourism may be ranged such concepts as non-reductive materialism,[51] transcendentalism, phenomenology, and emergent biology,[52] all in their various ways attempting to account for those aspects of human activity which have still to be incorporated satisfactorily in any holistic schema of psychopathology. At present these issues remain unresolved and necessarily a matter of personal bias. Meanwhile the contributions of scientific research continue both to consolidate the foundations of psychopathology and to open new fields of enquiry.

References

1 K. Jaspers, *General Psychopathology*, trans. J. Hoenig and M.W. Hamilton, 7th edn, Manchester, Manchester University Press, 1963.
2 J. Zubin, 'Scientific models for psychopathology in the 1970s', *Seminars in Psychiatry*, 1972, 4, 3: 283–96.
3 M. Oakeshott, *Experience and its Modes*, London, Cambridge University Press, 1978.
4 F. Mainz, *Foundations of Biology*, in *International Encyclopaedia of Unified Science*, vol. 1, no. 9, Chicago, Ill., University of Chicago Press, 1955.
5 J. Monod, 'The meaning of science', in W. Fuller (ed.) *The Social Impact of Modern Biology*, London, Routledge & Kegan Paul, 1971.
6 M.A.B. Brazier (ed.) *Brain Mechanisms in Memory and Learning: From the Single Neuron to Man*, International Brain Research Organization Monograph Series 4, New York, Raven Press, 1979.
7 T. Kuhn, *The Structure of Scientific Revolutions*, 2nd edn, in *International Encyclopaedia of Unified Science*, vol. 2, no. 2, Chicago, Ill., University of Chicago Press, 1970.
8 Commission on Terminology, 'Clinical and electroencephalographic classification of epileptic seizures', *Epilepsie*, 1969, 10, Supp. S.2.

9   R.V. Gjessing, *Contribution to the Somatology of Periodic Catatonia*, Oxford, Pergamon, 1976.
10 K. Menninger, *The Vital Balance*, New York, Viking, 1963.
11 See F. Kräupl Taylor, 'Dynamic psychology in relation to psychiatry', in M. Shepherd (ed.) *Handbook of Psychiatry*, vol. 5, Cambridge, Cambridge University Press, 1985, pp. 106–18.
12 H. Hartmann, 'Understanding and explanation', in *Essays on Ego-Psychology: Selected Problems in Psychoanalytic Theory*, London, Hogarth Press, 1964.
13 S. Fisher and R. P. Greenberg, *The Scientific Credibility of Freud's Theories and Therapies*, Hassocks, Harvester Press, 1977.
14 R.H. Cawley, 'Evaluation of psychotherapy', *Psychological Medicine*, 1970, 1: 101–3.
15 See R.H. Cawley, 'The principles of treatment and therapeutic evaluation', in M. Shepherd and O.L. Zangwill (eds) *Handbook of Psychiatry*, vol. I, Cambridge, Cambridge University Press, 1983, pp. 221–43.
16 M. Shepherd, M.H. Lader, and R. Rodnight, *Clinical Psychopharmacology*, London, English Universities Press, 1968.
17 F.A. Freyhan, 'Treatment-resistant or intractable?', *Comprehensive Psychiatry*, 1978, 19, 2: 97–101.
18 N.J. Legg (ed.) *Neurotransmitter Systems and their Clinical Disorders*, London, Academic Press, 1978.
19 A. Carlsson, 'Does dopamine play a role in schizophrenia?', *Psychological Medicine*, 1977, 7: 583–97.
20 J.W. Maas, 'Catecholamines and depression: a further specification of the catecholamine hypothesis of the affective disorders', in A.J. Friedhoff (ed.) *Catecholamines and Behaviour*, vol. 2, New York, Plenum, 1975.
21 See N. Kreitman, 'Epidemiology in relation to psychiatry', in M. Shepherd and O.L. Zangwill (eds) *Handbook of Psychiatry*, vol. I, Cambridge, Cambridge University Press, 1983, pp. 19–33.
22 M. Shepherd, 'Epidemiology and clinical psychiatry', *British Journal of Psychiatry*, 1978, 133: 289–98.
23 D. Rosenthal and S.S. Kety (eds) *The Transmission of Schizophrenia*, Oxford, Pergamon, 1968.
24 See David Mechanic, 'Social science in relation to psychiatry', in M. Shepherd and O.L. Zangwill (eds) *Handbook of Psychiatry*, vol. I, Cambridge, Cambridge University Press, 1983, pp. 69–79.
25 P. Alinstein, 'Theoretical models', *British Journal of the Philosophy of Science*, 1965, 16: 102–20.
26 S. Matthysse, 'Animal models of human cognitive processes', in I. Hanin and E. Usdin (eds) *Animal Models in Psychiatry and Neurology*, Oxford, Pergamon, 1977.
27 S. Matthyse and S. Haber, 'Animal models of schizophrenia', in D.J. Ingle and H.M. Schein (eds) *Model Systems in Biological Psychiatry*, Cambridge, Mass., MIT Press, 1975.
28 Carlsson, op. cit.
29 S. Matthyse, 'A theory of the relation between dopamine and attention', *Journal of Psychiatric Research*, 1978, 14: 241–8.
30 S. Matthyse, B.J. Spring, and J. Sugarman (eds) *Attention and Information Processing in Schizophrenia*, Oxford, Pergamon, 1979.
31 J.C. Lynch, V.B. Mountcastle, W.H. Talbot, and Y.C.T. Yin, 'Parietal lobe mechanisms for directed visual attention', *Journal of Neurophysiology*, 1977, 40: 362.

32 L.S. Squire, 'Amnesia and the biology of memory', in W.B. Essman and L. Valzelli (eds) *Current Developments in Psychopharmacology*, vol. 3, New York, Spectrum, 1976.

33 B. Maher, *Introduction to Research in Psychopathology*, New York, McGraw-Hill, 1970.

34 B.E. Ginsburg, J.S. Cowen, S.C. Maxson, and P.Y. Sze, 'Neurochemical effects of gene mutations associated with audiogenic seizures', in A. Barbeau and J.R. Brunette (eds) *Progress in Neurogenetics*, New York, Excerpta Medical Foundation, 1969.

35 B.E. Ginsburg, 'The role of genic activity in the determination of sensitive periods in the development of aggressive behaviour', in J. Fawcett (ed.) *Dynamics of Violence*, Chicago, Ill., American Medical Association, 1971.

36 P.A. Broadhurst, *Drugs and the Inheritance of Behaviour*, New York, Plenum, 1978.

37 B.E. Ginsburg, J. Yanai, and P.Y. Sze, 'A developmental genetic study of the effects of alcohol consumed by parent mice on the behaviour and development of their offspring', in *Research, Treatment and Prevention*, Washington, DC, NIAAA, 1975.

38 G. Racagni, F. Cattebeni, and R. Paoletti, 'A biochemical analysis of strain differences in narcotic action', in I. Hanin and E. Usdin (eds) *Animal Models in Psychiatry and Neurology*, Oxford, Pergamon, 1977.

39 E.C. Johnstone, 'Relationship between acetylator status and response to phenelzine', in J. Mendlewicz (ed.) *Genetics and Psychopharmacology: Modern Problems of Pharmacopsychiatry*, vol. 10, Basle, Karger.

40 B.E. Ginsburg, R.E. Becker, A. Trattner, J. Dutson, and S.R. Bareggi, 'Genetic variation in drug responses in hybrid dogs: a possible model for the hyperkinetic syndrome', *Behavioural Genetics*, 1976, 6: 107.

41 W.H. Gantt, *Experimental Basis for Neurotic Behaviour*, New York, Harper, 1944.

42 R. Lynn, 'Russian theory and research on schizophrenia', *Psychological Bulletin*, 1963, 60: 486–98.

43 I.M. Marks, *Fears and Phobias*, London, Academic Press, 1969.

44 H.R. Beech and M. Vaughan, *Behavioural Treatment of Obsessional States*, Chichester, Wiley, 1978.

45 Maher, op. cit.

46 W.R. Miller, R.A. Rossellini, and M.E.P. Seligman, 'Learned helplessness and depression', in J.D. Maser and M.E.P. Seligman (eds) *Psychopathology: Experimental Models*, San Francisco, Calif., Freeman, 1977.

47 R.A. Spitz, 'Anaclitic depression', *Psychoanalytical Study of the Child*, 1946, 2: 313–47.

48 R.A. Hinde and L. Davies, 'Removing infant rhesus from mother for 13 days compared with removing mother from infant', *Journal of Child Psychology*, 1972, 13: 227–37.

49 S.J. Suomi and H.F. Harlow, 'Production and alleviation of depressive behaviours in monkeys', in J.D. Maser and M.E.P. Seligman (eds) *Psychopathology: Experimental Models*, San Francisco, Calif., Freeman, 1977.

50 N. Bolton (ed.) *Philosophical Problems in Psychology*, London, Methuen, 1979.

51 J. Margolis, *Persons and Minds*, Boston Studies in the Philosophy of Science, vol. lvii, Dordrecht, Reidel, 1978.

52 W.H. Thorpe, *Animal Nature and Human Nature*, London, Methuen, 1974.

Chapter seven

Sir Aubrey Lewis – an Australian psychiatrist

Sir Aubrey Lewis was born in 1900 and died in 1975. He spent his first twenty-six years in Adelaide, then went to Britain and stayed there for the rest of his life, apart from one brief return visit. He planned to return to Australia after he retired, but unfortunately his wife died, and he was unable to make the journey.

I have tried to summarize his contributions to psychiatry by drawing on the four categories employed in British law to designate different forms of legacy: the specific, the general, the demonstrative and the residual. The general legacies are his writings and the research. The specific legacy is the Institute of Psychiatry, which at the time of Sir Aubrey's retirement was described by the University Grants Committee as probably the most academically brilliant, progressive and respected combination of clinical scholarship and critical integrity in the world.

His personal characteristics are part of the demonstrative legacy. To give you a notion of the measure of the man, here is an extract from a letter written shortly after Sir Aubrey's death by Sir Harold Himsworth, then Secretary of the British Medical Research Council.

I can't tell you how much I miss Aubrey. I had a tremendous respect for his intellect, and a great liking for him as a person. With the possible exception of Sir Isaiah Berlin, I know of nobody, certainly no near contemporary who could move with such ease among concepts at the frontiers of understanding.

For psychiatry, he was the right man at the right time. And above all he had the courage to be unpopular. I always felt safe and so did the MRC when he was about – and I always found him open-minded, unless he felt the work was shoddy. He was a great man in the real sense of that much-abused word...

Originally published in D. Copolov (ed.) *Australian Psychiatry and the Tradition of Aubrey Lewis*, Victoria, Australia, National Health and Medical Research Council, 1991, pp. 1–16.

Sir Aubrey Lewis's legacies are better known than his Australian connection, which has not received the attention that it merits. Shortly before he died he told me that his Australian background had contributed greatly to his achievements. His remark didn't mean a great deal to me at the time, because characteristically he did not elaborate on its significance. It wasn't until after his death, when I was able to examine some of his papers, that I came across his first publication, a paper not included in his collected works. It was written when he was ten years old and published as a prize essay, called 'My favourite season, Spring'. The final sentence reads: 'I am an Australian, and my essay is from an Australian point of view, which is not perhaps in concord with that of others who dwell on other parts of this globe.' That struck me as an unusual comment from a boy of ten and made me wonder about the way in which his achievements would be commemorated in his native country. Accordingly in 1976 I wrote to a former colleague of mine, who was living in Brisbane, and asked him about local plans. He replied, 'I wrote to the President of the Australian and New Zealand College of Psychiatrists concerning any moves to commemorate Sir Aubrey's death. To my astonishment I have received a letter in which he says, "I regret to say that I was unaware of his death. And I am quite sure that there are no moves of any sort in Australia to establish a memorial".' He added: 'I must confess that this ignorance astonished me, bearing in mind that the writer is the President of the Australian and New Zealand College, though in all fairness he does live in Western Australia, which is even more remote from the rest of the world than Brisbane!' The Scientific Programme Convenor of the Australian College wrote: 'It was good to hear that so much interest is being taken in Sir Aubrey Lewis and we are very pleased that he came from South Australia originally. But I really must point out that once he left here he never returned, and really the scene of his entire working life was in the United Kingdom.'

Two factors contributed to the lack of recognition of Aubrey Lewis's work in Australia: first, practically all his contemporaries had died and, second, he never revisited Australia during his postgraduate years. Helped by Professor Brian Davies, I collected the names of a number of people who knew Aubrey Lewis in his early days and wrote to them, collecting many fragments of information.

Before referring to these I think it might be helpful to know what Aubrey Lewis meant by saying he saw things as an Australian. If the child is really father to the man, we should direct our attention to the Adelaide of the early twentieth century, which boasted about 100,000 inhabitants; agriculture was booming and copper had been discovered. It was the commercial capital of South Australia and contained a cathedral, several churches and hospitals. But what was the milieu in which young Aubrey Lewis grew up?

Of the various accounts I found, two are relevant. The first comes from the autobiography of Stella Bowen, an Australian artist who seems to be quite little known here, perhaps because she, like Aubrey Lewis, left Adelaide in her twenties and did not come back.[1] She too travelled to Britain and made her reputation as a painter. The first chapter of her book is entitled 'Adelaide'. It covers the city and the life in it from her rebellious point of view at almost exactly the same time that Aubrey Lewis was growing up. A brief extract will convey its flavour:

> I have reconstructed Adelaide in my memory as a queer little backwater of intellectual timidity, a kind of hangover of Victorian provincialism. Isolated by three immense oceans and a great desert and strickened by recurrent waves of paralysing heat, it lies shimmering on a plane encircled by soft blue hills, pretty, banal and filled to the brim with an anguish of boredom.
>
> The life on sheep stations was the most characteristically Australian I ever saw. But in the town, except for the modifications imposed by the climate we were just pale imitations of something which was already moribund in England. We were in fact a suburb of England. And in Adelaide a girl's social popularity depended pretty exactly on her proficiency at tennis. Not to play tennis was unthinkable; it debarred you from almost all the daytime entertainment that there was. If you were a bad player, you nevertheless tried to run hard and to seem keen and if you were cheerful, humble and energetic you were tolerated. It was necessary to be tolerated because otherwise what would you do on Wednesdays and Saturdays, when everyone else would be at the Adelaide Oval, where the Lawn Tennis club had 16 lovely grass courts and everything was properly done? There were no men of leisure in Adelaide, everyone was in business who was not studying for a profession. The Australian brother was usually much less civilised than the Australian sister who has utilised her leisure to cultivate her person and her manners and even her mind. Brother would often be a pimply young simpleton, either too shy to speak or boisterously hearty. The few who weren't the good dancers and the good talkers, who were interested enough in femininity to be interesting themselves, behaved like lords of the earth, and had everything their own way. And what with test matches and interstate and intercollegiate football and cricket, as well as the international tennis, the Oval was the great centre of social life.

This picture also shows the childhood background of two Adelaide medical figures who were Aubrey Lewis's contemporaries. Both Howard Florey and Hugh Cairns were in precisely this social stratum of the city G. Macfarlane, Florey's biographer,[2] was primarily concerned with Florey's work as a scientist, but he does touch on some aspects of Adelaide at this time. He says, for example, that Florey's school life was of steady, dedicated progress, winning prize after prize. On the games field he was equally successful; he was a natural athlete and made every effort to excel. He played cricket, football and tennis for the university and became a double blue; he was able to give Davis Cup players a run for their money. And of course he became a Rhodes scholar because, as Macfarlane says, he had all the qualities required by the trustees – industry, determination, leadership, outstanding academic and athletic ability and the right social background. His character is not dwelt on, but some aspects of it are recognizable in the farewell letter he wrote to his fiancée on the eve of his departure to Britain, which begins, 'I'm not going to write you any sentimental slush, I don't think either of us are built that way. I see rather more in you. You may not be brilliant at your work, but you seem to have some sort of understanding of men and things.' This, according to Macfarlane, is the nearest approach to a love letter that Florey ever wrote. Anyone who ever met Lady Florey will realize that he completely missed the point because, as Macfarlane points out, Lady Florey was intensely ambitious and rated her medical career as far more important than affairs of the heart.

The pattern here was conventional, as was the case with Cairns who was also a Rhodes scholar, went to Oxford and became a member of Balliol College. He was a young man with striking good looks and physique, a fine oarsman who rowed for Oxford in the boat race, and eventually married the daughter of the Master of Balliol, so his career got off to a good start.

Aubrey Lewis's didn't. As the only son of an Orthodox Jewish watch-maker who lived in a small house in an unfashionable part of the city, he came from a very different background on the wrong side of the track. He went, not to the fashionable public school attended by Florey and Cairns, but to the local Catholic school, the Christian Brothers College. His school reports show him to have been a remarkably gifted child. The emphasis, however, was on the humanities. A contemporary says:

Aubrey was always a loner at school, because he was not the least interested in sport of any kind and so he never rushed in with the other boys. He didn't consider himself better than others, but he didn't think along the same lines or do the same things as most teenage boys. For example, out of a sense of duty he would regularly attend the football or cricket matches that the college was involved in, but he sat by himself on a seat at the side of the Oval and read a book throughout the match. I don't think he ever kicked a football or held a cricket bat in his hand.

Clearly, he lived rather apart. I was puzzled to know why somebody of this type should have gone into medicine, and put this question to a number of my correspondents. Two of the replies are of some interest. One is from a psychiatrist in Perth who knew him and knew Adelaide. He says:

There has always been a powerful and prominent, almost a dynastic, influence of medicine in Adelaide. It wouldn't be surprising that the aspirations of a clever man would draw him in this direction. Another reason for the choice of medicine may be perhaps in Lewis's position straddling the Jewish and Catholic cultures, the latter at least most certainly having so much of a ghetto mentality at that time. For the same reason that Jews have been said to choose to be their own entrepreneurs, for fear of discrimination when throwing in their lot with organisations such as commercial companies, universities etc., it has always been traditional for Catholics in Australia aspiring to higher things, to choose the professions, particularly medicine.

The other reason is rather more personal, from somebody who knew him quite well at the time, and who commented:

> If I can guess, from my knowledge of the Lewis family, it is probable that Aubrey's mother influenced his choice of career. She was tremendously proud of her brilliant son, and would have known that he was capable of attaining any dizzy heights. But in Australia, and certainly at that time, it was much more prestigious to be a doctor than to do arts – which lead to teaching or library work. Even a chair in English Literature would in her eyes not amount to as much as being a physician.

Once he had entered medical school we have rather more information. He spent much time editing the medical students' review, which he rapidly transformed. Howard Florey had been the previous editor and it is rumoured the Adelaide Post Office refused to handle the journal because of the obscenity of its content. When Aubrey Lewis took over it moved in a rather more sedate direction, buttressed by his own contributions.

Several contemporaries commented on his strikingly individual characteristics. Here are a few examples:

> I remember him well. He was different from most other medical students; he was very much an individual and looked different. I can remember his dark eyes and intense expression which was followed always by a quiet smile. He was editor of the student magazine and was also interested in theatre and cultural matters which was most unusual for a medical student at the time.
>
> He was what would now be called a loner, because he didn't mix freely with other people and he thought more deeply than the average medical student, indeed, much more deeply than most house surgeons and even the honorary staff at the time. He was a serious-minded medical student, well liked and respected.
>
> He took no part in sporting or social life, and considered sporting events a waste of time. All his interests were scholastic, and the time-honoured medical student pranks had no attraction. The only competitive

game I ever knew him play was chess, and of this he was very fond. During the whole of his internship, he could be found sitting before a chess board with a telephone transmitter in his hand playing a game with a colleague who was an intern at the Children's Hospital. As a student he really had a mastery of several languages besides English, and was interested in old books, particularly the early French and Spanish authors provided only that the volumes were in the original and not in translation. I remember him on one occasion reviling me for reading the English translation of *Don Quixote* and telling me how the beauty of the original was marred in translation.

He was a man of exemplary character based on a strict religious family background. He was very polite, well beyond the standard of the average medical student.

What were Sir Aubrey's own views? There is, fortunately, quite a lot of information because he wrote extensively, and his private papers contain a number of essays and ruminations. Two extracts carry some significance for my theme. The first comes from an essay on the value of literacy, which was published when he was twenty years old:

A doctor has to know human nature. Art in a similar way seeks to illuminate the difficult book of human nature, so that you may more clearly read by its light. It may be argued that this is really the function of psychology. The difference between literature and psychology is the difference between *King Lear* and an essay on filial ingratitude. Both, though very different, will be of value to the student of human nature. The confidence and respect of patients is essential to a doctor; to this end he must not only be a skillful physician or surgeon, but a gentleman – and in my view the terms are synonymous – a man of culture. It may be said that the qualities of a gentleman are not to be acquired. Supposing it to be otherwise, the example and friendship of gentlemen may do much to make a man a gentleman himself. And it is chiefly by means of literature that we can gain access to their lives and conversation. Close association with such gentlemen as Charles Lamb and Marcus Aurelius, Uncle Toby and Colonel Newcombe, who couldn't add a score of such names, does not leave a man as they found him. It's a rein upon the headlong, a spur to the clean spirit and we reject it at our peril.

When his contemporaries thought of him as a 'loner' they were not aware of this wide circle of friends and acquaintances. These were the gentleman that he was studying so avidly in the public library and at home, and it was from them that he began to shape his outlook and his thinking.

The second extract is quite different but equally relevant. The title of this essay is 'Quacks!', and the passage reads as follows:

The stronghold, the almost impregnable fortress of the quack is one built not by himself but by his dupe, and its name is human credulity. So long as men are willing to believe a thing to be true, although their reason judges it false, so long will the quack flourish. He knows well wherein his strength consists, and the scientific attitude of mind, scepticism if you like, is the one thing that he dreads. For a physician, an open mind is one of the most precious qualities we can be endowed with. One always feels inclined to say that the right time to poleaxe a man, especially a doctor, has come as soon as he shows sign of believing that whatever he learns, whatever he does, whatever he thinks must be right – and all who disagree should be put down; in short as soon as he has the symptoms of a form of scientific senility which is called obscurantism. Understandably the quack flourishes nowhere more than in the field of nervous diseases. Psychological medicine, fraught as it is with great possibilities, is only young as yet, and perhaps some day faith cures and related observations will cease to be the puzzling phenomena that they are at present.

For a young man of twenty this is a remarkable passage which is, I believe, the first reference to psychiatry in all his writings. It certainly does not indicate that he had a special interest in psychological medicine. His original interests took him in quite different directions. I wondered why a man of his considerable intelligence and wide cultural background should have chosen to specialize in a subject which was not at first sight so obviously attractive for his career. This question was put to him directly during a videotaped interview. He replied as follows:

I think my entry into psychiatry was fortuitous. I was at a university where there was a great deal of interest in anthropological research because the Aborigines were clearly a vanishing race and people wanted to make as many observations as they could on them. The presence of Wood Jones, an anatomist with wide interests who was particularly concerned with anthropology, contributed to stirring up the interest of people like myself. So I seized the opportunity of going on one or two expeditions and collecting some data concerning the dreams of Aborigines, many of whom came into the hospital where I was a student or a houseman. When two emissaries of the Rockefeller Foundation came to Adelaide to look for people who might be trained to make psychological observations of the Aborigines (because up till then the anthropological studies in this field had been psychometric) they were told of my existence and they asked me whether I would like to train as a psychologist. In order to equip me to study the Aborigines in detail, I agreed, though I recognised that it was in a sense wasting my medical education for me now to start on a fresh career as a research psychologist. Until then I had always thought of myself as having a bent towards neurology, and I thought of myself as following the usual Australian sequence of then coming to England, obtaining the Membership of the Royal College of Physicians, and then more neurology at Queen's Square and finally acquiring a practice as a specialist. However, this advent of the Rockefeller men of course deflected me and it was agreed that I should have a training as a psychologist. The difficulties arose because the Professor of Psychology in my university was really a philosopher and he had no liking, or indeed any tolerance, of the kind of psychology he knew was practised in America – academic experimental psychology instead of metaphysics, which he saw as the real business of the psychologist – so he refused to guarantee me a place in the university in his department on my return. This was the obvious way of arranging things, in accordance with the usual requirements of the Rockefeller Foundation that the university from which a man came should be prepared to give him a job on completion of his training. When the predicament was explained to the Rockefeller people they said they were prepared to transfer my fellowship from psychology to psychiatry. And so when I went to America it was to departments of psychiatry that I went. In a sense, therefore, I suppose I was not taking up psychiatry because it was my aim and ambition and purpose in life at that time but because it was fairly close to some other interests of mine which happened to fit in with the opportunity that was suddenly thrust before me . . . From then on, of course, I was psychiatrically coralled.

In my monograph[3] I have tried to summarize what Aubrey Lewis contributed to the theory and practice of psychiatry over the subsequent forty years. His own assessment of his achievements was recorded in another interview, when he was asked about his views on so-called Maudsley psychiatry:

AUBREY LEWIS: The connotation is partly positive and partly negative. Taking the negative side first [the Maudsley Hospital] is not a place that is dominated by psychoanalytic or cognate speculations or theories, and people recognise that and regard it therefore as in a sense hard-headed, perhaps supercritical, perhaps sceptical, but not pie-in-the-sky or ethereal. On the positive side, I should think that it is regarded as a centre where Maudsley psychiatry is concerned with empirical clinical methods strengthened by the results of research, which then enable theory to be formulated and eventually applied to practice. But I think it's chiefly in the balance that is observed in Maudsley psychiatry which is regarded by many in foreign countries as typical of the general English attitude in medicine, which is a balanced one, avoiding the extremes of enthusiasm and bold claims, but not settling down into a stagnant acceptance of things as they are. Whether it is right to regard those as English attributes or whether it's appropriate to designate the Maudsley, I don't know. I should think it probably is, so that when people are looking for a psychiatrist of a particular sort, they know that they are unlikely to get a man whose outlook is predominantly psychodynamic. Should they find such a chap he won't be a typical product of the Maudsley – he would be a sport. If they want a man who is interested in social psychiatry, or epidemiological psychiatry to fill a vacancy in an American unit they always turn to us. I think the statistical approach, the application of statistical methods to the testing of hypotheses, is also accredited to us, and I've no doubt that there are many people not knowing the inner relationship of the staff who would regard Professor Eysenck as a typical Maudsley psychiatrist. It's amusing to find that people regard him as a doctor and a psychiatrist and believe that his views are those held by the whole of the staff here. In the same way, the late Professor Hargreaves used to be annoyed when I would say to him, 'You people at the Tavistock say such and such,' and it was explained to me that the Tavistock Clinical had a great diversity of opinions and people. In the same way I suppose it's true here that although to the outside world we seem like a monolithic structure of sceptics and cautious observers and practitioners, we know ourselves to be less monolithic.

INTERVIEWER: In some sense I suppose you've seen the development of social psychiatry as a way out of the dilemma of the organic and the dynamic approaches. Wouldn't it be true to say that?

AUBREY LEWIS: I wouldn't have said it was a dilemma. I think that there is a proper place for the dynamic and the organic approaches, but the social side of psychiatry is so obtrusive at every point, and has been in the history of psychiatry at all times that I don't see how it's come to be suggested as it has, except that the methods of investigation are ill-formed and the whole of sociology is still embryonic. If it weren't for that I think the crying need for better knowledge of the social aspects of psychiatry would have been fully recognised, whether you speak from the standpoint of the law or from the standpoint of we'll say, drug-taking, drug addiction, or the conditions within which a certain form of mental disorder appear to be generated or fermented. You can see the social importance, important social considerations staring you in the face, and my own concern in particular was given a fillip after the setback in 1930, when there were a lot of unemployed people. With the help of Miss Galloway I made a study of their psychiatric condition. Letitia Fairfield, who was then at the London City Council, gave us a list of people who were supposed to be the hard nuts who couldn't be cracked, the core of unemployability. But as soon as conditions improved, back they went to work. Social enquiry has become more and more the concern of the Medical Research Council Unit and other groups here; it's impossible to draw a sharp line between social and psychological. Often when I suggested to Professor Eysenck that there was a need for a social researcher here he would put the view that the psychologist was quite capable of carrying out any of the social psychological enquiries that were needed, which were much the same as sociological and when you look at the blurred outlines of these behavioural sciences of psychology, sociology, anthropology, you can see that a case can be made for the right of any of the people coming from any of these disciplines to attack problems which, I suppose, broadly can be thought social problems.

Aubrey Lewis in his Australian context is important to contemporary Australian psychiatry. Here it is useful to take a broad view. Some years ago there was a very interesting paper in *Science*, written by a historian of science who addressed himself to the general question of 'importance' in the scientific field.[4] He asserted that three criteria are often confused in estimating the importance of major figures in the history of scientific thought. The first is the indispensability of what they wrote or said, regardless of its effect, judged simply as a stage in the development of our present knowledge. From this point of view, to earn a place in history a person need only be the first to discover the material or express the idea in question. Medical history is riddled with the names of such people. The second criterion is the effect of an individual's contribution on other thinkers and non-thinkers which, unlike the first, requires publication, recognition and sometimes misinterpretation. The third is the extent of personal indispensability, something which is much more difficult to judge. These two criteria bring us back to the demonstrative and residuary legacies of Aubrey Lewis. They are much less tangible and can best be illustrated by what was said of him shortly after his death, by the British Association of University Teachers of Psychiatry:

> Sir Aubrey Lewis raised the standing of psychiatry in a profession when eminence was unmistakable, and above all he saw to it that a number of very able men and women entered the speciality after first having their own spurs as physicians. It is not the formation of the Royal College of Psychiatrists, but the creation of a body of well-educated doctors and medical scientists that has led to the influence of psychiatry in medical and social councils. And he enabled us all to bask in his achievement. Everyone who came in contact with this man was altered by the experience; for most of us he was, and will have been, the only great man that we have met. Those who did not have that contact may derive a little comfort from the experience of his many pupils who try to pass on his lessons.[5]

What were these lessons? The first of them goes back to that essay that he wrote at the age of twenty, in which he mentioned the importance of scepticism, which he identified with scientific thought. The word 'scepticism' has acquired pejorative overtones, but in its philosophical context it is a very respectable notion; it simply means to look at or inspect. Aubrey Lewis was fond of quoting the phrase, 'that if a man begins with certainties, he ends in doubt, but if he's content to begin with doubt, he may end in certainties'. His approach to teaching, which has been widely described as Socratic, was by means of this searching method of question and answer. Unless the student were very careful he would find himself talking nonsense, after having started from what seemed to be a perfectly logical premise. Lewis's view was that this approach was indispensable in a subject that was so riddled with doubts and difficulties as psychiatry where a premium is to be placed on clear thought from the outset.

The second lesson was perhaps best summed up by the notion of integrity. When he wrote about his own teacher, Adolf Meyer, Lewis laid particular emphasis on Meyer's moral and intellectual integrity and his conception of the humane aims of psychiatry. These qualities struck anyone who knew Aubrey Lewis personally. He was a very scrupulous, honest man, sometimes to the embarrassment of his colleagues. He was also a great lover of the classics and he would have endorsed the judgement of the younger Pliny, in a letter which was written in AD 79. The Romans were as well aware of the general issues relating to human conduct as we and, as Pliny remarked: 'Nobler spirits seek the reward of virtue, in the consciousness of it rather than in popular opinion. What we call fame should be the result and not the purpose of our conduct and if for some reason it fails to follow there is no less merit in cases where it was deserved.'

This verdict could certainly have been applied to Aubrey Lewis. He was a man who abjured all forms of publicity and, when I was told the other day by a journalist that he was a man who could have done with a public relations representative, I could think of no comment that would have horrified him more. His personal qualities reinforced his professional abilities and made him a model for people who knew him. It is all very well to talk about how difficult it is to practise psychiatry, to expatiate on the need to integrate a wide range of disciplines in a clinical framework, but it is rare to find somebody who combines these complex functions in their own activities. Most impartial observers who knew Lewis and saw him in action would have recognized that the task was feasible and have acknowledged his underlying determination of purpose. In his description of Florey and Cairns, Macfarlane writes:

> In all Australians who go overseas there is just a touch of the old pioneer spirit, and this attitude of mind obvious to visitors is quite un-European. It doesn't strike Australians as peculiar until they themselves visit Europe. Men like Florey absorbed it naturally and the more readily, because it harmonised with their pleasures in overcoming difficulties.

This was equally true of Aubrey Lewis. He encountered immense difficulties in setting up the Institute of Psychiatry, and in establishing the sort of base from which this enterprise became possible. But, in true Australian fashion, he was not deflected by all the practical and personal obstacles.

Finally I will refer to one of the last papers that Aubrey Lewis wrote, which touches directly on what we have been hearing about the unit named after him.

> Psychiatry has received much public attention in the last three decades and the importance of mental health has been recognised with increasing readiness. It's therefore easy to infer that the demand for more knowledge and effective treatment of mental health is already being impressively met. But this in my opinion is to overrate the scientific and clinical gains of the last two or three decades upon which the expectation is based. These gains have been substantial, but not of a kind to justify immediate hopes of any so-called breakthrough, which will provide cures for many of the major mental disorders. Sober appraisal of our recent history suggests that research must be our first concern even though there is room for more extensive application of present knowledge.

Among the many documents that have come my way recently is a mental health discussion paper which was presented to the Australian Health Minister's Advisory Council at the end of 1989. It contains the clear statement of a principle, 'that governments and professional organisations support and encourage mental health research, through a range of appropriate initiatives, including training in research, methodology, increased funding and targeted programmes'. I have no doubt that Aubrey Lewis would have endorsed the spirit of that recommendation, and that he would have been delighted to learn that an Australian research unit dedicated to this subject had been associated with his name.

References

1   S. Bowen, *Drawn from Life*, London, Virago Press, 1984.
2   G. Macfarlane, *Howard Florey*, Oxford, Oxford University Press, 1979.
3   M. Shepherd, 'A representative psychiatrist: the career, contributions and legacies of Sir Aubrey Lewis', *Psychological Medicine*, Monograph Supplement 10, Cambridge, Cambridge University Press, 1986.
4   M. Sirimu, *Science*, 28 Aug., 1955, 477.
5   Anon., 'Aubrey Lewis – an appreciation', *Newsletter of the Association of University Teachers of Psychiatry*, Feb. 1975, 2–4.

Chapter eight

The legacies of Sir Aubrey Lewis

In the autumn of 1975 I was asked to address the American Psychiatric Association at its annual meeting, with the specific request that the lecture be devoted to Sir Aubrey Lewis, who died a few months earlier that year. Since on such occasions an invited speaker is usually entitled to choose his own topic I was moved to question the reasons for so pointed a suggestion, especially as I knew that while Sir Aubrey's reputation in the USA had always been high among knowledgeable observers of the British scene, to most American psychiatrists his work had been largely unknown and in some centres it had been blatantly misunderstood. His status there was epitomized in the American *Psychiatric Dictionary*, where he is included as almost the only twentieth-century British figure in the following exiguous entry:

> Lewis, Sir Aubrey (1900–1975) Australian-born psychiatrist who joined the staff of the Maudsley Hospital (London) in 1928; Professor of Psychiatry at the associated Institute of Psychiatry, which under his direction became an international center for teaching and research.[1]

Just a bare six facts, one of which, as we shall see, is glaringly incorrect.

I learnt from my enquiries that after his retirement in 1966 Sir Aubrey's reputation had begun to grow in North America. The appearance of his collected papers in 1968 had opened the eyes of a wide readership, and attracted many appreciative notices. Among these reviews I would single out the long essay entitled 'A man for all reasons' by one of Sir Aubrey's former students, the child psychiatrist and psychoanalyst, Professor E.J. Anthony, who had emigrated from Britain to the USA in the late 1950s.[2] His assessment went beyond the books to the man and his achievement.

Based on the ninth Aubrey Lewis Lecture at the Institute of Psychiatry, London, November 1985. Originally published in *A Representative Psychiatrist: The Career, Contributions and Legacies of Sir Aubrey Lewis*, Psychological Medicine Monograph Supplement No. 10, Cambridge, Cambridge University Press, 1987, pp. 21–30.

He is the administrator with a mission – to create a great scientific institute – an educator of genius who imparts not the product but the art and craft of his science; he is already part of psychiatric history and something of a legend in his own time.

Professor Anthony made it clear that there were lessons to be learnt from a contribution which transcended national boundaries when he concluded that in the USA 'a Maudsley trend was in the making and that many well-established psychodynamic centres were undergoing a curious change of heart and personnel'.

It seemed to me, then, that two factors had prompted my invitation: a desire for information, coupled with a feeling on the part of my hosts that they had missed out on something. Americans, as Henry James made unforgettably clear, are notoriously averse to missing out on anything, and to try and satisfy their curiosity I did my best to assemble the basic facts concerning Sir Aubrey's career and contributions.[3] There proved to be more material than I had anticipated, much of it irrelevant to my immediate purpose. When, therefore, I was asked for a second time to devote an eponymous lecture to Sir Aubrey Lewis I felt that not only would it be wholly appropriate to this memorial day, but also it would be possible and fitting to do so without repetition by taking up the final theme of my earlier lecture, which had to do with what I identified as Sir Aubrey's legacies to his successors.

By analogy with English legal practice, I allocated these legacies to four categories: the demonstrative, the specific, the general, and the residuary. I did so then in order to suggest that they might help resolve the sense of what had been called the 'crisis and confusion' so evident among American psychiatrists at the time. A decade later I suspect that they are still more relevant to our own concerns. Originally I was able to devote to them little more than a brief mention. Today I should like to consider them in more detail. Let me take each in turn.

The demonstrative legacy

As the demonstrative legacy I designated the way in Aubrey Lewis 'showed how some of the most stubborn problems presented by psychiatry can be tackled through open-minded research on a very broad front'. I was not referring to the results of that research – the clinical and biological investigations, the studies of genetics, medical history, and, above all, the social enquiries – which are embodied in his published work, so much as to the less tangible features of his personal style, a topic which merits a word in its own right, the more so since as there are already relatively few colleagues who will have had direct contact with him in his prime.

'Le style, c'est l'homme même.' That Sir Aubrey subscribed to this notion was made clear in 1939 in a speech delivered at the presentation of a portrait

135

to his predecessor, Edward Mapother. Tributes on such occasions are mostly ephemeral, but this one, scribbled hastily on an LCC envelope, has survived among his papers. This is part of what he said:

> You will no doubt feel that in identifying Dr Mapother with the Maudsley much that we appreciate most is left out. His loyalty to his associates, his high sense of professional duty, his wit, his penetrating flair for spotting what is genuine and what is sham and frothy.... You can't separate a man from what he makes. You can't conceive of a great architect apart from his building. What was finely written in St Paul's about Christopher Wren is true of all great builders, whatever their medium. Behind the style is the man because the man's style is in his work, and Dr Mapother's work at the Maudsley has shown qualities that put him among the great architects of psychiatry in this century.

Much of this could be said of Aubrey Lewis, who resembled Mapother in many ways. His was a vigorous and vigilant presence, very different from that of those many contemporary specimens of *homo academicus* of whom it has been said that 'The absent-minded professor has given way to the absent professor, the public figure whose round of committees, conferences and trusts means that he sees more of air-hostesses than of students.'[4] Aubrey Lewis was not absent-minded and was rarely airborne. He was a down-to-earth professor whose impact on his students tended to be direct and considerable. There must be several hundred senior psychiatrists with vivid memories of the experience, well illustrated by the example of the young, now middle-aged, man from a faraway, semi-totalitarian country, who was involved as an expert witness on the mental state of the murderer of a prominent political figure. After several hours of gruelling cross-examination by the public prosecutor he was asked how he had acquitted himself so well. 'I used to present patients to Professor Lewis at Monday morning case conferences', he replied. In another vein, many students would have surely endorsed the experience of a well-known British ethanologist, who spoke of a single encounter with Aubrey Lewis as 'a sort of Jamesian experience', from which he emerged 'knowing that he would then and there travel to America and learn how to treat alcoholism'.[5] Which he did.

Not all his contemporaries reacted so positively, however, and Professor Anthony, as befits a psychoanalyst, developed the point when discussing the writings:

> It is extraordinary how little of Sir Aubrey's life comes out in these addresses.... This impersonality, this 'cool and critical intellect', this objectivity, this balanced point of view, and this *lack* of rancour make Lewis a perfect figure for projection. Accordingly, generations of students and colleagues have developed varying degrees of transference in relation

to him, some seeing him as one of the wisest, shrewdest, most perceptive individuals to emerge from British psychiatry since the last war, whilst in the minds of others he has become a powerful, manipulating grey eminence obsessed with making his own point of view prevail.[6]

In retrospect it is possible to appreciate the significance of this observation. There are on record a host of tributes to Aubrey Lewis's humanity, his integrity, and what C.P. Blacker called his essential kindness.[7] At the same time the astringent self-disciplined aspects of his personality which dominate Ruskin Spear's portrait clearly made their mark and his own lack of rancour was not always reciprocated, especially by some of his more senior colleagues. One long-standing associate, for example, described those same published papers which had so impressed Professor Anthony, as 'liable to put young doctors off [psychiatry] for 200 years' in a prominent journal edited by another.[8] There are pointed descriptions of him as primarily an organizer,[9] and an educator,[10] and even as a psychologist manqué,[11] and as a man who 'often opposed progress and generally left the personal treatment of patients to others'.[12] As recently as 1984 a two-volume reference work published in this country summed up this feeling of what Professor Anthony would probably term 'ambivalence' in the following entry:

A British psychiatrist born in Australia. He was Jewish and religious but never visited Israel. Intellectuality was used as a protection for his shyness. Of outstanding erudition and intelligence, anxiety prevented him from embarking on the unpopular and hazardous road of real creativity. He destroyed ideas with wisdom and purpose but rarely rebuilt. He taught by threat and only those who survived could learn. When relaxed he had great charm and had a real capacity for communication with the unthreatening patient. Lewis was essentially kindly with a great sense of moral purpose, the highest standards, and an immense and enduring sense of humour. After World War II he became the architect of the clinical and teaching programme at the Institute of Psychiatry, the Maudsley Hospital, London.[13]

Perhaps the most obvious judgement on such comments was expressed with antipodean bluntness by one of Lewis's compatriots: 'his detractors did not stand far enough away from those easily pluckable bunches of sour grapes'.[14] My purpose in disinterring these comments from the Lethe to which they belong, however, is not to rake over dead ashes or to provide one more example of the well-established maxim that public figures cannot please all of their contemporaries all of the time. It is, rather, to highlight the professional and personal style characterizing Lewis's demonstrative legacy. This was manifested by an apparent disregard of personal considerations that was so evident and so sustained as to have led many colleagues to assume that he was unaware of the issues. In this they were wholly mistaken. His private war-time letters make it clear that even then he was fully cognizant not only of the identity and motivations of his critics but also, more significantly, of the futility of trying to persuade them to put the general wood before the personal trees and of the need for that self-restraint, which, according to Goethe, is the sign of true mastery. With regret, but quite without rancour, he seems very early to have determined to follow his own star in the company of what was at first a very small number of colleagues who shared his objectives.

This behaviour pattern is unusual among psychiatrists but it is the hall-mark of many medical scientists of outstanding distinction. Here is a description of one of them:

> He could be brusque, sometimes brutally direct, seldom complimentary, and never flattering. Nevertheless, it was his personality that captured so many able young research workers, who had initially been attracted by his scientific reputation. What they found in him was an infectious vitality: great physical energy combined with an independence of mind that seemed to open mental windows and let the fresh air of realism clear away stuffy academic pomposities. Above all they gained something of his own attitude to research, the sense of purpose, the excitement of discovery (which he seldom expressed in words), and the will to work. And he gave them confidence. Despite his disparagement and seeming pessimism, they felt that like a good ship's captain, he was always in control, and knew exactly where he and they were going. Like a good captain, too, he treated his crew fairly and well. He knew (and cared) far more about their personal difficulties and troubles than most of them ever realised, and his offhand manner concealed an unsuspected sensitivity.[15]

This passage was written not about Aubrey Lewis, but about another Adelaide man, Howard Florey, just two years older, who also came to England in the 1920s to make his mark. The profile is recognizably similar, however, and goes some way to account for the reputation that Lewis acquired among his younger associates. Far from his putting them off psychiatry for 200 years, he – like Florey – made the subject appear an exciting challenge and helped steer their energies and ambitions into appropriate channels.

The basic qualities of such men are, of course, innate but perhaps some part of the achievement is attributable to the soil as well as the seeds. Lewis and Florey – and, one might add, Hugh Cairns – were medical men of a comparable mould, none of them much concerned with the number of buttons on the cuff, all of them having spent their formative years in a small, south Australian town. There are few descriptions of Adelaide at the turn of the century, but one of the more revealing is to be found in the autobiography of the artist, Stella Bowen. 'We were', she writes, 'a suburb of England, ... there were no men of leisure. Everyone was in business who was not studying hard for a profession.'[16]

Perhaps it is not fanciful to suggest that the mid-Victorian spirit of these same men was reflecting the shade of Colonel Light, who laid out the city of Adelaide in the 1850s, and on whose commemorative plaque is written his epitaph: 'I am delighted with my enemies for vilifying me so roundly for my plans. That way at least posterity will be certain that Adelaide is my creation alone.'

Aubrey Lewis would never have expressed himself in these terms, but the remark is in keeping with his style. Before looking at his own plans more closely I think it instructive to re-examine his general legacy, namely the writings.

The general legacy

Aubrey Lewis once remarked that he had never had time to write a book. He wrote many papers, the majority of which have been published in three volumes, where the reader will find the fruits of his research and his considered opinions relating to a wide range of topics.[17] They are, however, far from all that he wrote. At the end of his bibliography, it is stated simply that 'in addition to signed work, there are numerous reviews and editorials'. These include a host of unpublished lectures, book reviews, reports, annotations, and obituaries. Much of this material is little known because it is scattered and mostly unsigned, but it constitutes an indispensable guide to an understanding of the size and scope of his general legacy.

The medical journalism appears to have originated in the early 1930s with his work for *The Lancet*, to which he became a principal adviser. Later his activities spread to other journals. By way of example I would mention his book reviews, which numbered several hundred, the vast majority anonymous. Far too little attention is paid to the function of the good book reviewer: this is, as David Lodge has pointed out, 'to monitor and disseminate information about the endless production of new ideas and artefacts, on behalf of the rest of us, who will never have the time, opportunity or will to encounter them all directly'.[18] The truth of Lodge's judgement is well illustrated by Lewis's book reviews in *The Lancet*, the *British Medical Journal, Brain, Nature*, the *Eugenics Review, Medical History*, the *British Medical Bulletin*, the *Journal of Neurology, Neurosurgery and Psychiatry*, the *British Journal of Medical Psychology*, the *American Journal of Psychiatry, The Times Literary Supplement*, the *New York Review of Books*, and several other journals. The subject-matter included not only a stream of specialized topics but also historical themes, medical ethics, ethology, anthropology, and the history of ideas, all of them in direct or indirect relation to psychiatry. Several are full-scale scholarly essays, packed with arcane allusions and quotations drawn from a remarkably wide variety of sources. Here, for example, is an extract from his review of *La Terre du Remords*, a French translation from the Italian original by the Professor of the History of Religions in Rome, dealing with tarantism, viewed as an expression of how Christianity confronted pagan resistance:

There are two obvious approaches to the analysis of tarantism – through psychiatry and through cultural anthropology.... Similarities abound between it and such cults as those of the Sudanese with their bo..., the Haitian voodoo, of the Ethiopians with their zar in which people possessed by an evil spirit have been exorcised by music and dancing. Similarities abound also at a different level between it and the effects of a venomous bite as understood by the Greeks, with their concept of the oistros, the maddening gadfly, and their notion (described for us by Nicander) of the mental effects of a spider bite. The role assigned to the music and dancing in the myth comes at times close to the modern scene in Apulia. It is, for example, with music that Eurydice is to be brought back after she has been killed by a venomous bite, and it is by the same means that people who are sick and disturbed in mind are to be restored to normal mind, then as now. The anthropologist has no difficulty in adducing numerous customs of the broad pattern so boldly portrayed in Salente.[19]

The earlier editorials and annotations are of interest in other respects. At all times he emerges as a stickler for accuracy. In a letter to the editor of *The Lancet*, for example, he writes

I was shocked at your alteration of 'forgo' to 'forego'. There is a nice footnote on p.19 of the *Rules for Compositors and Readers at the University Press, Oxford*, which tells how Gladstone was corrected about his 'correction' and showed a characteristic obstinacy, even in defeat.[20]

On issues of substance he was unflinching. As early as August 1933, in an editorial devoted to German eugenics, he referred to

The odious forms in which the social spirit of Germany is now manifesting itself, by persecution and chauvinism. The policy is highly integrated. Its espousal by these German physicians and geneticists may in part be attributed to their explicit preference for a form of society in which intelligence and humanity are less respected than ruthless devotion to the state.[21]

His comments on the mind of Adolf Hitler[22] and the case of Rudolf Hess[23] are no less forthright.

But perhaps the principal interest of this material lies in the demonstration it provides of the way in which he was rehearsing some of the topics to which he was to make so important a contribution during the post-war years. On taking up the chair of psychiatry in 1946, he did not, as Professor Anthony suggests, 'spring fully equipped from the head of Jove'. These occasional writings, in conjunction with his letters, make it clear that he had been cogitating on the work that needed to be done for the previous fifteen years. Thus on teaching, he stated roundly in an editorial written in 1935, 'the teaching of psychological medicine as a whole is becoming more and more plainly a necessary part of medical education'[24] and by 1943 he had developed this theme with special reference to post-graduate training.[25]

His views on the social dimension of psychiatry began with his pre-war studies on unemployment and were consolidated by his extensive experience of war-time planning. It was there that he first clearly developed the notion of neurosis as 'the very type and paradigm of social illness' and reached the conclusion that 'it is clear that mental health is too large a matter of public concern to be treated otherwise than as an essential part of the public health service'.[26] Looking ahead to the problems of the future, in 1944 he wrote a prescient editorial on the problem of ageing, a topic which is now recognized as a major issue but whose importance he was one of a very few to foresee so accurately at the time.

> With them [the elderly] it is not a question of rehabilitation, but of adjustment: jobs must be found adjusted to their now limited powers, and they must adjust themselves to their changing condition, without that sharp break called retirement, which is at first often welcomed as marking release from the burden of earning and working, but later often regretted as the beginning of an unfriended, melancholy, slow and aimless tedium. It is better that something should be asked for from the aged so long as it is not more than they can contentedly give; 'ne poltulantur sed ne quantum possumus quidem cognimur' is Cato Major's complaint in the De Senectate, and it may be hoped that social medicine and industry will take heed of it, provided always that in positions where freshness is all, the old are not left to clog and petrify affairs; for we have it on wise authority that men of age object too much, consult too long, adventure too little, repent too soon, and seldom drive business home to the full period, but content themselves with a mediocrity of success. Although admittedly life can only be lived forward, we have Kierkegaard's authority...that it can only be understood backward.[27]

And perhaps of most relevance to this occasion, there is an editorial in 1935 on psychiatric research in which he alluded with approval to the view of his distinguished namesake, Sir Thomas Lewis, that research must start from the actual problems of disease and must return thereto, though the methods be borrowed from other sciences. Research in psychiatry by those who know nothing of psychiatry is apt to be fruitless because irrelevant.... The supporting sciences must be the means of fresh advance and the guarantee of its stability.[28]

Among the supporting sciences he listed physiology, genetics, pharmacology, endocrinology, virology, psychology, sociology. He goes on: 'these are not merely hopeful fantasies.... The results are still few because the problems are unusual and difficult.'

A characteristically positive, pragmatic comment to introduce his specific legacy.

The specific legacy

It is generally conceded that the building in which we are meeting, and which houses the activities being discussed today, is the specific legacy, the particular brain-child of Sir Aubrey Lewis. In one sense the institution speaks for itself through the mouths of its scientific workers, but they hold differing views on its overall function. Here I am concerned with what it represented to its founder, an objective that can best be achieved by a brief glance at the growth and development of the concept of the research institute in the field of the life sciences.

The establishment of such institutes is not much more that 100 years old, dating back to the Koch Institute in Berlin, the Lister Institute in London, and the Pasteur Institute in Paris. Though the Rockefeller Institute in New York enlarged the scope of its activities to include a small selection of scientific topics with medical implications, these institutions and their many successors tended to concentrate on non-clinical basic science focused on specific areas of enquiry. Furthermore, their administrative structure was originally related to but separate from university bodies. In 1958 the history of their role in the advancement of medicine was sketched in a Linacre lecture by Sir Charles Harington, then director of the MRC National Institute for Medical Research which opened in 1920.[29] He concluded by defining what he called an 'unsolved problem' for the future, namely whether 'we might, by forming institutes for clinical research and associating or combining them with laboratory research institutes, forge weapons for the advance of medical science more powerful than any we might possess'. Harington might have been more confident of solving his problem if he had taken note of developments in psychological medicine. As Lawrence Kolb pointed out in the first Aubrey Lewis Lecture, an early unsuccessful attempt to found a psychiatric research institute had been made in New York as early as 1896 but the major influence on developments in this direction were to come from Germany.[30] 'The nature of psychiatry', wrote Emil Kraepelin in 1917, is such that questions which are constantly being formulated can be answered only on the basis of evidence supplied by a number of auxiliary disciplines; clinical observation must be supplemented by thorough examination of healthy and diseased brains, the study of heredity and degenerative diseases, the chemistry of metabolism, and serology. Only exceptionally well-trained specialists possess competency in each particular field... only a well-planned and comprehensive programme of research can bring us closer to the goal which we are striving to attain.[31]

In that same year the German Institute for Psychiatric Research in Munich was formally established. This was first located in the laboratories of the university neuropsychiatric hospital and some rented premises before becoming part of the Kaiser Wilhelm Society for the Advancement of Science in 1924. Four years later it became an Institute of Basic Research in a new building supported not only by local funds but also by the Rockefeller Foundation of New York. This in turn became a Max Planck Institute in 1954. Though Kraepelin himself had wished to include a clinical department as an integral part of the Institute, the first beds were not made available until 1922 and the Max Planck Institute did not receive its own clinic until 1966.

The debt of this Institute of Psychiatry to Kraepelin's vision has often been acknowledged. It was Kraepelin's idea of a psychiatric hospital specializing in early treatment, research, and teaching that impressed Henry Maudsley sufficiently to make his offer of £30,000 to the London County Council and persuaded Sir Frederick Mott to move his laboratories to the newly named Maudsley Hospital in 1923. The notion of an Institute, however, was first advanced by Edward Mapother in 1930, when he approached the Rockefeller Foundation for financial assistance to set up what was, by the standards of the day, a large-scale project, namely an institute with a professional clinical director and no fewer than six senior workers.

It is also noteworthy that the Rockefeller Foundation played a part in the creation of both pioneer institutes. A key figure in this initiative was Dr Alan Gregg, the director of the medical sciences division, who was influential in the introduction of psychiatry into American medical schools during the inter-war years. Gregg was that rare phenomenon, an idealistic man of affairs, with clear-cut ideas on medical institutes and much practical experience to support them. In his essays on the subject he defines a medical institute as an 'institutionalised task force' whose 'greatest and deepest need... is to be needed' and which, when successful, is characterized by an

atmosphere of expectancy springing from the expectancy on the part of individuals not merely that each will do his expected task but that in some way not yet clear each will bring to the work of the Institute something distinctly and peculiarly his own and, at his good time, will add something unique to what may be expected of one in his position.[32]

Gregg goes on: 'To create an institute to meet a need that is widely felt and readily formulated requires no mean abilities; to institute an organization to meet a need not yet perceived by most men calls for quite exceptional talents.'

It should be noted that Gregg speaks of a leader, not a director. The distinction is crucial, as I discovered some years ago when serving on an external committee specially appointed by the Biological-Medical Section of the Max Planck Society to assess the organization and prospects of its Psychiatric Institute. What we found, in brief, was that while there was much attention devoted to the occupancy, role, and function of the director-ship, there was little linkage or integration between the clinical and theoret-ical institutes and almost no collaborative work. Since then, despite our recommendations, the gap has widened; the two institutes have separated and Kraepelin's dream has been shattered.

This unfortunate train of events underlines the significance of Aubrey Lewis's concept of an institute, a concept in which two considerations are paramount. The first of these was the distinction he drew between leading and directing. On countless occasions I have had to explain to bemused foreign visitors that, *pace* the *Psychiatric Dictionary*, the Institute did not have and never had had an executive director. To the inevitable question – 'What about Professor Lewis?' – I tried to answer that his influence was exercised by his moral and intellectual authority, *de facto* rather than *de jure*, that administratively he was never more than *primus inter pares*. No one person, he always maintained, can possibly master the many disciplines now required for progress in psychiatry and, in consequence, no one person has the right to exercise authority over his colleagues. What he provided was less obvious, a living illustration of Alan Gregg's judgement that

> The best leaders of scientific institutes whom I have known had only this in common: they made their values known and felt throughout the organ-isation...what a leader transmits is the quality and the variety of his values, for he is quick to recognise and encourage in others those qualities, purposes, and interests that seem most significant to him.[33]

The second premiss was Lewis's stated belief that 'the distinction between "basic" and "applied" science is an arbitrary and shifting affair, depending as much on the intention and motive of the scientist and the vantage ground from which he works as on the nature of his research'.[34] His insistence on this principle ensured the constant provision of what are sometimes called bridge workers and bridge concepts. This was a goal which he pursued tirelessly and at every level, whether forging clinical links with the late

Geoffrey Harris's endocrinological research programme, incorporating basic research workers in the department of psychiatry, or siting the canteen next to the library in order to encourage personal contacts.

Such activities reflected his awareness of the several fissiparous forces which can damage and even destroy a research institute, forces that operate within departments, between departments, and at the clinical/non-clinical junction. Throughout his career he did his best to cement the unity of the Institute by generating and sustaining that atmosphere of expectancy to which Alan Gregg referred. The emphasis on cohesion, rather than on bricks, mortar, and magnification, was at the core of his specific legacy.

The residuary legacy

Finally, we come to Aubrey Lewis's fourth, residuary legacy, which in law is the remainder of a person's property after all other legacies have been paid. This consists primarily, I suggested, in the provision of a model for his successors, in the same way as he suggested was the case with Henry Maudsley. In his Maudsley Lecture of 1951 Lewis indicated the relevance of this legacy by developing a fantasy of Henry Maudsley's being brought back to inspect and comment pointedly on the contemporary scene.[35] It would be a foolhardy man who attempted to repeat this exercise with Lewis but fortunately it is unnecessary, for in 1970 he wrote a little-known piece on the state of psychiatry in 1984.[36] It is worth recalling some of his predictions.

Limited advances, he suggested, could be expected in the spheres of psychopathology and psychological processes, in the more selective use of pharmacotherapy, the development of brain science, the construction of models derived from information theory, and a tighter view of social deviation. The spirit of his opinions, none the less, endorses Lewis Thomas's observation that practitioners of most clinical sciences have progressed from a state of total ignorance to one in which they are aware of their own ignorance. His views on the broader, communal aspects of mental disorder are of particular interest in view of recent developments:

probably the shift of psychiatric care for acute illnesses to the general hospitals will have taken place; the mental hospitals will have passed through a phase of being unable to attract enough staff – medical, nursing, and social – and will have been reprieved and refurbished after a painful reduction in their number; and enlargement of community services for the mentally ill and mentally defective will have gone forward, within limits set by the availability of suitable recruits and the stage of knowledge about effective measures of education and rehabilitation.[37]

And, perhaps, most significantly:

By 1984 medical students will be getting a much better grounding in the social sciences and in the clinical principles and methods of investigation appropriate to psychological medicine; and much of the work now falling to the psychiatric specialist will be competently dealt with by the general practitioners, in whose post-graduate training psychiatry will play a large part, commensurate with the frequency of psychological problems.[38]

The accuracy of these prophetic comments compels us to consider his major conclusion:

Psychiatry has received much public attention in the last two decades and the importance of mental health has been recognised with increasing readiness: it is therefore easy to infer that the demand for more knowledge and effective treatment of mental ill-health will have been impressively met by 1984. But this is to over-rate the scientific and clinical gains of the last twenty years, upon which the expectation is based. These gains have been substantial, but not of a kind to justify immediate hopes of a 'break-through' which will provide a cure for schizophrenia, an effective means of preventing melancholia, or a quick remedy for obsessional neurosis. Sober appraisal of our recent history suggests that research must be our first concern, even though there is room for more extensive application of present knowledge.[39]

This statement has acquired still more force in view of the shadows that have fallen on the face of psychiatry since it was written. It is not always recalled that the favourable public esteem in which the discipline came to be held in this country in the post-war period was relatively recent. As late as 1951 it was possible for the prime minister of the day, Sir Winston Churchill, to write a memorandum to Sir Edward Bridges, the then head of the civil service, remarking that 'the public, rightly or wrongly, is critical of psychiatry'.[40]

It is pertinent to recall that 1951 was the year of the Festival of Britain, when the nation was urged to throw off the last vestiges of wartime austerity and welcome new ideas. Among these, the popular dissemination of psychiatric concepts rapidly became a prominent feature via the mass media as well as through a vulgarizing literature. In 1975, shortly after Aubrey Lewis's death, *The Times* newspaper carried a complacent profile entitled 'The age of understanding: the success story of British psychiatry' by the then president of the Royal College of Psychiatrists.[41] In 1981 Professor Colin Blakemore chose to devote his Aubrey Lewis Lecture to the theme of 'Psychiatry and society', beginning with the assertion that 'Psychiatry is public property. It is, like no other area of medicine, thought about, agonised over, discussed and criticised by people who have no direct contact with it as a medical discipline either as practitioners or sufferers.'[42]

Yet in retrospect this very acceptance has to some extent rendered the discipline a victim of its own apparent success. It is one thing to demarcate a territory, another to occupy and cultivate it. The claims of the more enthusiastic proponents of psychiatry have not gone unchallenged. In the past decade there have been murmurings of disquiet along a wide spectrum of opinion, extending from the general press to the high priests of neuroscience. Essentially they are all raising the question which has been elegantly posed by the Master of Balliol College: namely, in what does the expertise consist within a discipline which claims to be scientific but where it proves 'uniquely hard to draw the line between matters of fact and matters of value'?[43] The doubts have spread to representatives of psychiatry itself. In the USA there has been animated discussion of its malaise and even of its impending demise.[44] 'Psychiatry in jeopardy' was the subject chosen by the outgoing President of the Royal College of Psychiatrists as the topic of his farewell address in 1984,[45] and some of the concerns of the general medical profession were voiced in a recent *Lancet* editorial entitled 'Psychiatry: a discipline that has lost its way'.[46]

This is not the first time that the foundations of the discipline have been assaulted. Similar views were widely expressed 100 years ago in North America during the course of what the medical historian, Charles Rosenberg, has called the crisis of psychiatric legitimacy.[47] This he attributed to three factors: first, that psychiatry is 'shaped by social values and needs and consequent decisions of social policy to a far greater degree than most other specialities in medicine'; second, 'the vexed and unresolved relationship between psychiatry and general medicine'; and third, the 'discontinuities within the internal structure of the psychiatric community itself'.

In his professional activities and in his writings Aubrey Lewis was constantly aware of the need to confront all three factors. The first two were incorporated in his conception of psychiatry as a branch of social medicine, a view which was broad enough to incorporate most of the issues involved. With regard to the third he was sufficiently concerned by the internal strains within his discipline to single them out in the course of a late essay on the principal obstacles to psychiatric progress. 'The onlooker', he concluded,

> may conclude that the achievements outweigh the deficiencies. He is, however, not well placed to judge; in so private and complex a matter the onlooker does not see most of the game.... The psychiatrist is obviously better informed than the onlooker about what is going on in treatment and research; it does not follow that he sees it steadily or whole.... A consensus of psychiatrists can be obtained on many arguable and knotty matters, but only if the psychiatrists whose opinions are being canvassed have had similar specialist education and background.[48]

The truth of this contention was amply confirmed by the responses that I obtained from a group of representative psychiatrists from various countries and backgrounds, who were invited to indicate their views on the nature of their profession.[49] The differences between many of them proved to be fundamental, reflecting disagreements which indicate the scientific immaturity of the discipline as well as the dogmatism of its proponents. The practical importance of such wide differences of outlook has been strikingly illustrated by the radical administrative action which had to be taken three years ago in one major European centre, where it was ruled that in the face of irreconcilable ideological disputes, the psychiatric facilities would have to be formally divided into three separate sectors: a psychological component for outpatients, a social component for the community at large, and a small biological component for in-patient research, each functioning autonomously under a director with a radically different outlook from that of his colleagues.

Here is another, disturbingly fissiparous trend within the body of psychiatry, to be placed alongside those to which I have already alluded. As indices of disintegration they would have horrified Sir Aubrey Lewis, whose massive sense of cohesion was founded partly on robust psychobiological foundations and partly on another, less overt but equally important substratum, to which he referred in an unpublished report for the WHO Regional Office for the Eastern Mediterranean on 'Dilemmas in psychiatry'.[50] These dilemmas turn out to be principally moral, ethical, and intellectual, the last of which he identified as a psychiatrist's philosophical background:

> Nobody in psychiatry can do without a philosophical background, but very often it is an implicit and not an explicit one. If you consider the history of psychiatry, you can see that philosophical factors have weighed very heavily indeed in determining its direction and course. We need to acknowledge and reckon with this when we are trying to establish a truly sound, scientific discipline of psychiatry.[51]

Aubrey Lewis's professional outlook was closely linked to a philosophical standpoint, one which I think falls most appropriately into the category of what Margaret Wiley has called creative scepticism, a tradition which runs from Montaigne via the neo-Platonists through David Hume and his successors.[52] This tradition differs from that of flat Pyrrhonic disbelief by virtue of an open-minded tolerance, an incessant demand for evidence, and a consistent awareness of the distinction between first and final causes. Henry Maudsley exemplifies these characteristics in his theoretical writings, but Aubrey Lewis was able to go beyond theory into practice. Perhaps the nearest he came to explicating this achievement was in the course of an interview after his retirement with Dr D.L. Davies, who asked him directly what he saw as Maudsley psychiatry. His answer is revealing:

The connotation is partly positive and partly negative. Taking the negative side first, it is not a place that is dominated by too many psycho-analytical or cognate speculations or theories. People recognise this characteristic and regard it therefore in a sense as hard-headed, perhaps hypercritical, perhaps sceptical, but not pie-in-the-sky or ethereal. On the positive side I should think empirical methods strengthened by the results of research which enable theory to be formulated and eventually applied to practice. But I think it's chiefly in the balance that is observed in Maudsley psychiatry. This is regarded as typical of the general British attitude in medicine, which is a balanced one, avoiding the extremes of enthusiasm, bold claims on the one hand, and on the other not settling down with a stagnant acceptance of things as they are.[53]

It is this sense of balance – controlling an unusual combination of intellectual drive, of ambition, tenacity, and vision – which characterizes Aubrey Lewis's residuary legacy, and it was most evident during what Marley has called the 'golden age' of his professorial tenure.[54] He did so, however, without mentioning the worm in the complimentary apple for unfortunately Golden Ages, as the Greek poet Hesiod first pointed out nearly 3,000 years ago and as history has repeatedly confirmed, tend to be short-lived and, unless great care is exercised, to be followed by epochs of Silver and Brass, each worse than its predecessor and eventually deteriorating to Iron Ages, in which – as the poet says – men 'never rest from labour and sorrow by day, and from perishing by night; and the gods shall lay sore trouble upon them'.[55] With linguistic modifications this might be taken as an early description of the plight of more modern research workers and academic administrators, beset as they are by the twin deities of economy and redundancy to sacrifice what they can on the altar of financial cuts and cost-effectiveness. And should they work in the field of mental disorder they cannot fail to bear in mind Aubrey Lewis's warning that

> What happens in research . . . will reflect the state of our society, its values, its overriding concerns. If our society regards the improved mental health of its members as a major object of endeavour, this will have its effect on psychiatric research.[56]

He might well have added that in turn the results of psychiatric research will have their effect on society. A glance at current programmes of legislation does not provide reassurance about the priority accorded to mental health in most countries, including contemporary Britain. None the less, priorities are susceptible to change, never more so than when influenced by evidence of progress and success. For this reason alone the need to build constructively on the foundations laid with such care by Sir Aubrey Lewis is more urgent than ever. Meanwhile, on a commemorative occasion, we may fittingly recall his achievements, acknowledge his bounty, and reflect on the implications of his legacies.

References

1 R.J. Campbell, *Psychiatric Dictionary*, 9th edn, Oxford, Oxford University Press, 1981, p. 352.
2 E.J. Anthony, 'A man for all reasons', *Psychiatry and Social Science Review*, 1969, 3, 9: 6–11.
3 M. Shepherd, *The Career and Contributions of Sir Aubrey Lewis*, London, Bethlem Royal and Maudsley Hospitals, 1977.
4 *The Times Literary Supplement*, 1985, p. 462.
5 *Lancet*, 'Edward Lincoln Williams' (obituary), 1969, ii: 1, 430.
6 Anthony, op. cit., p. 7.
7 C.P. Blacker, unpublished obituary speech.
8 E. Stengel, 'Book review: *Inquiries in Psychiatry* and *The State of Psychiatry* by Sir Aubrey Lewis', *British Journal of Psychiatry*, 1968, 114: 127–9.
9 E. Slater, 'Autobiographical sketch', in J. Shields and I.I. Gottesmann (eds) *Man, Mind and Heredity*, Baltimore, Md, Johns Hopkins University Press, 1971, p. 15.
10 *Lancet*, 'Aubrey Julian Lewis' (obituary) 1975, i: 288.
11 H. Gibson, *Hans Eysenck*, London, Peter Owen, 1981, p. 76.
12 W. Sargant, 'Eat all the humble pie you can', *World Medicine*, 1975, 18 June: 22–3.
13 J.G. Howells and M.L. Osborn, *A Reference Companion to the History of Abnormal Psychology, A-L*, London, Greenwood Press, 1984, pp. 546–7.
14 J.D. Russell, 'The late Professor Aubrey Lewis – a personal appreciation', unpublished paper delivered to the Congress of the Royal Australian and New Zealand College of Psychiatrists, Adelaide, 1976.
15 G. Macfarlane, *Howard Florey*, Oxford, Oxford University Press, 1979, p. 363.
16 S. Bowen, *Drawn from Life*, London, Virago, 1984, p. 25.
17 A. Lewis, *The State of Psychiatry* and *Inquiries in Psychiatry*, London, Routledge & Kegan Paul, 1967; *The Late Papers of Sir Aubrey Lewis*, Oxford, Oxford University Press, 1979.
18 D. Lodge, 'Rabbit reviewer', *Encounter*, 1984, July/August: 65.
19 A. Lewis, 'Tarantism: St Paul and the spider', *Times Literary Supplement*, 1967, 3, 400: 345–7.
20 Unpublished private letter to the editor of *The Lancet*.
21 *Lancet*, 'Eugenics in Germany' (leading article) 1933, ii: 297–8.
22 *Lancet*, 'The mind of Hitler' (leading article) 1940, i: 36.
23 *Lancet*, 'The case of Rudolf Hess' (annotation) 1945, ii: 750.
24 *Lancet*, 'Teaching on medical psychology' (leading article) 1935, i.
25 *Lancet*, 'Psychiatric training' (leading article) 1943, ii: 294–5.
26 *Lancet*, 'Psychiatrists in harmony' (leading article) 1945, i: 758–9.
27 *Lancet*, 'The problem of ageing', 1944, ii: 569.
28 *Lancet*, 'Research in psychiatry' (leading article) 1935, i: 1,223–4.
29 C. Harington, 'The place of the research institute in the advancement of medicine', *Lancet*, 1958, i: 1,345–51.
30 L.C. Kolb, 'The Institute of Psychiatry: growth, development, and future', *Psychological Medicine*, 1970, i: 86–95.

31 E. Kraepelin, *One Hundred Years of Psychiatry*, trans. W. Baskin, New York, Citadel Press, 1962; first published in German in 1917.
32 A. Gregg, 'Medical institutes', *Canadian Medical Association Journal*, 1954, lxx: 449–53.
33 ibid.
34 A. Lewis, 'Empirical or rational? The nature and basis of psychiatry', *Lancet*, 1967, ii: 1–9.
35 A. Lewis, 'Henry Maudsley: his work and influence', *Journal of Mental Science*, 1951, 97: 259–77.
36 A. Lewis, 'Health in 1984: changes in psychiatric methods and attitudes', *New Scientist*, 1964, 21, 423–4.
37 ibid.
38 ibid.
39 ibid.
40 W. Churchill, quoted by Bridges.
41 M. Roth, 'The age of understanding: the success story of British psychiatry', *The Times*, 10 February 1975, p. 8.
42 C. Blakemore, 'The future of psychiatry in science and society', *Psychological Medicine*, 1981, 11, 1: 27–37.
43 A. Kenny, 'The psychiatric expert in court', *Psychological Medicine*, 1984, 14: 291–302.
44 E.F. Torrey, *The Death of Psychiatry*, Radnor, Pa, Chilton Book Co., 1974.
45 K. Rawnsley, 'Psychiatry in jeopardy', *British Journal of Psychiatry*, 1984, 145: 573–8.
46 *Lancet*, 'Psychiatry: a discipline that has lost its way' (leading article) 1985, i: 731–2.
47 C.E. Rosenberg, 'The crisis in psychiatric legitimacy', in G. Kriegman, R.D. Gardener, and D.W. Abse (eds) *American Psychiatry: Past, Present and Future*, Charlottesville, Va, University Press of Virginia, 1975.
48 A. Lewis, unpublished manuscript.
49 M. Shepherd (ed.) *Psychiatrists on Psychiatry*, Cambridge, Cambridge University Press, 1982.
50 A. Lewis, 'Dilemmas in psychiatry', Mental Health Report for the Eastern Mediterranean, unpublished, 1961.
51 ibid.
52 M.L. Wiley, *Creative Sceptics*, London: Allen & Unwin, 1966.
53 A. Lewis, unpublished interview with D.L. Davies, 1967.
54 E. Marley, 'Sir Aubrey Lewis: the Golden Age of a career', *Journal of Psychiatric Research*, 1983: 93–9.
55 Hesiod, in *Works and Days*.
56 A. Lewis, *Research and its Application in Psychiatry*, Glasgow: Jackson, 1963.

Chapter nine

The origins and directions of social psychiatry

Though the term 'social psychiatry' is now widely employed, it remains controversial and poorly defined. In some measure this confusion derives from the word 'social', whose uses and misuses Alfred Grotjahn recognized seventy years ago:

> Unfortunately, this adjective is at present frequently misapplied, particularly by physicians and representatives of private welfare agencies. Thus, for instance, 'social' never means simply useful in our economic sense because many things are economically useful without deserving the attribute 'social'. Also, the word is not identical to 'beneficial for the lower socio-economic classes' because that would apply as well to a soup kitchen or an out-patient department, and no sociologist would consider either to be a social institution.... And the 'social physician' is a regrettable term which hopefully will never replace the simple welfare physician. In view of such linguistic abuses one should remember that the word 'social' derives from the Latin word 'socius' and always relates to society, community, or mutual benefit association.[1]

To maintain, as one professor of social psychiatry has recently done,[2] that his subject is 'part of social medicine' is to do no more than delegate the task of definition, for social medicine itself has been a hotly debated topic among physicians since the expression was coined by Guérin in 1848 and introduced into Germany by Virchow in the same year.

In Europe, that revolutionary period affected medicine along with most other forms of human activity, and Virchow captured the spirit of the times when he wrote in his journal *Medizinische Reform* that 'Die Ärzte sind die natürlichen Anwälte der Armen und die soziale Frage fällt zum grossten Teil in ihre Jurisdiktion'.

Originally published in *Integrative Psychiatry*, 1983, Sep.–Oct.: 86–8. Translations of various quotations from the original German are by Dr and Mrs Lothar Kalinowsky.

The six principles

The early statement by Virchow is a pointer to one of the two main roots of social medicine, namely the representation and expression of the humanitarian tradition in medical practice. For a clear exposition of the other, scientific sources of the discipline, it was necessary to await the six principles enunciated by Grotjahn in his *Soziale Pathologie* sixty years later. These are as follows:

1 *Prevalence* The significance of illness from a social point of view is primarily determined by its frequency. Medical statistics are, therefore, the basis of any sociopathological consideration because statistics study human disease manifestations in terms of their biological differences such as age and sex as well as their social differentiation.

2 *Clinical characteristics* An illness acquires social significance not only from its frequency but also from its most frequent manifestations, the characteristics of its clinical pathology. But, in the typical case, an illness does not present itself as being largely caused by, or causative of, social circumstances. It is, therefore, essential that, beyond the clinical and anatomopathological picture, a pathological condition be studied to determine its typical sociopathological form.

3 *Aetiology* The most important relationship between a disease process and social conditions lies, of course, in the aetiologic area. Most useful aetiologic studies adhere to the following scheme: (a) The social conditions create or favour disposition toward the illness. (b) The social conditions may directly cause or transmit the cause of disease. (c) The social conditions influence the course of the illness.

4 *Outcome* Not only are disease processes influenced by social circumstances, but they also, in turn, influence social conditions – particularly, population shifts, military strength, and work efficiency. Especially does disease outcome exert a sociological influence. The outcome can be (a) death, (b) cure, (c) crippling, (d) lingering illness, (e) predisposition toward other disease, and finally (f) degeneration, i.e. producing an inferiority transmissible to offspring.

5 *Treatment* If diseases have significance for the life of a society, no less does their elimination by medical means if that is at all possible. A fifth point for our consideration must, therefore, be whether an illness with social significance may actually be influenced by social changes.

6 *Prevention* How can we prevent disease or influence its course by social measures? The answer lies in social hygiene measures that can be extended to, and applied by, the entire population.

In contemporary terms these objectives would be seen as the objectives of epidemiologic investigation, whether devoted to the study of disease on the one hand or of the medical needs of society on the other.

The humanitarian element

A parallel development can be traced in the course of social psychiatry since it was first introduced as a hybrid discipline by Southard in 1917.[3] From the eighteenth century onwards the humanitarian element was to be found in the attempts to link mental disorder with a variety of social factors – war, industrialization, poverty, over-civilization – with the aim of improving conditions by means of social reform.

An adequate analysis of this process, as George Rosen has pointed out, calls for an understanding of the sociology of knowledge as well as the history of psychiatry and a recognition of the melioristic view of social psychiatry as an instrument of human engineering.[4] In the opinion of one of the best-known contemporary advocates of this position, for example, the term designates 'an "elastic" concept, to include all social, biological, educational, and philosophical considerations which may come to empower psychiatry in its striving towards a society which functions with greater equilibrium and with fewer psychological casualties'.[5]

For medical representatives of this brand of social psychiatry the more extravagant extensions of psychodynamic speculation have provided a theoretical base since the 1920s.[6] In particular, the widespread adoption of group psychotherapeutics in the Second World War led to the nebulous but pervasive idea of the 'therapeutic community' which has been so widely linked to social aggregates of all varieties, ranging from the family to institutions to the community at large. The global influence of these ideas was reflected in the activities of the World Health Organization and in 1959 an Expert Committee on Mental Health went so far as to define social psychiatry as 'the preventive and curative measures which are directed towards the fitting of an individual for a satisfactory and useful life in terms of its own environment'.[7]

Scientific studies

So much for social psychiatry as a humanitarian enterprise. The scientific study of the social aspects of psychiatry can be traced independently to the work of nineteenth- and early twentieth-century clinicians. Just over 100 years ago Henry Maudsley wrote: 'It seemed proper to emphasize the fact that insanity is really a social phenomenon, and to insist that it cannot be investigated satisfactorily and apprehended rightly except it be studied from a social point of view.'[8]

By the early years of this century the truth of this observation was fully recognized in France and, especially, in Germany, as exemplified by Aschaffenburg's *Handbook*, published in 1915, and the work of Wilmanns, Kronfeld, and Birnbaum. Its full development, however, was to depend on the systematic application of the epidemiologic method which has been the particular contribution of the Anglo-Saxon workers.[9]

The most outstanding examples of this approach to individual disorders so far have been the studies by Goldberger on pellagra[10] and Gajdusek on kuru.[11] The wider implications of the approach were most clearly defined by the British psychiatrist, Sir Aubrey Lewis, who founded the first research unit explicitly devoted to social psychiatry.[12] It is perhaps significant that this unit had been in existence for ten years before Lewis, recognizing as he did the ambiguous nature of the concept, would accept social psychiatry as a term that could be regarded as conferring sufficient scientific respectability on its research programme.

The cornerstones of Lewis's conception of social psychiatry were three-fold: first, the application of the principles of epidemiology to the problems under investigation, using the general population as well as the clinic and the laboratory for information and experiment; second, the identification of the social aspects of established clinical concepts for study whenever possible (rehabilitation, for example, becomes 'treatment from the social point of view', and handicaps are redefined as 'measurable symptoms relevant to social conduct'); third, the need to draw on the methods and constructs of the social sciences without losing sight of their limitations. In Lewis's own words, 'the social side of psychiatry is so obtrusive at every point and has been in the history of psychiatry at all times, that I cannot see how it could have been so neglected if the methods of investigation had been better formed. In particular, the field of sociology is still embryonic.'

From opinion to achievement

This view of sociology has not, of course, been accepted by the sociologists themselves, especially in the United States. After a period of mounting interest during the 1920s Brown went so far as to claim in 1934 that 'The field of social psychiatry embraces all abnormal forms of social adjustments, made by individuals and groups as well. Like social psychology, social psychiatry is a division of sociology.'[13] And as late as 1948 Warren Dunham claimed the subject as 'a creation of sociologists to designate the interest of certain of their numbers who are doing research in the field of personality disorder'.[14]

Though this attempt to annex the territory of social psychiatry in terms of a mixture of cultural anthropology, interpersonal theory, and psychoanaly-tic speculation has proved sterile, several social scientists have employed the epidemiologic method legitimately since Durkheim's early study of suicide. Dunham's own study on the ecology of schizophrenia in Chicago is a model of its type. While epidemiologic, investigation, as a prominent medical sociologist has observed, is a form of research which he and his colleagues have been doing all their professional lives,[15] in itself it does not constitute a licence for the absorption of social psychiatry into the maw of the social sciences.

Fortunately, the discussion has passed from the realm of opinion to that of achievement. There is now a considerable body of work to demonstrate that Grotjahn's six categories of the frequency, form, causation, outcome, therapeutic efficacy, and prevention of mental disease are all susceptible to scientific investigation. Furthermore, the significance of this work, whether it be conducted by the medical or the social investigator, is now recognized by the administrator, the clinician, and the research worker. As such it broadens the framework of the discipline of psychological medicine, within which social psychiatry takes its place as an indispensable component.

References

1   A. Grotjahn, *Soziale Pathologie*, 3rd edn, Berlin, Springer, 1923.
2   J.K. Wing, 'Innovations in social psychiatry', *Psychological Medicine*, 1980, 10: 219–30.
3   E.E. Southard, 'Alienists and psychiatrists', *Mental Hygiene*, 1917, 1: 567–71.
4   G. Rosen, 'Social stress and mental disease from the 18th century to the present: some origins of social psychiatry', *Millbank Memorial Fund Quarterly*, 1959, xxxvii, 1: 5–32.
5   M. Jones, *Social Psychiatry in Practice*, Harmondsworth, Penguin, 1968, p. 80.
6   E.H. Hare, 'The relation between social psychiatry and psychotherapy', in S.H. Foulkes and G.S. Prince (eds) *Psychiatry in a Changing Society*, London, Tavistock, 1969.
7   World Health Organization, 'Social psychiatry and community attitudes', Technical Report Series no. 177, Geneva, World Health Organization, 1959.
8   H. Maudsley, *The Pathology of Mind*, London, Macmillan, 1879.
9   M. Shepherd, 'Epidemiologische Psychiatrie', in K.P. Kisker, J.-E. Meyer, C. Müller, and E. Strömgren (eds) *Psychiatrie der Gegenwont*, vol. III (2nd edn), Berlin, Springer, 1975, pp. 119–49.
10 J. Goldberger, *D.E. Lamar Lectures*, Baltimore, Md, Williams & Wilkins, 1927.
11 D.C. Gajdusek and V. Zigas, 'Clinical, pathological and epidemiological study of an acute progressive degenerative disease of the central nervous system among natives of the Eastern Highlands of New Guinea', *American Journal of Medicine*, 1959, 26: 442–69.
12 M. Shepherd, 'From social medicine to social psychiatry, the achievement of Sir Aubrey Lewis', *Psychological Medicine*, 1980, 10: 211–18.
13 L.G. Brown, 'Social psychiatry', in L.L. Bernard (ed.) *The Field and Methods of Sociology*, New York, Long & Smith, 1934.
14 H.W. Dunham, 'Social psychiatry', *American Sociological Review*, 1948, 13: 183–7.
15 D. Mechanic, 'Problems and prospects in psychiatric epidemiology', in E.H. Hare and J.K. Wing (eds) *Psychiatric Epidemiology*, London, Oxford University Press, 1970.

Chapter ten

Healing in perversion

TORURE: 'the art or process of inflicting severe pain, especially as a punishment, so as to extort confession, or in revenge'. This is an impersonal dictionary definition of an unpleasantly personal topic, one which Voltaire saw as important enough to include in his *Philosophical Dictionary* of 1769 to underline its significance for the society of the day:

> The Romans inflicted torture only on the slaves, but the slaves were not reckoned to be human. Nor does it appear that a judge ... regards as a fellow man the haggard, pale, broken individual who is brought before him dull-eyed, with a long dirty beard, covered with the vermin that have been preying on him in the dungeon. He gives himself the pleasure of putting him to major and minor torture, in the presence of a surgeon who feels his pulse until he is in danger of death, after which they set to again ...

Until recently Voltaire's condemnatory views have been expressed by a relatively small minority, even though the twentieth century can claim some of the most savage examples of human barbarism in recorded history. On Human Rights Day in 1972, Amnesty International began its campaign against the systematic use of torture by governments, and in the following year published its disturbingly well-documented *Report on Torture* (Duckworth, 1973).

The *Report* included a full account of the medical and psychological aspects of torture and demonstrated by means of a survey that 'torture has virtually become a world-wide phenomenon and that the torturing of citizens regardless of sex, age, or the state of health in an effort to retain political power is a practice tolerated by others in an increasingly large number of countries'. The topic has since attracted mounting attention

Originally published in *Nature* 318, December 1985, 'Healing in perversion' is a review of E. Stover and E.O. Nightingale (eds) *The Breaking of Bodies and Minds: Torture, Psychiatric Abuse, and the Health Professions*, New York, W.H. Freeman, 1985.

and concern, though it was not until December 1984 that the Convention against Torture and Other Cruel, Inhuman or Degrading Treatment or Punishment was adopted by the United Nations General Assembly.

The psychological and psychiatric evidence, concluded the Amnesty *Report*, points to the existence of the potential to torture in *Homo sapiens*. Voltaire, who recognized torture as one aspect of the destructive element in man, would not have been surprised by these findings, while clinical observations have indicated that John Cowper Powys's admission that he could not remember a time 'when sadistic thoughts and images did not disturb and intoxicate me' is unusual more by virtue of its frankness than by its content. Further, torture carries its own appeal. Writing of perhaps the most distressing scene in world literature, the blinding of Gloucester in Shakespeare's *King Lear*, Wilson Knight remarked shrewdly that, 'The sight of physical torment to the uneducated brings laughter.' And with the laughter goes a form of pleasure, widely exploited by pornographers and wholly unrelated to educational status.

The Breaking of Minds and Bodies, published under the auspices of the American Association for the Advancement of Science, should help carry the campaign against torture a stage further. Its subtitle, however, *Torture, Psychiatric Abuse, and the Health Professions*, is more informative than its title. The book is in two parts, one concentrating on general issues and the other on psychiatric practices in the Soviet Union, each containing five articles by various authors with several case histories, along with editorial commentaries and three appendices providing codes of ethics, an inventory of relevant organizations, and a selected bibliography. Much of this information is familiar and, indeed, three of the articles have appeared elsewhere. The principal purpose of the book, however, is not so much to record the activities of repressive governments as to explore how they have 'enlisted the aid of medical practitioners in suppressing dissent and what steps need to be taken to prevent such professional complicity, and ultimately, to end the abuses themselves'.

The message is all the more timely inasmuch as the involvement of the medical profession has not always been acknowledged. The medical profession, nominally devoted to the preservation of health and the saving of life, places great store on the ethical conduct of its members, as epitomized in the International Code of Medical Ethics, adopted by the World Assembly of the World Medical Association in 1949, which states categorically that 'Under no circumstances is a doctor permitted to do anything that would weaken the physical or mental resistance of a human being except from strictly therapeutic or prophylactic indications, imposed in the name of his patient.' In fact, as the evidence makes clear, medical practitioners continue to disobey this injunction, actively or passively, in many countries. Voltaire's pulse-taking physician, far from giving succour to the victims of torture, was participating in the process.

Why does this occur? The book focuses on psychiatrists in the Soviet Union, whose well-documented activities occupy a major part of the text. By employing their mental hospital system to coerce dissident but mentally healthy citizens and perverting clinical concepts for the purpose, the Russians have provided a new variation on an old theme. But anyone who has had contact with medical representatives of this system cannot fail to recognize, along with the cynical, unscrupulous apparatchik, the sincere, if misguided, believer in an ethical system codified in the Physician's Oath of the Soviet Union which, after mentioning the health of man and the care of disease, goes on to state: 'I will in all of my actions be guided by the principles of communist morality, ever to bear in mind the high calling of the Soviet physician, and of my responsibility to the people and the Soviet state.'

This chilling sentence draws attention sharply to the need for account to be taken of more than one set of ethical guidelines when assessing professional behaviour. As Heijder has pointed out (see *Professional Codes of Ethics Against Torture*, published by Amnesty International in 1976), such conduct is affected by a least four factors: political systems, public opinion, organizational units, and individual codes of morality. The nocuous doctor, like the immoral priest or the crooked lawyer or the dishonest scientist, is the product of all these forces, whose balance determines the answer to the question posed by a distinguished German-Jewish refugee who had left Germany early in 1933 after finding most of his colleagues at the university clinic dressed in Nazi uniform the day after Hitler's accession to power – in the event of such circumstances in this country, he would ask, how many of your colleagues would be wearing civilian clothes?

Clearly it is unnecessary to postulate a Joseph Mengele in the vast majority of those uniformed physicians. The central issue is how far association with or acceptance of any system which employs or condones torture in any form is compatible with a medical ethos which must be preserved if the profession is to maintain its public status and its self-respect. Stanley Milgram's disturbing experiments on obedience and disobedience in response to authority reinforce the fragility of personal conscience in conflict with social pressures and reinforce the verdict of the Amnesty *Report*, namely that 'The prevention of torture . . . lies not in medical research but in political and legal remedies.' The value of this book resides in its contribution to the heightening of public awareness and the facilitation of official action.

Chapter eleven

The case of Arise Evans:
a historico-psychiatric study

Introduction

There is now a growing body of agreement on the common interests shared by the discipline of history with the study of human psychology, normal and abnormal. The links with aberrant conduct and motivation are perhaps the most apparent, and much information about the grosser forms of morbid behaviour in earlier epochs has come from the work of those medical historians who have concerned themselves with the development of psychiatry. Most of their work has understandably been focused on the theories and practices of earlier observers, not all physicians, confronted with the recognized mental illnesses of their day. There has also been a long-standing interest in the 'pathographic' study of particular individuals or types of individual, though a distinction may be drawn here between the earlier, exploratory studies in this field[1] and the more speculative interpretations favoured by some modern 'psycho-historians'.[2]

While such lines of enquiry are fundamental to the delineation of the clinical elements of psychological medicine, it must also be recognized that psychiatry, as Ackerknecht has pointed out, is more than a medical speciality.[3] In his outline of the broad area of general psychopathology, Karl Jaspers identified human history as 'the final field of investigation for psychopathology' because, as he said, 'the science of psychopathology no longer confines itself to the material found in institutions; it looks instead for material transmitted from the past and for psychic phenomena which the present offers outside hospital.'[4]

For work of this type the investigator is inevitably confronted by the need to take account of the historical sociology of mental disorder, a field of enquiry which has been defined as 'the place of the mentally ill . . . in societies at different historical periods and the factors (social, psychological, cultural) that have determined it'.[5] Progress here, however, depends on the recognition of a fundamental issue of method which Rosen has characterized as follows:

With Christopher Hill. Originally published in *Psychological Medicine*, 1976, 6: 351–8.

One cannot investigate mental and emotional disorders historically without reference to the milieu in which aberrant behaviour occurs. Individuals and groups function within sociocultural systems which define and establish the boundaries of deviance and abnormality. This means that the historian must have a genuine understanding of the sociocultural system as the suitable but omnipresent arena in which behaviour, normal and abnormal, presents itself.[6]

None the less, despite their familiarity with the primary sources relating to particular epochs, only a minority of professional historians appear to have incorporated a psychological dimension in their professional activities. One of the few historical scholars to have tackled this question directly was Lucien Febvre who concluded that

> the historian cannot understand the functioning of the institutions in a given period or the ideas of that period or any other unless he has that basic standpoint, which I for my part call the psychological standpoint, which implies concern to link up all the conditions of existence of the men of any given period with the meanings the same men gave to their own ideas.[7]

Febvre himself distinguished between group psychology, specific psychology, and differential psychology. Henri Berr added social psychology as a potentially significant source of information for the reason that 'the comparative study of societies must lead to social psychology and to a knowledge of the basic needs to which institutions and their changing manifestations are the response'.[8] An illustration of this theme has been provided by Grob's historical studies of psychiatric institutions in Massachusetts,[9] while Keith Thomas has furnished an impressive demonstration of how seemingly 'irrational' behaviour can furnish material of great historical significance.[10]

Against this background, it has seemed to us worth examining the possible value of scrutinizing conjointly a minor figure from the mid-seventeenth century whose conduct and character raise issues of both historical and psychiatric interest. The man in question was Rhys Evans, generally known as Arise Evans, who was born near Barmouth in Merionethshire in 1607 and lived through one of the most turbulent periods of English history.[11] Since so many features of his adult years are bound up with his contemporary milieu, it becomes necessary to pay some detailed attention to the social and political events of the time.

The historical background

Charles I came to the throne of England in 1625. Between 1629 and 1640 he ruled without Parliament, more and more losing the confidence of those of his subjects who mattered in the country. In 1640 he was forced by financial necessity to call a Parliament, but failed to come to terms with it. In 1642 civil war broke out, and by 1646 the King was defeated. In 1649 he was executed and a republic proclaimed. The 1640s, between the collapse of one system of government and the establishment of another, were years of unprecedented freedom. The episcopal church collapsed, and with it church courts and the censorship. Hitherto proscribed sects came up from underground, met, and preached freely. 'Religious toleration' meant freedom of assembly and organization for the lower classes.

In the seventeenth century, as historians are more and more coming to recognize, most men and women still lived in a world of magic; God and the Devil intervened in daily life, comets and eclipses were signs and portents, witches, fairies, and prophets were to be met on all sides. Science was still not differentiated from magic, astronomy from astrology, chemistry from alchemy. Both Robert Boyle and Sir Isaac Newton studied alchemy seriously; Newton first took up the study of mathematics because of his interest in astrology. Fellows of the Royal Society believed that you could cure a wound by anointing the weapon that caused it; John Locke treated pain in the kidneys by burying the patient's urine in a stone jug; the King's touch was believed to cure scrofula. At a lower level, most villages had their 'cunning man', their white witch, whom you consulted about your love affairs, your lost property, or your health. Cunning men were cheaper than doctors or lawyers, more powerful than Protestant parsons who claimed few of the magical skills attributed to their Catholic predecessors.

It is easy to see why miraculous interventions in daily life were taken for granted in the seventeenth century. We believe in a law-abiding universe because in fact 'acts of God' are rarer than 300 years ago. Universal insurance, including social insurance, better and free medical services, and especially anaesthetics, no plague, houses made of bricks and therefore far less inflammable, winter feed for cattle, so that spring is no longer starvation time – all this has transformed ordinary existence. The traditional insecurity of medieval life had been intensified from the sixteenth century by the new insecurity of the capitalist market. Nationwide slumps like that in the clothing industry during the 1620s led to fiercer competition; new attitudes – 'a man may do what he will with his own' and 'the devil take the hindmost' – disrupted the low-level social security of the medieval village, though people were apt to blame witches for their misfortunes rather than economic forces.

One effect of the collapse of the censorship in the 1640s was an increase in the flow of alchemical and astrological books, and of almanacs which curiously combined a rather advanced Copernican astronomy with astrological prophecies about the course and outcome of the civil war. The English, wrote Thomas Fuller in 1655, are said always to carry 'an old prophecy about with them in their pockets, which they can produce at pleasure to promote their designs, though oft mistaken in the application of such equivocating predictions'. Bishop Hacket agreed: 'we English are observed to be too credulous of vain prophecies such as are fathered upon Merlin and no better authors'. The astrologer William Lilly in 1644 sold 1,800 copies of his *Prophecy of the White King* within three days of publication. Lilly's repeated predictions of defeat and a violent end for Charles I may have contributed to bringing about these effects. Lilly, wrote Arise Evans with the jealousy of a less successful rival, 'knows nothing, nor ever did know anything, but as the Parliament directed him to write'. Lilly's writings, said a more sympathetic witness, in 1651, a Member of Parliament, 'have kept up the spirits of the soldiery, the honest people of this realm, and many of us Parliament-men'. Parliament voted Lilly a pension of £100 a year: he was taken very seriously by ordinary people.

But men thought of politics mostly in religious terms. Puritan preachers called on their hearers to fight for Parliament against Antichrist; there was a general millennarian feeling, which extended from a cultivated Cambridge graduate like John Milton, who spoke of Christ as 'shortly expected King', to rank-and-file soldiers in the parliamentary army who thought that the Earl of Essex, their commander, was John the Baptist, and that Jesus would shortly join him. Stimulated by the collapse of old certainties, by this millenarian enthusiasm, by the possibility of meeting and discussing freely, there opened up an extraordinary vigorous and uninhibited discussion. This went on not merely among the educated classes who dominated politics in normal times but also among the rank-and-file of the parliamentary armies, and among lay 'mechanic preachers' and their congregations in London. Printing was cheap and easily accessible: an unprecedented outpouring of pamphlets accompanied and encouraged this discussion. There were few heresies, from manhood suffrage to communism, from free love to polygamy, which did not get discussed, and printed, in what we used to think of as Puritan England.

Something that was almost a new profession arose to take advantage of these favourable circumstances – the prophet, whether as interpreter of the stars, or of traditional popular myths, or of the Bible. It is therefore important for us to grasp the role of prophecies in popular psychology. In this world, holy men and women were treated with respect. Lady Eleanor Davies, though some thought her mad, won 'the reputation of a cunning woman amongst the people' because of the accuracy of her prophecies of doom for Charles I and his Queen. Oliver Cromwell listened to her courteously. The generals were alleged to have made political use of the prophetess Elizabeth Poole in the anxious weeks immediately before the trial and execution of the King. It was a great age for symbolical gestures, for acting out the message. Quakers 'went naked for a sign'; Thomas Tany symbolically burnt the Bible in St George's Fields; Abiezer Coppe charged so many coaches, so many hundreds of men and women of the greater rank, in the open streets with . . . my hat cocked up, staring on them as if I would look through them, gnashing with my teeth at some of them, and day and night, with a loud voice, proclaiming the day of the Lord throughout London and Southwark.

In 1652 during service in the chapel at Whitehall a lady stripped naked with happy cries of 'Welcome the resurrection!'

But we must remember, before we dismiss such manifestations too easily, that Descartes, Pascal, and Lord Herbert of Cherbury saw visions no less than George Fox. It was an age in which the miraculous was taken for granted; it was also an age of acute social and psychological pressures and strains; it was an age, too, in which men thought in symbols, whether in painting, in emblem literature, or (with Quakers and Ranters) in action.

Protestantism had encouraged reading the vernacular Bible. Careful study of the Bible naturally gives rise to questions about the end of the world. Scholarly Protestant comment on the prophetical books of the Bible was intended to put the science of prophecy on a rational basis, to escape from the emotions and hysteria of vulgar prophets. The Bible was the accepted source of all knowledge. If properly understood, the Biblical prophecies could liberate men from the blind forces which appeared to them as destiny. By understanding and co-operating with God's purposes men believed that they could liberate themselves from necessity.

Luther had thought that the world would not last 100 years. An official declaration of Queen Elizabeth's government in 1589 spoke of 'this declining age of the world'. James I, Sir Walter Raleigh, Sir Thomas Browne, and very many more; all thought the latter days were drawing on. Scholarly mathematicians and chronologers like John Napier (who valued his invention of logarithms not least because it would speed up his calculations of the number of the Beast in *Revelation*), Thomas Brightman, Joseph Mede – all agreed in expecting the climax of human history in the seventeenth century. Large numbers of their works were published in popular versions as soon as the Press was free after 1640. Widespread knowledge of this scholarly consensus was taken for granted by Puritan preachers in the 1640s. 'Many ministers of the Gospel', wrote the astrologer John Gadbury, 'and from their example many illiterate men and women, were constantly from the years 1647 to 1650 counting that the end of the world was come.' 'Though men be of diverse minds as to the precise term', declared a pamphlet of 1653, 'yet all concur in the nighness and swiftness of its coming upon us.'

This was the highly charged atmosphere in which men read and discussed the Bible. They came to it with no historical sense but with the highest expectations: they found in it a message of direct contemporary relevance. This attitude must have been shared by many of the victims of economic and political crisis who turned to the Bible for guidance in those perplexing years, in which for the first time in English history their betters called upon them to assume political responsibilities. The 1640s and 1650s were the great age of 'mechanic preachers', laymen like Bunyan interpreting the Bible according to their untutored lights with all the confidence and excitement of a new discovery. Such men applied biblical tests to the problems of their age with no idea of the difficulties of translation, nor of the historical understanding required. Add to this the widespread conviction that only the spirit of God within the believer can properly interpret the Scriptures, and we can sense something of the intense personal relevance of the Bible's message to those who studied it, whether they were mechanic laymen or university theologians.

To many people the execution of Charles I in 1649 seemed to make sense only if it cleared the way for the direct rule of King Jesus. Fifth Monarchists expected Christ to descend immediately to take his throne and liberate his saints to judge the world; less excitedly, but no less firmly, Quakers believed that Christ had already come, and was beginning to reign in all men. No wonder that by 1660 the men of property thought it was time to restore Charles II to the throne of his fathers in the interests of social stability; no wonder that old enemies of the bishops thought it was worth having them back again if that was the best way to bring the lower classes back under control. It was a long time before ordinary people were again as free to express themselves as they had been between 1640 and 1660.

The life of Arise Evans

Arise Evans was one of those who took advantage of this freedom. His father, a local parishioner of adequate means, died when he was aged 7 without leaving him an inheritance. Evans's mother soon remarried and the boy was apprenticed to a tailor in Chester, but his master subsequently became bankrupt. Meanwhile his mother's second husband had died. She married again and moved to Wrexham, accompanied by her son and third husband. Shortly afterwards he was again apprenticed in Chester.

These bare facts about his early years are contained in Evans's various writings.[12] His first recorded philosophy must have been made in adolescence, predicting as it does that England would suffer woe on the second Thursday after Midsummer Day, 1623. As on many subsequent occasions, he was proved wrong, to lose credit accordingly, and to justify himself unabashedly none the less. Thus in 1659 he commented retrospectively that

upon that very Thursday in that very year Oliver Cromwell presented a petition to King James touching the Fens in Lincolnshire and about Ely,...and as soon as King James took the petition his nose fell a-bleeding, that he swore it was an omen saying if he could tell how, he would hang that fellow that had given him that paper.

Although there is no evidence to suggest Cromwell's interest in this issue at that time, Evans maintained that 'the fire between King and country started that very day'.

In 1629 Evans set out for London to work as a tailor. After establishing himself in this trade he began to have 'visions' which foretold disaster to his country and his king. This knowledge impelled him to public action. He approached the court, the Earl of Essex, and even his king. His friends, his landlord, and his family regarded him as mentally deranged and during 1634 he was persuaded to return to Wrexham. In the following year, however, he was back in London, married, and with an undimmed determination to apprise the authorities of his prophetic knowledge. In August 1635 Evans was arrested and remained in prison for two years. He continued to undergo visionary experiences during this time and was eventually discharged on the grounds of mental disorder. He then returned to Wrexham where he remained for four years but in 1641 he came back to London, accompanied by his wife and a brood of small children.

At the outbreak of the civil war Evans's claim to divine knowledge spread to embrace many religious and political controversies of the day. Once more he was arrested, and this time he went so far as to state: 'I am the Lord thy God: thou shalt have none other God but me.' Despite his subsequent recantation, Evans was again sent to prison, though for a short time only and against the opinion of several ministers of religion who tried to have him certified insane. From this time onwards he appears to have been unmolested, and, indeed, to have enjoyed remarkable freedom in his behaviour and his writings.

Until 1647 Evans's attitude to the army was relatively benign but thereafter he switched his allegiance to the royalist cause. His first tract, published in 1652 and entitled *A Voice from Heaven to the Commonwealth of England*, advocates the support of Parliament and the army for the peaceful restoration of Charles II, whom he later described as 'a child of God and appointed to be the most eminent servant of Jesus Christ in all the world'. Throughout his writings this theme remains constant, allied to a denunciation of all opponents of such a reconciliation, whether from the Church or the violent wing of the monarchist party. Evans is for the most part sympathetic to Cromwell himself, though some of the Protector's supporters are severely castigated. He is harsh and malicious about his detractors, including rival prophets and astrologers. Like most lay preachers of the day, Evans made liberal use of the Bible in his political and religious pronouncements:

Afore I looked upon the Scripture as a history of things that passed in other countries, pertaining to other persons, but now I looked upon it as a mystery to be opened at this time, belonging also to us. I am as the Paul of this time; he was a mechanic, a tent-maker, Acts. 18:3. I am a tailor.

At times Evans indulged in curious and seemingly absurd views. Thus he foresaw the role of Charles II as a Messiah destined to convert the Jews and in a later pamphlet advocates the selection of a poor man, chosen by lot, to be the next king of England. None the less, he survived the interregnum unharmed and his views were quoted with some respect by proponents of both sides in the political struggle. Our last authentic glimpse of him is in 1660, fittingly enough requesting from Charles II a cure for a skin disease which, he records, responded to the royal touch. He died in some unknown year during the 1660s.

The clinical data

The primary data on which to base a clinical assessment of so remote a historical figure are exiguous. They consist in Evans's own descriptions of his feelings, thoughts, and behaviour, along with what can be gleaned of the impression which he made on his contemporaries. This information must be evaluated against the social and political background of the mid-seventeenth century.

No reliable information exists on Evans's family, childhood, or early years. From a clinical standpoint the facts available about his adult life raise two related but discrete questions: first, the significance of his subjective experiences and his behaviour during his early adult life; and second, the 'diagnostic category' which might be applied to him in the light of what we know of his subsequent career. These questions may best be considered separately.

First, Evans describes his core experiences very clearly. The following two passages are representative:

> when I came to my Chamber I laid my books upon the table, & fell upon my knees, went to prayer, and putting my whole strength and Faith to obtain, and fervency to ask the true light and knowledge of God's will concerning my self, I soon was out of breath and not able to utter a word though my spirits boiled within me, and being thus wearied to refresh myself I laid me down upon my bed, and as I in high Meditations or Contemplations did ascend in thoughts to Godward, being perfectly awake and sensible, a laudable sharp shrill, halting voice near mine ear, said to me go to thy book, whereupon apprehending the same voice to come from God, I suddenly started up and to the Table I went, where my Bible lay open, immediately fastening my eyes upon Ephes. 5.14. being these words, wherefore he saith, Awake thou that sleepest, and arise from the dead, and Christ shall give thee light ...
>
> ... as I lay upon the bed the third day in the morning expecting some sign of deliverance from God, there came in at the window a round Cloud, in colour like unto the Rain-bow, and it covered me, abiding upon me

about a quarter of an hour, and when it came upon me I was so revived as if I had eaten all the delicates in the world; and after a quarter of an hour the Cloud departed out at the window in the same manner as it came in, until it ascended out of my sight.

It may be remarked that such accounts, and the many others like them, cannot be deemed morbid in themselves. There are no features which are pathogonomic of mental disorder, and the details can be matched by those of many other individuals who have reported similar varieties of religious experience unassociated with any suggestion of insanity.[13] At the same time the intensity of the phenomena, Evans's consequent behaviour, and the reaction of other people to him, all indicate that he was unwell during this time:

And having so many visions upon visions to confirm the certainty of the judgement, I could not contain my knowledge, but was forced to declare to all that I had to do with. Then the people began to spend their various thoughts upon me, and though I spake as good sense and gave them as good reason for what I said as would satisfie men in other cases, yet many look upon me as a distracted man in regard of the impossibility of such alterations, and the desperate boldness of my affirmation, therefore they did fear to come with me, or hear these things from me, and accounting it a delusion, forbid me their houses.

Evans was not here exaggerating the social response to his ideas and his conduct. As mentioned above, during this early period of his life he was twice imprisoned, Bedlam having been suggested as an alternative to Bridewell on one occasion. His release from prison was on the grounds of mental illness, and his friends and family then prevailed on him to spend some years away from London in his native Wales. At this time the impression which he made on society was evidently that of a dangerous madman.

Second, from 1641 onwards Evans appears to have spent the next twenty eventful years in or around London. During this whole period, as his writings clearly attest, he continued to have 'visions' and his reactions to many of the political turmoils appear erratic by the standards of the day. None the less, his opinions no longer led to accusations of insanity or antisocial proclivities as his contemporaries – for example, Loveday, Gostelow, Ashmole – mention him and his views with respect, and not a few of his detractors took him seriously enough to level the charge of duplicity against him. More than 100 years after his death Evans's visions still constituted a controversial topic. They were then regarded as authentic by one eminent ecclesiastic, who was in turn accused of gullibility by his contemporaries, for Bishop Warburton spoke of Evans as not only 'a strange fellow' but also as 'an impudent knave' and John Jortin makes no reference to Evans's derangement but describes him pithily as a warm Welshman, and not disposed to be an idle spectator in so busy a scene. So he left his native country for London; and finding on his arrival there, that Inspiration was all running one way, he projected to make a diversion from the Round-heads to the Cavaliers, and set up for a Prophet of the Royalists... and he had a spice of what we seldom find wanting in the ingredients of a modern Prophet, I mean Prevarication.[14]

Jortin's verdict, based as it presumably was on the study of the politico-religiose content of Evans's writings, is comprehensible to the student of those tracts today. Many of Evans's opinions and judgements may well have been unusual, even by the standards of an unusual epoch, but they are hardly suggestive of mental disorder. The syntax and grammar are unexceptionable; the arguments, given their sometimes exotic premisses, hang together well. As to the 'visions', their primary function appears to have been the compounding of politics and the Bible in such a way as to furnish interpretations of events with one objective – namely, Evans's own infallibility. His technique under pressure was to appeal over the heads of his fellow mortals to a divine being to whom he alone had access. This dubious device is supported by recourse to harsh denigration of rival 'prophets', 'astrologers', and 'visionaries' (unless they are of his persuasion); to unctuous flattery of powerful persons; and to retrospective justification and choplogic when his predictions are not confirmed. Furthermore, amid all the froth and rhetoric, the tracts contain long passages of hard sense, some of which must have offended one or other powerful political faction. It says something for Evans's shrewdness and resilience that he was able to survive unscathed in view of his outspoken views on matters of central importance to the government.

What, then, can be made of such information in clinical terms? In some measure any answer must remain conjectural but the available evidence strongly suggests that Evans underwent some form of severe mental illness in early life. In form and content this might be regarded 300 years later as conforming most closely to one of the atypical functional psychoses described by Kleist as a 'revelatory psychosis'.[15] This illness is characterized by the appearance of 'autochthonous ideas' defined as

convictions and inspirations which regularly appear..., erupting suddenly without any intermediaries, casting a spell on the patient's thoughts and deeds: these 'revelations' as the patients often call them, seem to them to come from God, from angels, or from the *Weltgeist*, according to their particular outlook and religious beliefs. An extrapersonal and super-personal power is always experienced as the source of such revelations, which also often assume a sensory tone and are then described expressly as 'voices'.... The exaltation of personality by which the patient feels himself seized or enraptured, represents... an inflammation of his social outlook and of the religious feelings that push him towards supernatural forces.

As the outcome of a disorder of this type is towards remission, the diagnosis would not imply that Evans suffered from a chronic form of insanity for the remainder of his adult life. Neither what is known about his life nor the internal evidence of his writings would support such a contention. If any medical label can be applied to him in his later years, it is that of 'abnormal personality', which may or may not have been related to his original illness. Many of the findings of transcultural investigation have shown how closely this diagnosis is related to the sociocultural norms of a particular milieu. This conclusion can reasonably be extended to time as well as space, and, in his analysis of the part played by emotionally disturbed people in the radical sects of the seventeenth century, Rosen has emphasized that they were able to participate actively in their social environment 'as long as their behaviour was not considered evidence of undue psychological impairment and socio-cultural distortion'.[16] However, the evaluation of their conduct depended, in turn, on a *Zeitgeist* which was itself aberrant. In this historical epoch, as Tindall vividly points out,

England was lighted by the queer radiance of insanity and shaken by the regrettable demonstrations of the inspired. An abnormal atmosphere was the normal medium of the lay preachers, who accepted the theory of inspiration, admired anything, however curious, which they knew to be godly, and arranged their daily lives upon preconceptions which the rational must distrust. Their lives were odd but never uninteresting.[17]

Arise Evans might well have fared worse if he had lived in less troubled times.

References

1 W. Lange-Eichbaum, *Genie, Irrsinn und Ruhm*, Munich, Reinhardt, 1928.
2 G. Rosen, 'Psyche and history', *Psychological Medicine*, 1972, 2: 205–7.
3 E.H. Ackerknecht, *A Short History of Psychiatry*, New York, Hafner, 1959.
4 K. Jaspers, *General Psychopathology*, Manchester, Manchester University Press, 1963.
5 G. Rosen, 'Preface', in *Madness in Society*, New York, Harper, 1968, p. xi.
6 G. Rosen, 'Mental disorder, social deviance and culture pattern: some methodological issues in the historical study of mental illness', in G. Mora and J.L. Brand (eds) *Psychiatry and its History*, Springfield, Ill., Thomas, 1970.
7 L. Febvre, 'History and psychology', in P. Burke (ed.) *A New Kind of History: From the Writings of Febvre*, London, Routledge & Kegan Paul, 1973.
8 H. Berr, *The Nature of History*, London, Macmillan, 1970, p. 122 (quoted by A. Marwick).

9   G. Grob, *The State of the Mentally Ill*, Chapel Hill, NC, University of North Carolina Press, 1966; *Mental Institutions in America*, New York, Free Press, 1973.
10 K. Thomas, *Religion and the Decline of Magic*, London, Weidenfeld & Nicolson, 1971.
11 C. Hill, *Change and Continuity in Seventeenth-Century England*, London, Weidenfeld & Nicolson, 1974.
12 Arise Evans, *A Voice from Heaven to the Commonwealth of England*, 1652; *An Echo to the Voice from Heaven*, 1652; *To His Excellencie the Lord General Cromwell and his Honourable Councel of the Army*, 1653; *The Bloudy Vision of John Farley*, 1653; *The Euroclydon Winde Commanded to Cease*, 1654; *The Voice of Michael the Archangel to his Highness the Lord Protector*, 1654; *A Message from God... to his Highness the Lord Protector*, 1654; *The Voice of the Iron Rod to his Highness the Lord Protector*, 1655; *Light for the Jews*, 1656; *A Rule from Heaven*, 1659; *To the Most High and Mighty Prince Charles the II... an Epistle*, 1660; Arise Evans and W. Pennington, *Mr. Evans and Mr. Penningtons Prophesie*, 1655 (all titles were published in London).
13 W. James, *The Varieties of Religious Experience*, London, Longman, 1902; repr. London, Collins, 1960.
14 J. Jortin, *Remarks on Ecclesiastical History*, London, 1751, in the appendix, vol. 1, pp. 377–87.
15 K. Kleist, 'Uber zykloide, paranoide und epileptoide Psychosen und über die Frage der Degenerationspsychosen', *Schweizer Archiv für Neurologie und Psychiatrie*, 1928, 23: 3–37.
16 G. Rosen, 'Emotion and sensibility in ages of anxiety: a comparative historical review', *American Journal of Psychiatry*, 1967, 124: 771–84.
17 W.Y. Tindall, *John Bunyan: Mechanick Preacher*, New York, Russell & Russell, New York, 1964.

Chapter twelve

Epidemiology and clinical psychiatry

The Maudsley Bequest lectures have traditionally been intended for trainee psychiatrists. No previous lecture in the series has been concerned directly with epidemiology, and the trainee who seeks enlightenment in the British textbooks of psychiatry is likely to be disappointed or misled, for the standard view of the subject is epitomized in the statement which appears in their weightiest representative: 'In this field the epidemiological approach concerns itself with investigation of the frequency with which definable forms of psychiatric disorder occur in carefully delineated populations.'[1] While this aspect of the discipline is central to the interests of workers in the field of public health and administration, the notion of epidemiology as primarily an exercise in head-counting is unlikely to suggest the relevance of the discipline to clinical activities, especially if these are conceived as being focused primarily on the individual patient. In this lecture I propose to try and correct this impression and indicate the provenance and scope of epidemiology as a major branch of scientific inquiry which is indispensable to clinical psychiatry.

Epidemiology, meaning literally no more than 'on the people', is a term used in medicine to designate the study of populations rather than individuals. It is instructive to recall, as a point of departure, the remarkable monograph, *The Epidemics of the Middle Ages*, first published almost 150 years ago, in which J.F.C. Hecker traced the course and effects of three major calamities.[2] Two of them, the Black Death and the Sweating Sickness, might have been expected but the third, and in many ways most interesting, study is of an epidemic of disordered behaviour, the Dancing Mania, to which Hecker later added another example in the form of a long essay on Child-Pilgrimages. In these accounts Hecker makes no distinction between epidemics of infectious disease and those of morbid behaviour, whose cause he identified as an abnormal emotional state. This view was maintained by many influential medical scientists, not least among them Rudolf Virchow, and was not to be disputed until much later in the nineteenth century, when the rise of the germ theory and the establishment of bacteriological science

Based on a Maudsley Bequest lecture to the Royal College of Psychiatrists, London, February 1978. Originally published in *British Journal of Psychiatry*, 1978, 133: 289–98.

led to the claim that the notion of 'epidemic' be confined to the designation of infectious disease, based squarely on the establishment of host, agent and vector as the triad of key factors.

With the identification of individual organisms and the therapeutic use of antibiotics the trend became more pronounced and the terminological issue more acrimonious, the debate over words concealing, as so often, a major issue of substance which continued for some fifty years. As late as the early 1950s an eminent professor of bacteriology was moved to write to the *British Medical Journal*, condemning

> an undoubted debauchery of a precise and essential word, 'epidemiology', which is being inflated by writers on social medicine and similar subjects to include the study of the frequency or incidence of diseases whether epidemic or not. The right and, as I thought, obvious meaning of epidemiology is given by the shorter *O.E.D.* as 'the study of epidemics', and an epidemic is 'a disease prevalent among a people or a community at a special time, and produced by some special causes not generally present in the affected locality'. Therefore, to speak of the epidemiology of coronary thrombosis, or of hare lip, or diabetes, or of any non-epidemic disease is a debasement of the currency of thought. It is of no use saying that the word is being used in its wider sense. It has no wider sense.[3]

The snide reference to social medicine was understandable as a response to the challenge which had been issued by its first and foremost representative in this country John Ryle:

> Public health has been largely preoccupied with the communicable diseases, their causes, distribution and prevention. Social medicine is concerned with all diseases of prevalence, including rheumatic heart disease, peptic ulcer, cancer, the psychoneuroses, the psychoses and accidental injuries – which also have their epidemiologies and their correlations with social and occupational conditions and must eventually be considered in greater or less degree preventable.[4]

To support his contention in the field of mental disorder Ryle might have cited the example which illustrates *par excellence* the place of epidemiology in psychiatry, namely the contribution of Joseph Goldberger to the problem of pellagra. This outstanding but still surprisingly neglected work repays consideration in some detail.

Elucidation of pellagra: an impressive achievement

In the early years of the twentieth century pellagra was a disease which evoked great concern, especially in Italy and the southern states of North

America. Here is a brief description from an Italian textbook of mental diseases at this time:

> Pellagra is an endemic disease of remittent course, and generally afebrile, which sooner or later proves fatal. It is dependent upon a specific cause – namely, the eating of maize (commonly used in the form of polenta and pan giallo) that has been damaged by moulds. Its clinical picture is that of a cachexia from intoxication, and when fully established includes not only intestinal, gastric, and cutaneous symptoms, but also motor and psychic phenomena.[5]

Other authorities favoured other views, including genetic transmission and, above all, the spread by an unknown organism. In the USA two influential Commissions in 1911 and 1913 had declared themselves in favour of an infectious aetiology, and a year later Joseph Goldberger was assigned by the Surgeon-General to the task of identifying the organism and eradicating the disease.

Goldberger himself was then a professional epidemiologist in the US Public Health Service.[6] In this capacity he had rapidly acquired the reputation of an outstanding investigator and had made a number of important contributions to the elucidation of various infectious diseases, including yellow fever, dengue, typhus, measles, diphtheria and Schamberg's disease. In early 1914 Goldberger visited the State hospital for the insane in Jackson, Mississippi, knowing almost nothing about mental disorder. In June of the same year he published the first of his papers on pellagra. Only three pages long, it is entitled *The Etiology of Pellagra: the Significance of Certain Epidemiological Observations with Respect Thereto*.[7] The following extract demonstrates how he approached the problem in his own clear-sighted way:

> The writer desires to invite attention to certain observations recorded in the literature of pellagra, the significance of which appears entirely to have escaped attention.
>
> At the National Conference on Pellagra held in Columbia, SC, November 3, 1909, Siler and Nichols in their paper on the 'Aspects of the pellagra problem in Illinois' stated that certain facts would seem to indicate that the exciting cause of the disease is present within the institution (Peoria State Hospital), and added that 'at the same time no nurses, attendants, or employees have shown the disease'.
>
> The results of personal inquiry at some of our State asylums in which pellagra occurs confirm the reported observations above cited. Thus at the South Carolina State hospital for the insane, where Babcock (1910 Ann. Rept.) states that while cases of pellagra develop in patients who have been there for years, no case so far as the writer was able to ascertain has occurred in the nurses or attendants. It may be of interest to recall in this

connection that in his annual report for 1913 Babcock states that a total of about 900 pellagrins had been admitted to his institution during the preceding six years.

At the State hospital for the insane at Jackson, Miss., there have been recorded 98 deaths from pellagra for the period between October 1, 1909 and July 1, 1913. At this institution cases of institutional origin have occurred in inmates. Dr J.C. Herrington, assistant physician and pathologist, told me at the time of my visit of a case in an inmate after 15 and in another after 20 years' residence at the institution. No case, so far as I was able to learn, has developed in a nurse or attendant, although since January 1, 1909 there have been employed a total of 126 who have served for periods of from 1 to 5 years.

In considering the significance of such observations it is to be recalled that at all of these institutions the ward personnel, nurses, and attendants spend a considerable proportion of the 24 hours on day or night duty, in close association with the inmates; indeed at many of these institutions, for lack of a separate building or special residence for the nurses, they live right in the ward with and of necessity under exactly the same conditions as the inmates.

It is striking therefore that although many inmates develop pellagra after varying periods of institutional residence, some even after 10 to 20 years of institutional life and therefore, it seems permissible to infer, as the result of the operation within the institution of the exciting cause or causes, yet nurses and attendants living under identical conditions appear uniformly to be immune. If pellagra be a communicable disease, why should there be this exemption of the nurses and attendants?

To the writer this peculiar exemption or immunity is inexplicable on the assumption that pellagra is communicable. Neither 'contact' in any sense nor insect transmission is capable of explaining such a phenomenon, except on the assumption of an incubation or latent period extending over 10 to 20 years. In support of such an assumption there exists, so far as the writer is aware, no satisfactory evidence.

The explanation of the peculiar exemption under discussion will be found in the opinion of the writer in a difference in the diet of the two groups of residents. At some of the institutions there is a manifest difference in this regard; in others none is apparent.

The latter would seem to be a fatal objection to this explanation, but a moment's consideration will show that such is not necessarily the case. The writer from personal observation has found that although the nurses and attendants may apparently receive the same food, there is nevertheless a difference in that the nurses have the privilege – which they exercise – of selecting the best and greatest variety for themselves. Moreover, it must not be overlooked that nurses and attendants have opportunities for supplementing their institutional dietary that the inmates as a rule have not.

In this connection brief reference must be made to two other epidemio-logical features of pellagra. It is universally agreed (1) that the disease is essentially rural, and (2) associated with poverty. Now there is plenty of poverty and all its concomitants in all cities, and the question naturally arises – why its greater predilection for rural poverty? What important difference is there between the elements of poverty in our slums and those of poverty in rural dwellers? It is not the writer's intention to enter at the time into a detailed discussion of these questions; he wishes to point out one difference only. This difference relates to the dietary. Studies of urban and rural dietaries (Walt, Office of Experiment Stations, *Bulletin*, 221, 1909) have shown that on the whole the very poor of cities have a more varied diet, than the poor in rural sections. 'Except in extreme cases, the city poor...appear to be better nourished than the mountaineers of Tennessee.'

In view of the great uncertainty that exists as to the true cause of pellagra, it may not be amiss to suggest that pending the final solution of this problem it may be well to attempt to prevent the disease by improving the dietary of those among whom it seems most prevalent. In this direction I would urge the reduction in cereals, vegetables, and canned foods that enter to so large an extent into the dietary of many of the people in the South and an increase in the fresh animal food component, such as fresh meats, eggs, and milk.

From these initial observations Goldberger set out the implications of his own hypothesis. These were, in his own words, 'first, that a difference in diet as between pellagrins and non-pellagrins be demonstrable; second, that the disease must be curable by a proper diet; third, that it must be preventable by such a diet, and, fourth, that it may be experimentally produced by diet.' The way in which he proceeded to sustain these propositions is to be found in more than 50 papers which contain the essence of his work over the remaining fifteen years of his life.[8] First, he established that the distribution of early pellagra was related to dietary deficiencies in other institutions, notably orphanages. Then he showed that a diet of milk, eggs, meat, beans and peas prevented the occurrence of pellagra in institutions where it had been rife. And, to clinch the case, he went on to induce pellagra among the inmates of a prison by dietary deprivation, a procedure which would prob-ably upset the members of most ethical committees today.

Next, he moved from the institution to the community in his famous field survey of cotton-mill villages in South Carolina. This is one of the great examples of 'shoe-leather' epidemiology, which entailed fortnightly house visits to all members of the population from whom he obtained detailed socio-demographic, personal and dietary information. From the mass of data which he collected Goldberger was able to clinch the association between pellagra and low animal protein food (*not* corn), home food-supplies and, above all, selective poverty. Working with the economist, Edgar Sydenstricker, he constructed the 'ammain', a socio-economic unit for measuring variation in gross demand for articles of consumption which, they demonstrated, was significantly related to the incidence of pellagra. The detail of their painstaking inquiry is legendary:

(1) Statements were obtained from households as to the immediate source of every article of food entering into their half-month's supplies. Thus it was ascertained, for example, whether the fresh milk used by the household was produced at home, purchased from another mill worker's household in the village, or from some specific farmer, dairy or store, or donated by a relative, neighbour, or other person. In the event that a household had a source of supply not common generally to households in the village, inquiries were directed with a view to ascertaining the length of time the household had had such a supply, particularly with respect to the period after January 1, 1916.

(2) From farmers, hucksters, or 'peddlers' selling from house to house, statements were secured relating to the quantities sold, prices, frequency of selling, and character of produce sold since January 1, 1916.

(3) From managers and clerks in the stores, markets, and other retail establishments at which mill workers' households largely dealt, data were secured relating to (a) prices during the 15-day period and price changes during 1916; (b) sources of each food sold, whether direct from nearby farms or through middlemen from local agricultural territory or from other sections of the United States; (c) names of brands and quantities of the foods sold; (d) practices with respect to credit to mill workers' households, especially as affected by the amount of earnings by the mill workers.[9]

As the facts accumulated it became abundantly clear that the prevalence of pellagra was related to the availability of supplies of certain foods but that this in turn was closely influenced by the one-crop type of agriculture with its lack of diversification. Characteristically, therefore, Goldberger and Sydenstricker undertook what amounted to a full-scale economic analysis of tenant-farming in the cotton-producing area of the deep south. They concluded: 'The situation is manifestly one which calls for study with a view of working out practicable solutions of the economic and agricultural problems involved. In such study, however, the needs of health must be held in mind as of controlling importance.'

At the same time as he adopted this macro-sociological approach, however, Goldberger became increasingly aware of the need to study the micro-behaviour of individuals and family units, if only to account for the apparent exceptions to the general rule which he was formulating. The following passage illustrates how well he appreciated the role of personal factors:

Reference may be made to the group of factors that tend to determine the amount and proportion of family income available for the purchase of food, an example of which is the occurrence of sickness or injury, making an unusual draft on the family income. Related to such factors are the general spirit of the household with respect to thrift (which, when unwisely directed, may be harmful) and the intelligence and ability of the housewife in utilizing the available family income.

More tangible than these, and perhaps of more immediate practical importance in its effect on the household diet, is the difference among households with respect to the availability of food supplies.

Even granting what is not necessarily the case, that financial ability to provide may be assumed to be invariably synonymous with the actual provision of a good diet and that a liberal diet was actually available to the individual, it by no means follows that such diet was in fact consumed. For such assumption would totally ignore the existence of individual likes and dislikes, more or less marked examples of which may be observed at almost any family table.

Further, a great variety of causes may operate to bring about individual peculiarities of taste with respect to food. They may have their origin in the seemingly inherent human prejudice against the new and untried food or dish; they may date from some disagreeable experience associated with a particular food; they may arise as the result of ill-advised, self-imposed or professionally directed dietary restrictions in the treatment of digestive disturbances, kidney disease, etc.; they may originate as a fad; and in the insane they may arise because of some delusion such as the fear of poisoning, etc.[10]

And, as if all this were not enough, towards the end of his life, Goldberger took another, paradigmatic step. He abandoned the epidemiological method altogether because, as he pointed out, it had confirmed the hypothesis that pellagra was a deficiency-disease but had also reached the limits of its own potential. He therefore turned to the laboratory and the experimental method and set himself two different objectives: (a) to determine the pellagra-preventive action of various foods, and (b) to identify the nature of the specific deficiency involved. He had already disposed of the infection theory by injecting first Rhesus monkeys and then himself and his wife with biological fluids derived from pellagrins. Having gone on to establish an animal model in canine black-tongue he began by working on the hypothesis of an amino-acid deficiency, possibly tryptophan, then on the unknown pellagra-preventing factor in water-soluble vitamin B which was to be identified in 1937 as acotinic acid, of which tryptophan is a precursor.

This brief summary of one of the most impressive medical achievements of the century illustrates the role of epidemiology in one of its several spheres of application – the investigation of the causation of disease. Essentially it proceeded by establishing an hypothesis through observation, supporting it by ecological inquiry, tracing the multifactorial genesis of individual cases and then providing experimental confirmation. Not the least remarkable feature of the work is that Goldberger succeeded in combining what Griesinger had called the study of aetiology, i.e. the patterns of the associations of disease, with the study of pathogeny, i.e. the mechanisms of disease. In *sensu strictu* the epidemiologist addresses himself to finding causal factors rather than elucidating their mode of action. Goldberger did both, and eliminated a major scourge in the process.

This example is now more than fifty years old but, with the possible exception of kuru, it remains the most elegant demonstration of the way in which the epidemiological method can be applied to elucidate the causes of a neuro-psychiatric disorder. Why should this be so? The answer, I would suggest, is twofold. First, Goldberger was an investigator of exceptional ability and very few men of his calibre have concerned themselves with any aspect of mental disorder. Second, as a disease entity pellagra might be regarded as having been riper for investigation than the great majority of conditions which are included in the formal category of mental illness. Goldberger himself indicated as much when, towards the end of his life, he was made a financially attractive offer to direct a research unit for the study of dementia praecox. He took his time to consider the proposition, studied the current literature and then declined in a letter which gave his reasons: 'In five or more years I could probably find out nothing. Much work will be needed on the physiology of the central nervous system and on many collateral problems before dementia praecox can be understood.' After half a century these words remain still uncomfortably relevant to the contemporary situation.

But the role of epidemiology in psychiatry is far from confined to basic research. It has at least two other major spheres of application. One of these is in the sphere of the workings of health services which, important as they are, chiefly affect the administrative aspects of psychiatry. The other function of the subject, by contrast, concerns all trainee psychiatrists, namely its direct links with clinical psychiatry.

Clinical epidemiology in psychiatry

The transmission of mental disorder

This is historically the oldest sphere of epidemiological concern and activity, and extends to the current interest in so-called 'socially shared psychopathology'.[11] The induction of schizophreniform states with paranoid features, for example, is a well-recognized clinical phenomenon, described by various authors as 'communicated insanity',[12] 'folie communiquée'[13] or 'symbiotische Psychosen'.[14] Among the non-psychotic conditions, outbreaks of irrational behaviour, often loosely designated hysterical, have most often been described, sometimes affecting whole communities,[15] sometimes being confined to a particular institution.[16]

For many workers abnormal group behaviour has been accounted for in terms of the responses of more or less predisposed individuals to particular physical, psychological or social factors, a process which has been given such descriptively variegated names as 'imitation', 'collective disposition' and 'pluralistic emotional spread'. In the past a number of attempts have been made to analyse the phenomena within the framework of the classical epidemiological triad of host, environment and agent. As to the agent, it has been suggested that the morbid or exaggerated idea might be regarded as a noxious agent spreading the 'infection' in epidemics of aberrant beliefs.[17] A more concrete approach along similar lines can be provided when the agent in question is a physical substance such as a drug, and a clear demonstration of how epidemiological techniques can be applied to the spread of drug use within a community has been provided by de Alarcón.[18] Having demonstrated a sharp increase in heroin abuse among young people in one of two communities he showed that the incidence rate had increased after a latent period; further, he was able to determine the identity of the initiator of the epidemic and the approximate date of the first injection, and to demonstrate that the increase in number of cases was due to person-to-person contact. Figure 12.1 presents the trees of transmission which could then be constructed from the data.

The study of the 'host' has traditionally tended to belong to the geneticist. But, as Ødegaard has pointed out, it has not always been appreciated that 'In human population genetics epidemiological methods have to be introduced as soon as one proceeds beyond the study of individual pedigrees'.[19] Paradoxically, however, the geneticist's interest may well become more focused on the agent than the host since the modern view is that we must 'ask the question "what does this gene do to this individual?" in the same sense as the virologist inquires about the effect of a specific virus'.[20] It is significant that in recent years geneticists have come to speak of the 'transmission' of mental illness,[21] but the contribution of genetics to the clinician concerned with individual cases of mental disorder, as opposed to mental subnormality, still remains exiguous. In Lionel Penrose's words, 'When the classical work of Sjögren on amaurotic idiocy is compared with the monumental surveys of Rüdin and his school on psychosis, it is like comparing the movements of a cat with those of a rhinoceros'.[22]

In clinical practice every psychiatrist must, of course, clearly pay close attention to the environment, or milieu, in which morbid ideas can be transmitted and mental illness induced. On a large scale this has been well documented at times of social upheaval and natural disaster, when aberrant conduct and frank mental disorder are often prominent. Figure 12.2 tells its own story.[23] The detailed study of such phenomena, however, is usually

Figure 12.1 Transmission of heroin abuse in Crawley New Town

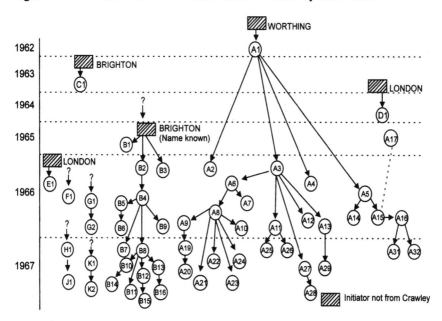

Source: R. de Alarcón, 'The spread of heroin abuse in a community', *World Health Organisation Bulletin on Narcotics*, 1969, 29: 17.

limited by chance and opportunity, as in the observations of Rawnsley and Loudon on the inhabitants of Tristan da Cunha whom they were able to study after a volcanic eruption, comparing their results with data obtained from a survey carried out twenty-five years before.[24]

More often the clinical study of environmental factors which bear on the transmission of mental disorder are on a smaller scale, and tend to be focused on the nuclear family. In the sphere of general morbidity the clustering of illness episodes within families has been well documented. This phenomenon has now been shown to apply to non-infectious disorders, including emotional illness. In a careful study extending over a period of two years, Brown was able to make a continuous assessment of two matched groups of families: one with and the other without a mother suffering from neurotic disability.[25] During the period of observation the neurotic women exhibited significantly more illness, physical as well as psychological, than their controls, and by the same criteria a similar difference was recorded for the husbands and the children of the index patients. The factors contributing to such family interaction are complex, including as they do genetic influence, assortative mating, sociocultural determinants and the intra-familial milieu, and though some relevant work has been carried out much more research is needed to estimate their relative significance.

Figure 12.2 Relation between trend of battle injury and neuropsychiatric admissions, selected divisions, Fifth US Army

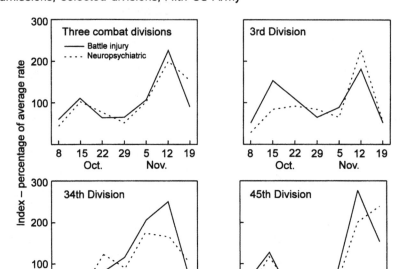

Source: A.J. Glass and R.J. Bernucci (eds), *Neuropsychiatry in World War II,* Washington, DC, Office of the Surgeon General, Department of the Army, 1966.

The phenomena of illness

(a) First among these may be placed what has been called the completion of the spectrum of disease.[26] In psychiatry the extension of epidemiological inquiries focused on the extramural dimensions of morbidity has radically modified our view of the nature and distribution of mental illness in the population at large. The model is indicated in Figure 12.3.

To elaborate on just one example. We now know from epidemiological inquiries that psychiatric illness in the community is composed largely of minor affective disorders.[27] From a clinical standpoint it is apparent that this large pool of affective illness not only extends the spectrum of the concept of such disorders but also bears pointedly on the aetiology of these illnesses and on the sterility of much work on their classification based on hospital cases. Further, it seems that in the middle-aged groups these disorders are associated with a raised expectation of physical morbidity, including major disease;[28] that the more chronic forms are also associated with long-term problems of social adjustment;[29] and that new

Figure 12.3 Coverage of sickness continuum achieved by the major sources of morbidity statistics

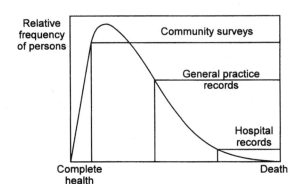

Source: G.W. Kalton, 'The contribution of research in general practice to the study of morbidity', *Journal of the Royal College of General Practitioners*, 1968, 15: 81.

episodes are often precipitated by events in the family and social orbit.[30] These findings are in conformity, both with the theoretical concept of 'illness-proneness' and with much recent work on the significance of life-change. They point to the need for co-ordination between mental health, general medical and social services in the management of patients with a consistently high experience of morbidity.

(b) Next we come to outcome and prognosis. Concerned as they are with the manifold associations of disease, the methods of epidemiological inquiry are central to the study of the natural history of mental disorders, a concept whose bearing on diagnosis and classification has been generally appreciated since the work of Kraepelin. The numerous follow-up studies of the schizo-phrenias, for example, have for the most part been conducted within the Kraepelinian framework and have tended to incorporate outcome as an axis for diagnostic classification in the absence of a clear aetiology and patho-genesis. Outcome has been defined in several ways, including the length of illness, the recurrence of attacks, the presence or absence of defect states and the chances of acquiring a hereditary disorder. These measures have in turn been related to such clinical features as abruptness of onset, the occurrence of particular symptoms, the pre-morbid personality and the body-build.

More recently, the impact of social factors on the course of schizophrenia has also been demonstrated in a series of epidemiological studies, focusing initially on mental hospital patients[31] and thence extending to the commun-ity through consideration of discharged patients and their families.[32] Research on institutionalism and schizophrenia has been supplemented by studies of discharged patients whose subsequent progress has been related to their type of living-group, their degree of emotional involvement with relatives, their occupational adjustment and the experience of stressful events. It seems clear that the course and outcome of schizophrenic illness are heavily influenced by social factors which have to be taken into account in assessing individual prognosis. These studies are important, not merely in that they render prediction more accurate but because they point to relatively specific social measures for improving the long-term outcome.

(c) Closely related to outcome studies are two other spheres of enquiry, each of which I can do no more than mention. The first is the actuarial assessment of individual morbid risk, either to calculate illness-expectancy among the relatives of patients with established mental disorder or to assess the risk for the patient himself in conditions where the occurrence of one or more previous attacks is held to influence the probability of future episodes.[33] The second is nothing less than the whole area of therapeutic evaluation by means of the controlled clinical trial, which is itself essentially no more than an exercise in applied epidemiology.[34]

(d) And finally – underlying all these endeavours – is the basic issue of the diagnosis and classification of mental disorder. For the epidemiologist, representing as he does what has been called the science of denominators, it becomes imperative to attain diagnostic precision to ensure that he can add or subtract or compare like with like. For the clinician, even though his primary concern be the individual case, this same objective becomes the springboard for his central function, which Sir James Spence has defined as 'the knowledge of disease as a predictable sequence of events, the understanding of which becomes the basis, the only basis, by which the process of disorder in the living patient can be rationally interpreted'.[35] And just as Molière's M. Jourdain is unaware of the fact that he is talking prose, so the clinician does not always appreciate that he is talking epidemiology. By way of illustration we may take two examples of the end-product of clinical assessment, the diagnostic formulation: 'A 19-year-old single student of good pre-morbid personality and a family history of affective illness, suffering from a depressive reaction to work and domestic stresses which should respond to medication and supportive psychotherapy'; and: 'A 45-year-old unmarried university professor with paranoid personality traits and a history of heavy consumption of alcohol who has developed delusional ideas of grandeur. No evidence of physical disease. Prognosis uncertain.'

Both statements, neither of them unusual of their kind, are impregnated with the epidemiological perspective which, if given due consideration, provides the trainee clinician with perhaps its most important contribution, namely a constant reminder of what he does *not* know about the individual patient under his care. With this awareness he can be both protected from self-deception and, perhaps, prompted to explore the general implications of the particular case, alive to the fact that while every patient is in some measure unique he also exemplifies Sir Aubrey Lewis's dictum that 'considered as an isolated unit, the behaviour of any single human being is much like a lost piece of a complete jigsaw puzzle carrying little meaning in itself'. The epidemiological approach does not, of course, embrace all issues of clinical significance. It would not, for example, furnish necessary information about biological mechanisms, therapeutic techniques or the art and ethos of the medical role. All of them depend, however, on a clear-sighted awareness of the logical infrastructure of the clinical method. This, I would maintain, is very close to epidemiology and in no branch of medicine is it needed more than in psychiatry.

References

1   E. Slater and M. Roth, *Clinical Psychiatry*, 3rd edn, London, Baillière, Tindall & Cassell, 1969, p. 776.
2   J.F.C. Hecker, *The Epidemics of the Middle Ages*, trans. B.G. Babington, 3rd edn, London, Trübner & Co., 1859.
3   A.D. Gardner, 'Debauchery of honest words', *British Medical Journal* (Correspondence), 1952, 1: 715.
4   J.A. Ryle, *Changing Disciplines*, London, Oxford University Press, 1948.
5   E. Tanzi, *Trattatto delle Malattie Mentali*, trans. W. Ford Robertson and T.C. Mackenzie, *A Textbook of Mental Diseases*, London, Rebman, 1909, p. 286.
6   R.P. Parsons, *Trail to Light*, New York, Bobbs-Merrill Co., 1943.
7   J. Goldberger, *The Etiology of Pellagra*, Public Health Reports, 1957, 29, 26: 1683.
8   M. Terris, *Goldberger on Pellagra*, Baton Rouge: Louisiana State University Press, 1964.
9   Goldberger, op. cit.
10 ibid.
11 E.M. Gruenberg, 'Socially shared psychopathology', in A.H. Leighton, J.A. Clausen and R.N. Wilson (eds) *Explorations in Social Psychiatry*, London, Tavistock Press, 1957.
12 D.H. Tuke, 'Communicated insanity', in *A Dictionary of Psychological Medicine*, vol. 1, London, Churchill, 1892, p. 240.
13 C. Lasègue and J. Falret, 'La folie à deux ou folie communiquée,' *Annales médico-psychologiques*, 1877, 38: 321.
14 C. Scharfetter, *Symbiotische Psychosen*, Bern, Huber, 1970.
15 H. Cantril, *The Invasion from Mars: A Study in the Psychology of Panic*, Princeton, NJ, Princeton University Press, 1940.
16 S. Benaim, J. Horder, and J. Anderson, 'Hysterical epidemic in a classroom', *Psychological Medicine*, 1973, 3: 366–73.
17 L.S. Penrose, *On the Objective Study of Crowd Behaviour*, London, Lewis, 1952.
18 R. de Alarcón, 'The spread of heroin abuse in a community', *World Health Organisation Bulletin on Narcotics*, 1969, 29: 17.
19 Ø. Ødegaard, in T. Kemp and G. Dahlberg (eds) *Proceedings of the First International Congress of Human Genetics*, *Acta Genetica et Statistica Medica*, 1957, 7, 2: 457.
20 J.A. Böök, *Causes of Mental Disorders: A Review of Epidemiological Knowledge*, New York, Milbank Memorial Fund, 1961.
21 D. Rosenthal and S.S. Kety (eds) *The Transmission of Schizophrenia*, Oxford, Pergamon Press, 1968.
22 L.S. Penrose, 'Psychiatric genetics', *Psychological Medicine*, 1971, 1: 265–6.

23 A.J. Glass and R.J. Bernucci (eds) *Neuropsychiatry in World War II*, Washington, DC, Office of the Surgeon General, Department of the Army, 1966.

24 K. Rawnsley and J.B. Loudon, 'Epidemiology of mental disorder in a closed community', *British Journal of Psychiatry*, 1964, 110: 830.

25 M. Shepherd, B. Cooper, A.C. Brown, and G.W. Kalton, *Psychiatric Illness in General Practice*, London, Oxford University Press, 1966, ch. 12.

26 J.N. Morris, *Uses of Epidemiology*, Edinburgh, Livingstone, 1957.

27 M. Shepherd, 'Beyond the layman's madness: the extent of mental disease', in J.M. Tanner (ed.) *Developments in Psychiatric Research*, London, Hodder & Stoughton, 1977, pp. 178–98.

28 M.R. Eastwood, *The Relation between Physical and Mental Illness*, Toronto, University of Toronto Press, 1976.

29 B. Cooper, 'Clinical and social aspects of chronic neurosis', *Proceedings of the Royal Society of Medicine*, 1972, 65: 19.

30 G.W. Brown and T. Harris, *Social Origins of Depression*, London, Tavistock Publications, 1978.

31 J.K. Wing and G.W. Brown, *Institutionalism and Schizophrenia*, London, Cambridge University Press, 1970.

32 G.W. Brown, E.M. Monck, G.M. Carstairs, and J.K. Wing, 'Influence of family life on the course of schizophrenic illness', *British Journal of Preventive and Social Medicine*, 1962, 16: 55.

33 E. Strömgren, 'Statistical and genetical population studies within psychiatry: methods and principal results', in *Proceedings of the First International Congress of Psychiatry*, vol. 6, Paris, Herman et Cie, 1950, pp. 155–92.

34 M. Shepherd, 'The evaluation of treatment in psychiatry', in P. Sainsbury and N. Kreitman (eds) *Methods of Psychiatric Research*, London, 1975, pp. 88–100.

35 J. Spence, *Lectures on the Scientific Basis of Medicine*, London, Athlone Press, 1954.

Chapter thirteen

Karl Jaspers: *General Psychopathology*

To begin with, a few facts. Karl Jaspers's *Allgemeine Psychopathologie* (*General Psychopathology*) was first published in 1913.[1] The author was then barely 30 years of age, working as a physician in the psychiatric hospital at Heidelberg. Two years later he moved away from medicine towards first psychology and then philosophy, the field in which he was to emerge as one of the outstanding figures of the twentieth century. He continued, however, to retain an interest in psychopathology, revising and expanding his book in several later editions. Within the German-speaking world it was at once recognized by leading psychiatrists as a unique achievement, a mountainous landmark in the history of the subject. If Jaspers's reputation was to decline in Germany between the two world wars, this is attributable chiefly to his outspoken, uncompromising resistance to national socialism. Philosophy for him was a public as well as a private concern, and it was his courageous political stand which led Hannah Arendt to describe him as a contemporary successor of Immanuel Kant.

Here, then, was a rare bonus for psychiatry. One of the foremost thinkers of the day, a trained physician, had spent a long enough period in the practice of the subject to write a major volume on its foundations. None the less, half a century was to elapse before an English version appeared,[2] during which time countless inferior books had been translated from the same language. With some exceptions, furthermore, its reception in the anglophonic countries has been respectful rather than enthusiastic, and in some quarters downright hostile. Here, for example, is the verdict of one influential British textbook:

> It is all over-simplified and though the phenomenology of psychiatric illness is described with great accuracy and detail, Jaspers fails to see that much of it is dependent on the institutional milieu in which the patients then lived. He therefore is unaware of some of the meaningful links, and 'real causes' like genetics which were considered proven at the

Originally published in *British Journal of Psychiatry*, 1982, 141: 310–12.

time the first edition appeared are no longer tenable. This work has however greatly influenced German psychiatric thinking and some who are unhappy over the logical inconsistencies of Freudian psychopathology or who would wish to subscribe to anything but Freud will find in Jaspers an adequate intellectual exercise. It will not help towards an apparent understanding of the apparent illogicalities and contradictions of emotionally toned behaviour and is therefore very dated and out of touch with modern advances in psychiatry.

As a former co-examiner of the author of this egregious assessment I can testify to its impact on would-be members of the Royal College of Psychiatrists.

There would seem to be three principal reasons for the lukewarm response to the anglicization of *General Psychopathology*. In the first place, it is not an easy work to read, concentrated in argument and diffuse in form, difficult enough in the original German and often understandably opaque in another language despite the heroic efforts of the translators who were faced with what the late Professor E.W. Anderson acknowledged as 'the difficulty and at times impossibility of rendering the author's subtle thought into concise and comprehensible English'. Without persuasive advocates it was never likely to appeal to a wide readership.

A second obstacle to the ready acceptance of the text is embedded in the passage cited above. By 1963, when the English translation was published, the word 'psychopathology' had become heavily coated with psychoanalytical encrustations. In contrast, the term is employed by Jaspers in a much wider sense. Its essence, he maintains, can emerge only from a composite framework constructed with 'the viewpoints and methods that belong to the world of the Humanities and Social Studies . . . since the methods of almost all the Arts and Sciences converge on psychopathology'. Further, in the later editions of his book Jaspers becomes increasingly critical of psychoanalysis which, he concluded, is a pseudo-faith, 'an enormous process of self-deception conditioned by the age we live in, which bewitches its victims, who find in it the satisfaction of their lives'. Not surprisingly, so negative a verdict has not endeared his views to the majority of psychoanalysts, whose powerful influence on psychiatric theory has rarely been challenged directly by so informed and penetrating a critic.

But perhaps the principal difficulty posed by the book for the reader is that of fitting it into a recognizable and familiar mould. *General Psychopathology* cannot be classified as a textbook. Rather, it should be regarded as an intellectual map, a guide to a series of separate but related areas of knowledge identified in the list of contents as Individual Psychic Phenomena, Meaningful Psychic Connections, Causal Connections of Psychic Life, the Conception of the Psychic Life as a Whole, the Abnormal Psyche in Society and History, and the Human Being as a Whole. Within this broad topography there are large uncharted territories, and the contours of the map are undergoing constant revision. The primary purpose of the work, however, is to furnish not an ordnance survey but a general overview designed, in Jasper's words, 'to develop and order knowledge guided by the methods through which it is gained – to learn to know the process of knowing and thereby to clarify the material'. The attainment of this objective depends primarily on the clarification of a host of concepts which are traditionally either ignored or over-simplified in the psychiatric literature. To do justice to such themes as the mind-body relationship, the role of scientific enquiry, the principles of classification, personality, the subjective–objective dichotomy, or the notions of health and disease calls for a familiarity with the history of ideas in other disciplines. It is here that Jaspers comes into his own, bringing a massive tradition of philosophy and social theory to bear on these perennial problems in relation to psychopathology.

To grasp the full significance of the achievement, however, the reader must be aware of the sources and the ways in which they have been adapted. The views of Kant, Kierkegaard, Nietzsche, Max Weber, and Jaspers's own later theorizing are as central to the construction of *General Psychopathology* as the work of Griesinger, Wernicke, Kraepelin, or Kurt Schneider; and some of the better-known specific concepts are openly borrowed from German thinkers, e.g. the emphasis on phenomenology derives from Husserl and the distinction between 'understanding' and 'explanation' from Dilthey. For this reason I always found extensive background reading essential when conducting seminars on the book.

General Psychopathology contains a complex admixture of exposition, psychological description, critique, and especially in the later editions, philosophical speculation. While the whole text is impregnated with Jaspers's holistic approach to his subject-matter, the neophyte is probably best advised to sample the text in fragments. He could, for example, profitably begin with the subsection on 'Delusion and awareness of reality' (pp. 93–102); move on to 'Pathological psychogenic reactions' (pp. 383–93); and, after contrasting the chapter on the 'Psychology of meaning' (pp. 301–13) with the 'Characteristics of explanatory theories' (pp. 530–4), examine the use made of this distinction in the assessments of Kretschmer (pp. 40–1), Wernicke (pp. 534–7), von Gebsattel (pp. 540–6), and Freud (pp. 537–40). Then, lest he should regard Jaspers as a distant, impersonal figure, he should turn to the important sections on psychotherapy, which have been published separately in book form,[3] in order to appreciate Jaspers's clear-headed humanism and his concern for the doctor-patient relationship, well illustrated in the following paragraph:

There are no scientific grounds for determining what kind of psychotherapist one will become nor the type which will be considered ideal. Certainly a psychotherapist should have a training in somatic medicine and in psychopathology, both of which have to be scientifically based. If he has no such training, he would only be a charlatan, yet with this training alone he is still not a psychotherapist. Science is only a part of his necessary equipment. Much more has to be added. Among the *personal prerequisites* the width of his own horizon plays a part, so does the ability to be detached at times from any value-judgement, to be accepting and totally free of prejudice (an ability only found in those who generally possess very well-defined values and have a personality that is mature). Finally, there is the necessity for fundamental warmth and a natural kindness. It is therefore clear that a good psychotherapist can only be a rare phenomenon and even then he is usually only good *for a certain circle of people* for whom he is well suited. A psychotherapist for everyone is an impossibility. However, force of circumstance makes it the psychotherapist's usual duty to treat everyone who may ask his help. That fact should help him to keep his claims to modest proportions.

To grasp fully the development of Jaspers's leitmotivs, however, it is necessary to become familiar with the structure of the whole text. One key example, which I have attempted to examine in detail elsewhere,[4] is the complex relationship between general psychopathology and the sciences. For Jaspers 'natural science is indeed the groundwork of psychopathology and an essential element in it but the humanities are equally so and, with this, psychopathology does not become in any way less scientific but scientific in another way'. The psychopathologist must, he claims, employ the scientific method and the scientific attitude, even when dealing with subjective experience or meaningful connections, but then he goes on:

Only when the biological aspects have been clearly distinguished can we proceed to discuss what essentially belongs to man. Whenever the subject studied is Man and not man as a species of animal, we find that psychopathology comes to be not only a kind of biology but also one of the Humanities.

From this springboard he elaborates the need for 'metaphysical understanding' as a philosophical position.

So, to conclude, an opinion: *General Psychopathology* remains the most important single book to have been published on the aims and logic of psychological medicine. Its scope and clarity, as Kurt Kolle has observed, provide nothing less than 'the criterion by which the qualification for psychiatry is tested'. For this reason alone it should be studied and assimilated by all psychiatrists in training. And by their teachers.

References

1 K. Jaspers, *Allgemeine Psychopathologie, Ein Leitfaden für Studierende, Arzte and Psychologen*, 1st edn, Berlin, Springer, 1913.
2 K. Jaspers, *General Psychopathology*, trans. from the German 7th edn by J. Hoenig and M.W. Hamilton, Manchester, Manchester University Press, 1963.
3 K. Jaspers, *The Nature of Psychotherapy: A Critical Appraisal*, trans. by J. Hoenig and M.W. Hamilton, Manchester, Manchester University Press, 1964.
4 M. Shepherd, 'The sciences and general psychopathology', in M. Shepherd and O.L. Zangwill (eds) *Handbook of Psychiatry*, vol. 1, Cambridge, Cambridge University Press, 1982.

Chapter fourteen

John Ryle

Dr Stockman: It is ignorance, poverty, ugly conditions of life, that do the
devil's work.

(Henrik Ibsen, *An Enemy of the People*, Act IV)

I first met John Ryle in 1944. Having recently taken the chair of Social
Medicine at Oxford he had initiated occasional socio-medical teaching and
demonstrations at the Radcliffe Infirmary for clinical students, of whom I
was one. Something of Ryle's reputation had preceded him, and we students
were curious to see how he compared with the many stars in our own
teaching galaxy who included Leslie Witts, John Stallworthy, Hugh Cairns,
Arthur Ellis, Chassar Moir, R.G. MacFarlane, Ida Mann, and, not least,
Ryle's long-standing colleague, Arthur Hurst.

It was evident at once that he was a man apart. Tall, erect, with a grave
courteous mien and the expression of a visionary, his striking appearance
made an instant impression on us all. The patient, a middle-aged woman
suffering from cardiac asthma, was about to be discharged from hospital.
Ryle listened attentively to the presentation before questioning her in some
detail about her symptoms. In view of her dyspnoea he did not examine the
chest and confined his physical assessment to the radial pulse, which he
asked us to compare with his own. We then retired to a side room where he
elaborated on his personal experience of anginal pain as well as on the
patient's cardiovascular condition before turning to her social history,
with special reference to her background, early environment, upbringing,
and domestic circumstances. Then came the prognosis. How, he asked, was
the patient going to cope with her disability at home? In response to my
profession of ignorance he suggested that I visit the home to see for myself.
Just before leaving he returned to the bedside for a few moments in private
with the patient herself.

Originally published as Introduction to J.A. Ryle, *The Natural History of Disease*, The
Keynes Press/British Medical Association, 1988, pp. xi–xix.

Shortly afterwards I found myself on a Saturday afternoon cycling along a side street in Cowley to learn something of the socio-medical significance of cardiac invalidism. Though obviously puzzled by the purpose of my visit, the patient was clearly glad to see me and was co-operative throughout. And as I took my leave she asked me to convey her thanks to 'the other doctor'; 'I shall never forget his kind words,' she murmured.

From then on I attended Ryle's teaching sessions whenever possible. He invited me to the Institute of Social Medicine and to his home. After qualifying I met him briefly on two or three occasions and heard him deliver the Maudsley Lecture in 1947. The appearance of his book, *Changing Disciplines*, in 1948 rekindled my interest in his ideas on social medicine in the setting of the National Health Service. His health, however, was failing and he died in 1950 at the age of 60.

John Ryle was a member of an unusually gifted family. His grandfather and a paternal uncle were bishops; his father was a rationalist doctor with a philosophical bent who contributed to the Aristotelian Society. His younger brother was an eminent philosopher and one of his sons was a Nobel prize-winning astronomer. His father numbered among his forebears Sir Humphrey Gilbert and Thomas Dudley, and his mother several prominent Scotts.

He was born in 1889, one of ten children, and educated at Brighton College. His medical education, like his father's, was at Guy's Hospital. He was awarded the Treasurer's gold medal in 1912 and qualified in 1913. After resident appointments he served in the RAMC throughout the First World War, returning to Guy's as Medical Registrar in 1919 when he obtained the MRCP and an MD with a gold medal. In 1920 he was appointed assistant physician and demonstrator in morbid anatomy at Guy's Hospital where he worked until 1935. There he established a reputation not only as an outstanding clinician with a large and growing practice but also as an original clinical investigator, particularly of the gastrointestinal and cardiovascular disorders. His work on the fractional test-meal and the introduction of 'Ryle's tube' for taking samples of gastric juices gave him an international reputation and in 1925 he delivered the Goulstonian Lectures to the Royal College of Physicians on 'Gastric function in disease'.

He was elected FRCP in 1924 and from 1932 to 1936 was physician to His Majesty's Household. In 1932 he was Hunterian Professor of the Royal College of Surgeons. Throughout this strenuous period he was heavily involved in research and practice, the fruits of which were to mature in seventy-seven published papers. Thirty-four of these lectures and essays were brought together under the title of *The Natural History of Disease*, which appeared in 1936 and in a second edition in 1948.

Ryle describes his book as 'gleanings from the current experience of a general physician'. It merits re-reading on several counts. First, for its unpretentiously clear and elegant style: there are few tables and laboratory findings, but the text is spattered with reference to great clinicians of the past – Hippocrates, Hunter, Harvey, Heberden, Bright, Laennec, Osler. Second, for its meticulous accounts of disease states, including pain, peptic ulcer, renal and cardiac disorders, and various infections. Third, for the chapters in which he enunciates the principles underlying his work and outlook.

Essentially, Ryle identified with the notion of the physician as naturalist, a student of nature and biology rather than merely of disease. The spirits of Gilbert White, of Linnaeus, and of Darwin are constantly in evidence. 'There are', he comments, 'better inspirations to thoughtful medicine to be found in the Origin of the Species than in a modern textbook of bacteriology' (p. 432). He insists, however, that the study of *homo sapiens* must be conducted humanistically. Despite the title of the volume he stresses the importance of studying the natural history of man in disease as well as the natural history of disease in man and he observes that 'more than half of practical medicine is psychology' (p. 432). Emphasizing the need to cultivate 'a lively sympathy', he remarks that 'The embarrassed patient, like the wild bird, cannot be successfully studied if he is self-conscious or afraid' (p. 17). Physicians, he concludes, 'must needs observe the temperament, peculiarities and individual reactions of our patients and of their near relatives with a constant watchfulness if we are to preserve a just balance in the department of diagnosis, prognosis, and treatment' (p. 403). How well he translated this holistic approach into clinical practice is particularly well illustrated by his descriptions of the visceral neuroses, anorexia, angor animi, colonic spasm, and peptic ulcer.

Claiming as he did that symptoms, 'the purely subjective phenomena of disease', merit precedence over physical signs in the study of sick people (p. 69), Ryle was inevitably drawn to the observational method in clinical research, taking up the cudgels on its behalf against the complementary experimental approach associated with clinical science advocated at the time by Sir Thomas Lewis. He asserts that

> Research in clinical medicine is not pathological, bacteriological or biochemical research. These are concerned with the study of agents, the processes and the consequences of disease in man under the conditions of the laboratory, and often with the help of experiments in animals. Clinical science should rather be considered as a branch of the science of human biology. It studies the behaviourism of disease in man, or perhaps it would be more correct to say of man in disease. It observes, records, and, when possible, measures the processes of disease as they occur in the living subject, and within certain limitations it may control, modify or reproduce these processes for purposes of detailed study. (p. 407)

It followed that in the 1930s Ryle was cautiously critical of the new model of the research physician being initiated by the Medical Research Council, expressing concern lest the trainees should be deprived of the experience of a broad cross-section of diseases and their manifestations. And a self-portrait is surely reflected in his comment on the attributes of these hybrids.

> In the selection of candidates credit should be given for a broad earlier education and particularly for some grounding in philosophy, logic or psychology as against purely technical abilities or an uninterrupted scient- ific education from the school period. Qualities as physician or naturalist should be allowed at least as strong a claim as qualifications for research in other spheres. A scholarly heredity should, by Galtonian doctrine, be considered a very distinct advantage. (p. 414)

Such characteristics might well be regarded as ideal for an academic posi- tion. None the less, it came as something of a surprise to his contemporaries when in 1935, at the early age of 46, Ryle accepted the Regius Chair of Physic at Cambridge. The reasons, it would appear, were partly to relieve him of the intolerable strain on his health placed by his huge clinical commitments and partly because he was beginning to entertain doubts about the path along which he had been progressing so successfully. In place of the glittering prizes of the medical establishment – an ever-growing private practice, the presidency of the Royal College of Physicians, public honours and titles – he chose, as his Inaugural Lecture makes clear, to try and create the conditions for 'a renaissance in Medicine'.[1] A leading article in the *British Medical Journal* devoted to *The Natural History of Disease* commented that the move to Cambridge augured well for the development of academic medicine in Britain.[2]

It was not to be. At first the course continued smoothly enough. He quickly built up a department of gifted and productive workers, and in 1935 he became a member of the Medical Research Council. The following year he was appointed Physician Extraordinary to the king and in 1939 he delivered the Croonian lecture of the Royal College of Physicians, of which he had become a censor. None the less, Ryle did not fit easily into the slow-moving, inward-looking, complacent milieu of pre-war Cambridge. His view of disease in terms of human biology was leading to a growing awareness of human ecology and of the impact of environmental factors on health and morbidity. He slowly underwent a profound re-evaluation of his fundamen- tal beliefs in coming to consider the implications of his clinical philosophy for social action.

Alongside his abiding interest in clinical medicine Ryle began to engage in socio-political activities. Before the Second World War he helped organize Spanish relief and work for medical refugees. He renounced his pacifist credo and shortly after the outbreak of the Second World War he stood unsuccessfully as a parliamentary candidate for Cambridge University as an Independent Progressive, referring pointedly in his election address to 'the furtherance of social and educational reforms and the better promotion of the health of the nation' and to an 'insistence on the proper maintenance of the social services and a fairer distribution of the burdens of war as between the well-to-do and the poorer classes'.[3] A little later he enrolled in the Emergency Medical Service, first as an administrator and later as a consultant adviser in medicine to the Minister of Health, and returned during the Blitz to work at Guy's for a while, living in a workman's flat near the hospital. From 1941 he began to work for the newly formed Anglo-Soviet Medical Committee, and in that same year he published a small book, entitled *Fears May Be Liars*, which expresses his humanistic faith and its value as a support in an epoch of helplessness and despair.

The strenuous war-time activities took a heavy toll of his physical resources and in 1942 he suffered a coronary thrombosis. Shortly afterwards he made another unexpected decision in accepting the newly created chair of Social Medicine at Oxford where he initiated an ambitious programme of socio-medical enquiries. He justified this step in a passage written some years later:

Some of my friends have rebuked me for leaving the clinical fold. I reply in effect that I have merely taken the necessary steps to enlarge my field of vision and to increase my opportunities of aetiological study. My allegiance to human medicine is in no whit broken. I wish I could convey to them and to others some of the sense of stimulation and rejuvenation that my close association with statisticians and medical social workers and with men and women in the public health and industrial health services has brought to me. Thirty years of my life have been spent as a student and teacher of clinical medicine. In these thirty years I have watched disease in the ward being studied more and more thoroughly – if not always more thoughtfully – through the high power of the microscope; disease in man being investigated by more and more elaborate techniques and, on the whole, more and more mechanically.... With aetiology – the first essential for prevention – and with prevention itself the majority of physicians and surgeons have curiously little concern.[4]

Why social medicine? Since the term was introduced by Guérin in 1848 the concept has undergone many vicissitudes.[5] Its origins lie among the roots of the public-health movement which in Britain can be traced to the work of such men as Edwin Chadwick, William Farr, Thomas Southwood Smith, and John Simon. On the European mainland the tradition was rather different but Alfred Grotjahn's notion of social hygiene, as Major Greenwood pointed out,[6] has much in common with Ryle's concept of social medicine, which he saw as 'a direct development and expansion of clinical medicine'; this, 'as its name implies, clearly has a main concern with the group as well as the individuals composing the group'.[7] In this respect social medicine overlapped with traditional epidemiology, though with a new emphasis on the emergent field of non-infectious disease. Ryle, however, went beyond the narrow confines of medical theory and practice in emphasizing his concern with 'the idea of medicine applied to the science of man as *socius*' and its links with social policy:

> It may properly be argued that many of the social evils, so widely manifest by disease, which have been cited above call not for medical action but for drastic social and economic reform. For these the electorate through their representatives, and not the doctors (as doctors), must become responsible. But who unearths and exposes the evils and their secondary effects? The factual evidence, the socio-medical experience, the statistical data – all of which must continue to be provided by the doctors and their scientific associates and field workers and particularly by those whose concern is rather with the social than with the individual aspects of disease. Whether in this basic manner, or more immediately as an educator of opinion, or incidentally in the course of his daily professional activities, we have reached a time in which 'the physician (to quote Professor Sigerist) must assume leadership in the struggle for the improvement of conditions'. Without research and teaching in social medicine to guide him he cannot faithfully fulfil his mission.[8]

In the 1940s social medicine was very much in vogue. It figured prominently in the writings of prominent medical figures,[9] and in Sir William Goodenough's influential Inter-Departmental Committee on Medical Education.[10] At the time, as Webster has pointed out,

> social medicine seemed to offer the key to the transformation of medicine and health care... The emergence of social medicine reflected increasing dissatisfaction with existing agencies of preventive medicine... Social medicine provided a convenient banner around which the medical intelligentsia flocked... although the term social medicine attracted interest before 1939, its general currency was due to the wartime mentality. Social medicine was consistent with the ethos of rational planning for victory and for postwar reconstruction.[11]

Ryle was a natural leader of this movement, whose cause he espoused in a volume entitled *Changing Disciplines*, which was published in 1948. His premature death cut short his efforts, however, and the enthusiasm for social medicine was tempered by the changes in the economic and cultural climate of later post-war Britain. The perennial question of the relation of medicine to society was answered in a different way by a subsequent generation. Ryle's Institute was closed and within a few years the term 'social medicine' was out of fashion. A recent historiographical essay significantly employs the past tense in questioning 'What was social medicine?'.[12]

So what, in retrospect, did John Ryle achieve? In some measure, the answer to this question depends on the perspective in which his life and work are viewed. To some observers he failed in his objectives, as the concluding sentence of the entry in Munk's Roll makes clear:

His influence on current and future thought was considerable, but these practical projects were only successful in part, for though he had sincerity, unselfishness, understanding and humility, as well as charm, he also had some of the idealist's limitations.

Many others saw him as the embodiment of the Victorian gospel of the 'Sanitary Idea',[13] summed up by George Eliot's Dr Lydgate as 'the most direct alliance between intellectual activities and the social good'. Relatively few of the men and women devoted to this cause, however, were practising physicians; their concerns were derived rather from politics, administration, social theory, basic science, statistics, epidemiology, or public health. John Ryle brought to their ranks the background and viewpoint of clinical medicine which helped to provide a focal point for these diverse interests. In so doing he illustrated well the truth of his philosopher brother's observation that 'medicine' is the name of a somewhat arbitrary consortium of more or less loosely connected enquiries and techniques'.[14]

But over and above his place in the evolution of his discipline Ryle owed his position to his personal qualities. A shrewd and experienced medicine watcher, Alan Gregg of the Rockefeller Foundation, commented after Ryle's visit to New York in 1947:

The impression he left wherever he went was of course strongly coloured by the distinction of mind, of bearing and of character which had characterised him always...my own estimate of John Ryle as a person and as a pioneer in British Medicine is such as to leave me a bit impatient with those who did not acknowledge him more promptly, and completely as a great leader...a good many of those he met here (the USA) were not quite equipped to appreciate his qualities and the quite extraordinary beauty of balance he achieved in the conduct of his own life, and I doubt not, in the lives of his patients.[15]

Ryle's friend and colleague, the distinguished neurologist Sir Charles Symonds, who was not prone to exaggeration, went further:

He was a truly remarkable man, in his presence distinguished, in his manner kindly, in his heart pure and in his spirit great. But there was something more than this, some undefinable quality, endearing and sublime, which raised him above the stature of ordinary men.[16]

This 'undefinable quality' would appear to have been a form of the religious temperament so memorably described by William James. Ryle's influence on his contemporaries may be attributed in part to his personal charisma, provided it be recalled that in Max Weber's original use of this now much-overworked term charisma (the gift of grace) was a theological conception, ultimately inexplicable but potent in its effects and tending to invest its owner with a particular form of authority. Ryle's professed faith was that of an agnostic humanist, but humanism, as R.H. Tawney insisted, 'is the antithesis not of Christianity but of materialism'.

How far Ryle's *religio medici* can be sustained in an imperfect world remains to be seen. Meanwhile we have his writings. None of these is more impressive than *The Natural History of Disease*, a classic in its own right, and there are many who will endorse the verdict of an eminent British general practitioner, writing nearly fifty years after its first appearance:

> John Ryle's book is amazingly relevant today. He gives excellent clinical descriptions... it is on more general issues such as diathesis, prognosis and on the physician as naturalist that I recommend anyone who has never seen it to read the book, and those who have to re-read it.[17]

References

1 J.A. Ryle, *The Aims and Methods of Medical Science*, Cambridge, Cambridge University Press, 1935.
2 Leading article, 'The physician as naturalist', *British Medical Journal*, 1936, 1: 890–1.
3 J.A. Ryle, *To the Parliamentary Electors of the University of Cambridge*, Cambridge, Habbakuk, 1940.
4 J.A. Ryle, *Changing Disciplines*, Oxford, Oxford University Press, 1948.
5 I. Galdston, *The Meaning of Social Medicine*, Cambridge, Mass., Harvard University Press, 1954.
6 M. Greenwood, 'Social medicine', *British Medical Journal*, 1946, 1: 117–19.
7 J. Ryle, 'Social medicine: its meaning and its scope', *British Medical Journal*, 1943, II, 4,324, 633–6.
8 As above, note 7.
9 Lord Horder, 'Social medicine: the appeal of the Common Man, in I. Galdston (ed.) *Social Medicine: Its Derivations and Objectives*, New York, Commonwealth Fund, 1949, 277–94
10 Report of the Inter-Departmental Committee on Medical Education, London, HMSO, 1944.
11 C. Webster, 'The origins of social medicine in Britain', Society for the Social History of Medicine, *Bulletin*, 1986, 38: 52–5.
12 D. Porter and R. Porter, 'What was social medicine? An historiographical essay', *Journal of the History of Sociology*, 1988: 90–106.
13 A. Briggs, 'Public health: the "sanitary idea"', *New Society*, 15 February 1968: 229–31.
14 G. Ryle, *The Concept of Mind*, London, Hutchinson's University Library, 1949, p. 323.

15 A. Gregg, unpublished correspondence, 1951.
16 C. Symonds, 'John Alfred Ryle', *Guy's Hospital Report*, 1950, 99, 4: 209–22.
17 J. Fry, 'Ryle's *Natural History of Disease*', *Journal of the Royal College of General Practitioners*, 1981, 31: 757.

Chapter fifteen

Urban factors in mental disorders: an epidemiological approach

Introduction

The process of urbanization has been a major factor in the development of *homo sapiens*. As in so many spheres of knowledge, Aristotle had the first word when he wrote: 'Men come together in the city to live; they remain there in order to live the good life.' Since then, as Lewis Mumford has documented in his magisterial survey,[1] the city has played a major role in history as the centre of some of man's most civilizing achievements. At all times, however, a delicate balance has existed between the advantages of urban life, with its rich and stimulating environment, and the cost exacted in terms of poverty, unnatural living conditions, and adverse environmental pressures. Summing up a substantial body of opinion, one twentieth-century observer has concluded that to live according to nature,

> we should pass a considerable time in cities for they are the glory of human nature, but they should never contain more than 200,000 inhabitants; it is our artificial enslavement to the large city, too enormous for human dignity, which is responsible for half our sickness and misery.[2]

This chapter examines the scientific overtones of this assertion in respect of mental disorder.

The coincident arrival of industrialization and modern medicine in the early nineteenth century led to several attempts to build on the Rousseau-esque notions of a simple life in natural surroundings, paving the way for the view of an environmental concept of health based on favourable social as well as individual conditions. A sanitary ideal was developed by many social reformers who believed in hygiene as a way of life. Identifying dirt, poverty, and overcrowding as causes of disease, they naturally focused attention on the city. In Germany these ideas were developed prominently by Max von Pettenkoffer in his lectures on 'The health of a city' that contain an account

Originally published in *British Medical Bulletin*, 1984, 40, 4: 401–4.

of the measures introduced successfully into Munich, which included even the planting of trees and flowers because of their supposed aesthetic effects on the mental health of the population.

In Victorian England the sanitary movement also led to such measures as the foundation of the Health and Town Association and the Public Health Act. Its essence is perhaps most vividly exemplified by the famous address delivered by Benjamin Ward Richardson to the Health Section of the Social Science Association in 1875. Aiming 'to show a working community in which death...is kept as nearly as possible in its proper or natural place in the scheme of life', Richardson presented an idealized view of a community in terms of health issues and, significantly, he concluded that social control of the environment was the key to prevention, an objective which took precedence over curative treatment.

Utopian though it may seem now, it was the spirit of the early sanitarians which paved the way for the laying of the foundations of urban sociology. And it was from the work of men like Booth, Weber, Tönnies, Park, and Simmel, all pioneers of the sociological discipline, that there emerged an intense preoccupation with fact-finding and quantification. Not the least significant result of these endeavours was the realization that the definition of a city is itself an issue. The demographers were quick to stress the importance of numbers, density, and heterogeneity, but these factors alone do not indicate that the urban ecosystem is a complex physical, biological, and psychosocial admixture which includes such diverse elements as climate, noise level, crowding, pollution, occupational specialization, and a constant adaptive struggle with stimulus overload.[3] Many studies have now demonstrated that the marked variation between the populations of urban aggregates or societies represents the resultant of a wide variety of factors. For the purpose of scientific enquiry, epidemiology, the quantitative study of health in populations, is the method *par excellence* of studying the pathological aspects of that variation, as I propose to illustrate.

Effects of urbanization on health

The simplest demographic level is that of medical geography. In the United Kingdom the routine collection of national statistics has made it possible to compare both mortality and morbidity rates by residential districts. The results demonstrate that urban dwellers are considerably less healthy than their country cousins, with the exception of the risk for traffic accidents.[4]

The use of such crude indices for mental disorder, however, is unfortunately limited by problems of ascertainment and of definition. Mental disorders are traditionally subdivided into the two broad categories embodied in the International Classification of Disease, namely the psychoses on the one hand and the neuroses and personality disorders on the other, although the distinction between them is not as sharp as has been maintained. In addition, a third category of distress and sub-clinical reactions has to be included. For convenience, each may be considered in turn.

The psychoses

However they may be defined, the psychotic illnesses are more severe, more socially disruptive, and more likely to lead to institutional care than any other forms of mental disorder. During the nineteenth century they were seen by several social commentators as diseases of 'civilization' and were located in large cities. As late as 1903 William Alanson White could write:

> The savage in his simplicity does not know what it is to suffer from the cares and worries which are the daily portion of the European, and it is little wonder that the latter, beset by all manner of disappointments and vexations, should more frequently break down in mind than his less gifted brother.[5]

The compilation of morbidity statistics derived from mental hospitals opened the door to quantitative investigations like that of Goldhamer and Marshall, who were able to show in their monograph, *Psychosis and Civilisation*, that industrialization had not apparently influenced the first admission rates to the Massachusetts mental hospitals for the hundred years after 1840.[6] Here, it should be emphasized, they were testing indirectly the hypothesis that the strains and stresses associated with increasing industrialization centred in cities would lead to an increase in insanity. With a wider range of mental hospitals, more direct comparisons have become possible. Most of them record a larger urban than rural rate of first admissions, but the influence of nosocomial factors may well influence these figures which, further, take no account of those cases which fail to enter institutions. Accordingly, more sophisticated modern investigators have adopted an ecological approach based on detailed surveys of whole communities and areas, chosen for their contrasting characteristics whenever possible.

One of the best-documented and most relevant of these studies was conducted by Eaton and Weil who studied the community of Hutterites, a Protestant sect in the USA who live in colonies organized to ensure a pastoral, law-abiding style of life far removed from the cut and thrust of urban existence.[7] Eaton and Weil's conclusions are as follows:

> Our findings do not confirm the thesis that a simple and relatively uncomplicated way of life provides virtual immunity from mental disorders.... Psychoses and other forms of mental disorder were found to occur with regularity in the Hutterite population. Their existence in so secure and stable a social order suggests that there are genetic, organic and constitutional elements which predispose a few individuals to mental

breakdown in any social system, no matter how protective and well-protected it may be ... a mental health Utopia is probably impossible.

At the same time they noted that the Hutterites engaged in very little antisocial activity and that their children were rarely disturbed emotionally, a point to which I shall return.

But the possible associations of urban life and mental illness cannot be confined to relatively crude contrasts of this type. The modern town or city is composed of heterogeneous sub-communities and these lend themselves to intra-urban comparison. The model for this type of enquiry was established in Chicago, the major American centre of urban sociology, where Faris and Dunham carried out their classical pre-war study, *Mental Disorders in Urban Areas*,[8] based on an analysis of first-admission rates to hospital from different areas of the metropolis. Their key finding arose from the distribution maps concerning schizophrenia and manic-depressive psychosis which showed that while the pattern formed by the distribution of the manic-depressive psychoses was essentially random, the schizophrenics were concentrated in the poorest, most disorganized areas of the city (Figures 15.1 and 15.2). The results led to the concept of 'insanity areas', comparable to

Figure 15.1 Areas of residence (shaded areas) in the city of Chicago with high first-admission rates to hospital for schizophrenia in persons aged 15–19 years by 1930 census tract

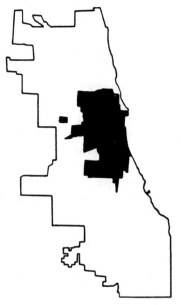

Source: R.E.L. Faris and H.W. Dunham, *Mental Disorders in Urban Areas*, 2nd edn, New York, Hafner, 1960.

Figure 15.2 Areas of residence (shaded areas) in the city of Chicago with high first-admission rates to hospital for manic-depressive psychoses in persons aged 15–64 years by 1930 census tract

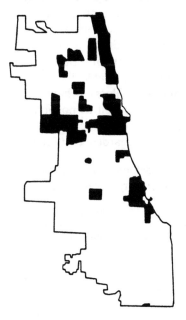

Source: R.E.L. Faris and H.W. Dunham, *Mental Disorders in Urban Areas*, 2nd edn, New York, Hafner, 1960.

Clifford Shaw's 'delinquency areas', and generated a number of questions, the most significant of which concerned the rival claims of the 'breeder' and 'drift' theorists in relation to schizophrenia. Though this debate now seems to have been decided in favour of the 'drift' or 'social selection' hypothesis it has stimulated a host of careful studies of the social and familial correlates of schizophrenia in different cities and different forms of urban life, all of them based on epidemiological and ecological methods of study.[9] Perhaps the most suggestive result of this work to date has been the notion that the outcome of schizophrenic illnesses is better in developing than in developed countries, a difference reflecting the more stressful impact of the westernized urban environment on the course of the condition.[10]

'Minor' psychiatric illness

The application of the epidemiological approach to the study of the 'minor' psychiatric disorders faces two problems from the outset. In the first place, only a small proportion of these conditions lead to contact with an institution, so that the use of administrative hospital statistics cannot be employed in their enumeration. Second, their identification, assessment, and classification all pose a host of unresolved problems, many of which have been illuminated by the information obtained from the general practitioners who assume responsibility for the care of the majority of these patients. In the United Kingdom with its comprehensive health service, it becomes possible to study the primary-care population and the results have shown that psychiatric morbidity constitutes a major segment of the presenting conditions.[11] A National Morbidity Survey, furthermore, has shown marked urban-rural differences (Table 15.1)[12] but here it is necessary to take account of variations in illness behaviour and diagnostic practices among general practitioners as well as possible variations in the patterns of disease. There is also a clear difference in the consultation rates for peptic ulcer, a condition sometimes regarded as stress-induced.

Table 15.1 Urban–rural differences in general-practitioner consultation rates (from 1st National Morbidity Survey, England and Wales)

Diagnosis	Consultations per 1,000 per year				
	Conurbations	Other towns, populations			Rural districts
	> 100,000	50,000– 100,000	< 50,000	
Psychoneurotic disorders	32	32	25	27	23
Peptic ulcer	15	18	15	14	10
All causes	610	593	607	582	567

Source: General Register Office, op. cit.

It must be acknowledged that the value of surveys of this type, however carefully conducted, is limited by their static, cross-sectional data. A more dynamic study has been mounted by Muñoz and his colleagues in the Spanish community living in the Baztan valley of Navarra.[13] The population of 8,750 inhabits three areas whose socio-demographic features could be characterized as 'urban', 'rural', and 'isolated', according to their respective life-styles. In this area migration from the less to the more urbanized district is an ongoing process, and a representative sample of subjects was studied in all three areas by means of a two-stage approach – an initial screening with a standardized questionnaire of established reliability, followed by detailed interviews. The key findings demonstrate a positive association between place of residence and neurotic illness, the rates diminishing from 'urban' via 'rural' to 'isolated' areas. The raised urban morbidity, it should be further noted, was significantly associated with males and females characterized as single, aged 15–24 years, unskilled, and with poor social and education levels. Support is therefore provided for an association of these phenomena with the process of urbanization which raises the question of

Figure 15.3 Per cent of schoolchildren with neurotic or conduct disorders (deviance) in the Isle of Wight (IOW) and an Inner London borough (ILB), 1975

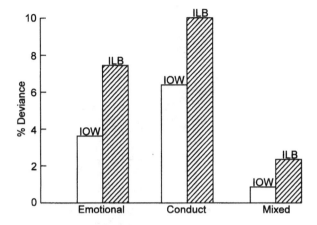

Source: M. Rutter, 'The city and the child', *American Journal of Orthopsychiatry*, 1981, 51: 610–25.

whether 'selection' or 'stress' – the equivalents of 'drift' and 'breeder' – may be responsible.

This issue has been examined in greater detail by Rutter and his colleagues in their comparison of the mental health of schoolchildren in the rural Isle of Wight and an Inner London borough.[14] Using a two-stage approach, these workers demonstrated a highly significant excess of neurotic and conduct disorders in the urban areas (Figure 15.3). They were also able to relate four factors causally to these differences both between and within the areas: these are family discord, parental deviance, social disadvantage, and school characteristics. In several respects their findings confirm the background features identified by West as important correlates of delinquent behaviour: low family income, large family size, parental criminality, low intelligence, and poor parental behaviour.[15] These factors make up a sub-culture in which other anti-social forms of conduct – e.g. drug-taking, attempted suicide, theft – also occur in the late adolescent and early adult years,[16] and which contrast sharply with the patterns of Hutterite life. Precisely what constitutes these categories of behaviour has still to be determined, but the evidence to date suggests that physical factors like genetic predisposition, coincident physical morbidity, and malnutrition play a relatively minor role compared with psychosocial influences.

Distress and sub-clinical disorders

The definition and identification of these disorders touches on the borderland between illness and deviant behaviour which lends itself to

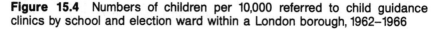

Figure 15.4 Numbers of children per 10,000 referred to child guidance clinics by school and election ward within a London borough, 1962–1966

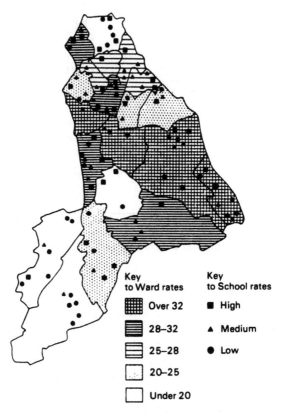

Key to Ward rates

▦ Over 32
▤ 28–32
▤ 25–28
☐ 20–25
☐ Under 20

Key to School rates

■ High
▲ Medium
● Low

Source: D. Gath *et al., Child Guidance and Deliquency in a London Borough,* Institute of Psychiatry Maudsley Monograph 24, Oxford: Oxford University Press, 1977.

micro-epidemiological enquiry, in which various environmental influences are studied independently. A few examples may be taken to illustrate the method. In one of our own studies, the site of enquiry was a single London borough within which the patterns of child guidance and delinquency rates were mapped within the smaller, more homogeneous areas defined by election wards (Figure 15.4).[17] Detailed statistical analyses based on socio-demographic features of the districts and the social characteristics of the schools pointed to a complex set of relationships. The best predictor of child-guidance referral proved to be the probation rate of the school, followed by the proportion of persons living in shared households, the proportion of foreign-born residents, and the rate of migration.

To render this type of analysis clinically useful, however, it is necessary to examine personal responses as well as group associations. Thus, while earlier clinical studies of urban living conditions have suggested that residents of high-rise flats, and especially the mothers of young children, are particularly prone to psychiatric disorder,[18] more recent epidemiological work with control groups has indicated the importance of vulnerable individuals, though there is undoubtedly a high degree of expressed dissatisfaction among the young mothers which may serve as the precursor of a depressive reaction.[19]

A comparable state of affairs emerged from our own study of the effects on mental health of another largely urban hazard, namely aircraft noise.[20] Here the areas of the city were subdivided geographically by noise levels and a survey of some 6,000 people was conducted to render comparisons possible. In the event, noise was found to be associated not with overt mental disorder but with the so-called 'annoyance' of the population, a state of subjective discomfort associated with such symptoms as nervousness, headaches, insomnia, tiredness, and irritability. To establish the causal links between annoyance and mental disorder, it proved necessary also to take account of noise sensitivity, a psychophysiological factor which varies markedly between members of the general population and was significantly related to both covert psychiatric morbidity and annoyance. With regard to one noxious urban factor, therefore, epidemiological investigation has succeeded in demonstrating that mental disorder is related to predisposition and reactivity as well as to direct causation, depending less on the intensity of any single factor than on the confluence of noxious factors on 'vulnerable' or 'high-risk' members of the population. If the quality of life becomes unbearable there is a transition from annoyance and dissatisfaction to dysthymic states and then to a frankly psychiatric symptom-pattern.

Conclusion

So much for this brief overview of the epidemiological approach to psychiatric morbidity in the urban milieu. Clearly the list of potential noxae can be widely extended to include a host of other pollutants but in all cases the objective is the same: to identify adverse factors in the environment and demonstrate their effect on mental health. But what then should be done? In asking this question we are proposing, implicitly or explicitly, that environmental changes may be desirable and by so doing we leave the protected harbour of medical and scientific enquiry for the choppy waters of social administration. The theory of public health is rooted in epidemiology, but its practice depends on political action. In the sphere of physical illness, the pattern has been established for the control of infectious diseases and is now being adapted to tackle such major issues as lead pollution, accident prevention, smoking, and other disorders related to life-style. So far, relatively little direct action has been taken because of the risks of mental disease but it is worth noting that the United States Appeals Court has ruled that electricity can no longer be generated by the reactor at the Three Mile Island site in Pennsylvania until it has been shown that the mental health of the population will not suffer as a consequence.[21] The implications of this decision for social policy may be profound, not least because it signifies an awareness of the impact of an environmental pollutant on psychological well-being. As such, it underlines the practical as well as the theoretical significance of the epidemiological approach to mental disorders.

References

1   L. Mumford, *The City in History: Its Origin, its Transformations and its Prospects*, Harmondsworth, Penguin, 1961.
2   C.V. Connolly (Palinurus, pseud.) *The Unquiet Grave: A Word Cycle*, London, Arrow Books, 1961.
3   S. Milgram, 'The experience of living in cities', *Science*, 1970, 167: 1,461–8.
4   Office of Population Censuses and Surveys, *The Registrar General's Statistical Review of England and Wales for the Year 1971*, London, HMSO, 1973.
5   W.A. White, 'The geographical distribution of insanity in the United States', *Journal of Nervous and Mental Disease*, 1903, 30: 257–79.
6   H. Goldhamer and A. Marshall, *Psychosis and Civilization*, Glencoe, Ill., Free Press, 1953.
7   J.W. Eaton and R.J. Weil, *Culture and Mental Disorders: A Comparative Study of the Hutterites and Other Populations*, Glencoe, Ill., Free Press, 1955.
8   R.E.L. Faris and H.W. Dunham, *Mental Disorders in Urban Areas: An Ecological Study of Schizophrenia and Other Psychoses*, 2nd edn, New York, Hafner, 1960.
9   L. Levy and L. Rowitz, *The Ecology of Mental Disorder*, New York, Behavioral Publications, 1973.
10 World Health Organization, *Schizophrenia: An International Follow-up Study*, Chichester, Wiley, 1979.
11 M. Shepherd, B. Cooper, A.C. Brown, and G. Kalton, *Psychiatric Illness in General Practice*, 2nd edn, Oxford, Oxford University Press, 1982.
12 General Register Office, *Morbidity Statistics from General Practice*, vol. 1 (General) by W.P.D. Logan and A.A. Cushion, Studies on Medical and Population Subjects no. 14, London, HMSO, 1958.
13 J.L. Vázquez Barquero, P.E. Muñoz, and V. Madog Jaúregui, 'The influence of the process of urbanization on the prevalence of neurosis: a community survey', *Acta Psychiatrica Scandinavica*, 1982, 65: 161–70.
14 M. Rutter, 'The city and the child', *American Journal of Orthopsychiatry*, 1981, 51: 610–25.
15 D.J. West, *Present Conduct and Future Delinquency: First Report of the Cambridge Study in Delinquent Behaviour*, London, Heinemann, 1969.
16 I.H. Mills and M.A.M. Eden, 'Social disturbances affecting young people in modern society', in G.A. Harrison and J.B. Gibson (eds) *Man in Urban Environments*, Oxford, Oxford University Press, 1977, p. 217.
17 D. Gath, B. Cooper, F. Gattoni, and D. Rockett, *Child Guidance and Delinquency in a London Borough*, Institute of Psychiatry Maudsley Monograph 24, Oxford, Oxford University Press, 1977.
18 N.C. Moore, 'Psychiatric illness and living in flats', *British Journal of Psychiatry*, 1974, 125: 500–7.

19 G.W. Brown and T. Harris, *Social Origins of Depression: A Study of Psychiatric Disorder in Women*, London, Tavistock, 1978.
20 A. Tarnopolsky and J. Morton-Williams, *Aircraft Noise and Prevalence of Psychiatric Disorders*, Research report, London, Social & Community Planning Research, 1980, p. 460.
21 Editorial, 'Can change damage your mental health?', *Nature*, 1982, 295: 177.

Chapter sixteen

The only metaphysical man: a re-examination of Otto Rank

Otto who? To many students of contemporary psychoanalysis the name of Otto Rank (1884–1939) is unlikely to figure among its most prominent exemplars. He was, the more knowledgeable would probably assert, an unimportant renegade who wrote about the trauma of birth and emigrated to the USA where he was regarded as a controversial, solitary figure, now largely forgotten.

The facts of the matter are more complex and much more interesting. Otto Who's surname was in fact Rosenfeld, not Rank, and his background differed from that of the founding fathers of psychoanalysis in several respects. He was the youngest son of a poor Viennese immigrant Jewish family; his father was an uncultivated artisan of modest means and unsympathetic disposition. In his diary the boy summed up his childhood: 'I grew up, left to myself, without education, without friends, without books.' He was a sickly youth, of diminutive stature, and unprepossessing appearance ('the short Dr Caligari body, the uneven teeth' were to impress a later admirer), whose life was changed at the age of 15 by that curious emotional cataclysm which overwhelms certain gifted adolescents, sweeping them towards a lifelong preoccupation with ideas and the inner life. The diaries, written between his eighteenth and twenty-first year, record the efforts of a born intellectual working as a locksmith in conditions of material poverty and drawing on books, music, and theatre to help discover an identity. At the age of 19 he symbolized his aspirations by formally renouncing his religious faith and adopting a non-Jewish surname that was borrowed, significantly, from a character in Ibsen's *A Doll's House*.

The strain was clearly considerable. It led to a consultation with the family doctor, Alfred Adler, who introduced the youngster to first the writings and then, at the age of 21, to the person of Sigmund Freud. For the next twenty years Rank was to play a central part in the psychoanalytical movement. In his capacity as salaried secretary of what became the Vienna Psychoanalytic Society from 1906 to 1915, and then as editor and publisher

---

Originally published in *Encounter*, November 1985, pp. 53–5.

of several journals, he proved himself an indispensable and indefatigable worker, his leader's closest associate in the movement and seemingly his master's voice. His role was well defined and acknowledged by one of his colleagues in the 'inner circle':

> Rank would have made the ideal private secretary, and indeed he func-
> tioned in this way to Freud in many respects. He was always willing, never
> complained of any burden put upon him, was a man of all work for
> turning himself to any task, and he was extraordinarily resourceful. He
> was highly intelligent and quick-witted.

But this long period of apparent subservience concealed Rank's own indi-
vidual development. The little outsider, without a medical qualification, socially inferior, largely self-educated, began to mature. He obtained a doctorate in his spare time, treated patients, and wrote incessantly on psychoanalytical topics with an evident bias towards artistic activity, myth, and legend. His early works include such studies as *The Don Juan Legend, The Double, The Incest Motif*, and *The Myth of the Birth of the Hero*.

Marriage and his experiences during the First World War further increased Rank's self-confidence and sense of independence, and in 1924 he emerged as his own man with the publication of *The Trauma of Birth*, a book which not merely modified but challenged some of Freud's central tenets. Stern disapproval and a brief period of reconciliation were followed by the inevitable sentence of excommunication. Rank and Freud met for the last time in 1926, and Rank's name and work were thenceforward virtually expunged from the official history of the psychoanalytical movement. In Ernest Jones's biography of Freud, Rank is said to have developed 'psych-otic manifestations that revealed themselves in, among other ways, a turning away from Freud and his doctrines'.[1]

Like so much in that fanciful book, the interpretation fails to fit the facts. On leaving Vienna, Rank continued to work as a psychotherapist, though of an increasingly heterodox type, in Paris and New York, eventually settling in the USA where he achieved success despite initial difficulties and eventually became something of a cult figure. During this phase of his life he met and treated several prominent people, among whom the writer Anaïs Nin was the most significant. He eventually divorced his first wife and married his devoted secretary. Towards the end of his life he discovered Mark Twain, and even signed some of his letters 'Huck'. Any possibility of his becoming Otto Finn, however, was erased by his early death at the age of 55.

This material may be found, not without difficulty, in *Acts of Will*, E. James Lieberman's long, sprawling biography.[2] Here is an example of Dr Lieberman's style:

It was a titanic hour: Henry 'phoned Anaïs excitedly that night and penned a fourteen-page letter to her the next day. The gangling Brooklyn refugee felt that the little Viennese analyst had probed his core. Miller, 41 and working on the *Tropic of Cancer*, was carried to his second wife, June, who could be equally comfortable in bed with a woman, with Henry, or with both. For a time she and Anaïs were fast friends who commiserated about Miller; they intermittently succored and shook his large but vulnerable ego.

The book is repetitious, poorly constructed, and unsophisticated to a degree. Much of the narrative is taken up with Freud and his followers, whose backbiting and infighting were seemingly fuelled by the jealousy and ill-will that characterize most sectarian squabbles and contrast so pointedly with the pretentiousness of their claims to understand human nature. Lieberman's heavy-handed presentation is particularly out of place in attempting to catch the essence of a man so elusive and secretive as Otto Rank.

Fortunately there is to be found a far more vivid portrait in the pages of Anaïs Nin's journals.[3] Encased as she was in her narcissistic world, this remarkable woman, like Lou Andreas-Salomé before her, was drawn by the bugle-call of Eros to become for a time a camp-follower of the psychoanalytical battalion. She brings Rank to life in a single passage:

Background: Books, shining and colorful books, many of them bound, in many languages. They form the wall against which I see him. Impressions of keenness, alertness, curiosity. The opposite of the automatic ready formula and filing-away. The fire he brings to it, as if he felt a great exhilaration in these adventures and explorations. He gets a joy from it. It is no wonder he has evolved what he calls a dynamic analysis, swift, like an emotional shock treatment. Direct, short-cut, and outrageous, according to the old methods. His joyousness and activity immediately relieve one's pain, the neurotic knot which ties up one's faculties in a vicious circle of conflict, paralysis, more conflict, guilt, atonement, punishment, and more guilt. Immediately I felt air and space, movement, vitality, joy of detecting, divining. The spaciousness of his mind. The fine dexterity and muscular power. The swift-changing colors of his own moods. The swiftness of his rhythm, because intuitive and subtle. I trust him. We are far from the banalities and clichés of orthodox psychoanalysis.
I sense an intelligence rendered clairvoyant by feeling.
I sense an artist.

Anaïs Nin's relationship to Rank was a close one – 'from patient to Muse to lover', says the blurb more bluntly than Lieberman's clotted prose. She repaid her debt handsomely: 'Give back pleasure, music, self-forgetting for all that he gave me.' And she goes on:

I unleashed a flow of confidences. He had written poetry and plays, he had wanted to be a writer before he came into contact with Dr. Freud. I resuscitated a submerged part of Rank's personality. 'I have not talked about myself for thirty years or even before that.'

What will happen to this writer who lived mute and concealed behind the fact of the doctor?

Some months later, she answered her own question, concluding that the cause of his 'tragic personal life' was too little spontaneity, too much will.

What, in retrospect, are we to make of the man and his achievements? Within a psychoanalytical frame of reference Rank emerges as no more than another heresiarch, possibly occupying a special role as one of Freud's former favourites. His earlier books and papers are of some interest because of their attempts to extend Freudian theory to the realms of art and culture, but his writings now appear turgid in thought and expression, clearly rooted in the tradition of Nietzsche and Schopenhauer with a gloss of sexual psychopathology. Lieberman's description of him as 'the consummate eclectic' covers this phase of his career. His later work shows him attempting to develop his own ideas via *The Trauma of Birth, Truth and Reality, Modern Education, Art and Artist*, and the revealingly entitled *Beyond Psychology*. His posthumous influence was extended by the Otto Rank Association, which lasted from 1965 to 1982. Some of his ideas have been adopted and adapted by others, most notably by Arthur Janov.

The most significant aspect of Rank's career, however, was his steadily increasing disillusionment with the creed on which he had been nurtured. Towards the end of his life he would surely have endorsed Janet Malcolm's opinion that

The crowning paradox of psychoanalysis is the near-uselessness of its insights. To 'make the unconscious conscious' – the program of psychoanalytic therapy – is to pour water into a sieve. The moisture that remains on the surface of the mesh is the benefit of analysis.[4]

The last word comes most fittingly from Anaïs Nin:

I entered with impunity the world of psychoanalysis, the great destroyer of illusion, the great realist. I entered that world, saw Rank's files, read his books, but I found in the world of psychoanalysis the only metaphysical man in it: Rank.

References

1   E. Jones, *The Life and Work of Sigmund Freud*, Harmondsworth, Penguin, 1964.
2   E. James Lieberman, *Acts of Will: The Life and Work of Otto Rank*, New York, Collier Macmillan, 1985.

3   Anaïs Nin, *Journals*, ed. G. Stuhlmann, vol. 1, 1931–4, London, Quartet, 1970.
4   J. Malcolm, *In the Freud Archives*, London, Cape, 1984.

Chapter seventeen

What price psychotherapy?

'An undefined technique applied to unspecified cases with unpredictable results. For this technique rigorous training is required.' How much the uncomfortable truth embedded in this old, caustic definition of psychotherapy continues to raise professional hackles is well shown by the reactions to a 'meta analytic' assessment of published psychotherapeutic versus placebo studies published recently in *The Behavioral and Brain Sciences*, a journal which carries open peer commentary.[1]

The conclusion by Prioleau *et al.* – that 'the benefits of psychotherapy do not exceed those of placebo in real patients' – provoked a predictably sharp division of opinion among the twenty-three commentators. For some, the findings confirmed the non-specific nature of psychotherapy in most of its various guises; for others, they merely indicated the need for more and better investigations. One of the most thoughtful responses was that of the much respected Jerome Frank, whose conclusions reflect long research experience in the subject:

> With many patients the placebo may be as effective as psychotherapy because the placebo condition contains the necessary, and possibly the sufficient, ingredient for much of the beneficial effect of all forms of psychotherapy. This is a helping person who listens to the patient's complaints and offers a procedure to relieve them, thereby inspiring the patient's hopes and combating demoralisation.[2]

So bland a conclusion borders on the self-evident. Why, then, should another influential commentator, Brendan Maher, observe that Prioleau *et al.* 'must expect to be attacked with a vigour that will be relatively independent of the rationality of their conclusions'?[3] In the USA the immediate reasons have to do more with economics and medical politics than with the niceties of scientific enquiry. Psychotherapy there is big business, and its

Originally published in *British Medical Journal*, 1984, 288: 809–10.

exponents are mostly in private practice, where their income depends largely on third-party payments from medical insurance. As Maher points out, this state of affairs has already resulted in widespread lobbying for the inclusion of mental disorder in insurance policies and in extensive advertising through the mass media. In addition, because the practice of psychotherapy remains without firm professional credentials, understandable but unseemly competition has developed between rival groups of mental-health professionals – psychiatrists, psychologists, social workers, nurses, and counsellors of various persuasion.[4] And, since the recent move towards making federal funds for psychotherapy dependent on proof of efficacy and safety,[5] the suggestion that a psychotherapist is little more than a placebologist must be, in Maher's pithy phrase, 'as welcome as a tax auditor at a business lunch'.

The implications of this vigorous transatlantic debate for the National Health Service have been apparent for some time.[6] Some of them may be detected in discussions of the registration of psychotherapists[7,8] and of the justification for recognizing so amorphous an activity as a specialized form of medical practice within the structure of a publicly financed health service.[9] It is pertinent to recall a central point made by Sir John Foster in his report on scientology,[10] a form of psychotherapy to its founder, a brand of quackery in the eyes of many, and a religion according to the High Court of Australia. As Foster pointed out: 'those who feel they need psychotherapy tend to be the weak, the insecure, the nervous, the lonely, the inadequate, and the depressed'. With so large and vulnerable a section of the population seeking help it is hardly surprising that nostrums are offered by an increasing number of thaumaturgical, pastoral, and blatantly commercial systems laying claim in one way or another to be 'psychotherapeutic'.

Here may be the key to an understanding of why the heat generated by psychotherapeutic polemics cannot be attributed to professional, technical, legal, or financial considerations alone. In his massive historical and clinical study of psychological healing Pierre Janet included miracles, philosophy, moral guidance, hypnotism, suggestion, rest, isolation, 'mental liquidation' (a term which includes psychoanalysis), education, excitation, magnetism, and psychophysiological methods within the orbit of psychotherapeutics.[11] As Janet makes clear, when stripped of the pseudoscientific pretensions all forms of psychotherapeutic activity are responses to a widespread demand for reassurance, hope, and support, accompanied by a willingness to believe in what is being offered for the purpose. In short, they are responses to part of the human condition.

The doctor's dilemma was clearly identified by Daniel Tuke in his observations on the influence of mind on the body 100 years ago: 'scepticism in the physician is the best means of arriving at the truth: faith in the patient the best means of arriving at health'.[12] In theory the double-blind, placebo-controlled clinical trial goes some way towards resolving this conflict, but in practice, and despite much evidence,[13,14] the function of the placebo in medical therapeutics tends to be minimized: Goodman and Gilman, for example, devote three short paragraphs out of 1,700 pages to placebo effects, concluding that, 'Although the inert medication may be an effective vehicle for a placebo effect, the physician-patient relationship is generally preferable.'[15] But if, as Prioleau *et al.* maintain, the relationship is itself a form of placebo – if the medium constitutes the message – then the problems of evaluation become more complex. Several of the difficulties emerged from an ill-fated Medical Research Council trial in the early 1970s,[16] though other studies have since shown that at least some of the obstacles can be overcome.[17] Unfortunately, most of the major research bodies in Britain appear to fight shy of the topic, and the professional organizations, including the Royal College of Psychiatrists, have done little more than pay lip-service to the need for action. With its broader view of hygiene and its professed concern for the consumer, perhaps the new College of Health might be prepared to confront the issues more directly?

References

1 L. Prioleau, M. Murdoch, and B. Brody, 'An analysis of psychotherapy versus placebo studies', *The Behavioral and Brain Sciences*, 1983, 6: 275–85.

2 J.D. Frank, 'The placebo in psychotherapy', *The Behavioral and Brain Sciences*, 1983, 6: 291–2.

3 B. Maher, 'Meta-analysis: we need better analysis', *The Behavioral and Brain Sciences*, 1983, 6: 297–8.

4 T.G. McGuire, 'Markets for psychotherapy', in G.R. Vandenbos (ed.) *Psychotherapy: Practice, Research, Policy*, Beverly Hills, Calif., Sage, 1980.

5 P. London, and G.L. Klerman, 'Evaluating psychotherapy', *American Journal of Psychiatry*, 1982, 139: 709–17.

6 M. Shepherd, 'Psychoanalysis, psychotherapy, and health services', *British Medical Journal*, 1979, ii: 1,557–9.

7 M. Shepherd, 'The statutory registration of psychotherapists', *Bulletin of the Royal College of Psychiatrists*, 1980, 4: 166–8.

8 Report of Psychotherapy Section Executive Committee, 'Statutory registration of psychotherapists', *Bulletin of the Royal College of Psychiatrists*, 1983, 7: 190–5.

9 G. Wilkinson, 'Psychotherapy in the marketplace', *Psychological Medicine*, 1984, 14: 23–6.

10 J.G. Foster, *Enquiry into the Practice and Effects of Scientology*, London, HMSO, 1971.

11 P. Janet, *Les Médications psychologiques*, 3 vols, Paris, Alcan, 1919.

12 D.H. Tuke, *Illustrations of the Influence of the Mind upon the Body in Health and Disease*, 2nd edn, London, J. & A. Churchill, 1884.

13 M. Jospe, *The Placebo Effect in Healing*, Lexington, Mass., Heath, 1978.

14 O. Lindahl and L. Lindwall, 'Is all therapy just a placebo effect?', *Metamedicine*, 1982, 3: 255–9.

15 A.G. Gilman, L.S. Goodman, and A. Gilman (eds) *The Pharmacological Basis of Therapeutics*, 6th edn, New York, Macmillan, 1980.

16 J. Candy, F.H.G. Balfour, R.H. Cawley, *et al.* 'A feasibility study for a controlled trial of formal psychotherapy', *Psychological Medicine*, 1972, 2: 345–62.

17 R.B. Sloane, F.R. Staples, A.H. Cristol, N.J. Yorkston, and K. Whipple, *Psychotherapy versus Behavior Therapy*, Cambridge, Mass., Harvard University Press, 1975.

Chapter eighteen

Two faces of Emil Kraepelin

Eponymous lecturers are expected to make some reference to the person in whose name the lecture is being delivered. In this case my task has been facilitated by the fact that the first Mapother lecture was devoted to Edward Mapother himself. It was given by his successor, Sir Aubrey Lewis, who, as was his wont, furnished a comprehensive account of his subject, demonstrating how this remarkable man laid the foundations of the institution to which he devoted his professional life. Lewis's lecture, entitled 'Edward Mapother and the Making of the Maudsley Hospital',[1] provides a link with this one via the mention of the visit paid by Frederick Mott in 1909 to Emil Kraepelin's Forschungsanstalt in Munich, where he was so impressed by what he saw that he resolved to use Henry Maudsley's bequest to found a corresponding institution in this country. Edward Mapother was to assume a major responsibility for this large enterprise which he justified as follows:

> The only hope for the sort of dispassionate long-term research which psychiatry needs, is the creation of teams of career investigators...most of whom should not be primarily psychiatrists at all, but real experts in various branches of science, who have brought its technique to the service of psychiatry and then received enough training in this to enable them to see its problems...Then we should get progress, not pot-boiling.

Pot-boiling: Mapother was never shy of calling a spade a spade and, as we now know, his realistic foresight has been amply attested by the development and status of the Institute and the joint hospitals.

Admiring Kraepelin as they did, Maudsley and Mott and Mapother would certainly have wished to do him honour at the special meeting organised in 1987 as one of the events celebrating the 700th anniversary of the founding of the University of Heidelberg. The symposium was devoted to schizophrenia and was held near the university psychiatric clinic where

---

Based on the 14th Mapother lecture to the Institute of Psychiatry, London, November 1994. Originally published in *British Journal of Psychiatry*, 1995, 167: 174–83.

Kraepelin first formulated many of the clinical concepts for which he is renowned. His name was invoked with reverence by most of the speakers and he figured prominently in the final summary of the papers by the octagenarian American psychologist, the late Joseph Zubin. Dr Zubin, who was something of a maverick, thanked the speakers for covering a wide spectrum of topics and then asked the solemn, predominately German audience what appeared to be a rhetorical question: 'What would Kraepelin have thought of this work?' His next question, however, was more disconcerting than rhetorical. 'Why don't we ask him?', he inquired, and proceeded to walk to the door, open it and call out 'Come in, Emil'. He then escorted an invisible figure – invisible at least to me – to a chair, and began a sort of ventriloquist's version of question and answer. The dialogue is reprinted in the published proceedings of the occasion in the form of a conversation between two characters, one called 'Interviewer', the other 'Emil'.[2] Here is a sample:

> EMIL: I am very happy about the progress you report on the revival and standardization of diagnosis of schizophrenia . . . I wonder, however, why you call the method neo-Kraepelinian. It seems to me that you have returned to the original Kraepelin system.
> INTERVIEWER: What led you to consider the importance of psychological tests as vulnerability markers?
> EMIL: I was a devoted disciple of Wilhelm Wundt, the founder of modern experimental psychology and my original career ambition was to follow in his footsteps. One day Wundt noticed that I was wearing a new ring on my finger and enquired 'Bist du verlobt?' I admitted that I was in love and was planning to get married. He looked at me with some astonishment and said 'You know, Emil, I cannot guarantee you a chair as Professor of Philosophy, and I wonder whether you are not taking responsibilities which you may find difficult to carry out'. Well, after this warning I felt compelled to take a post in the clinic when the next offer came. Thus not logic, but love, as it should, made the career decision for me.

Why recall this entertaining nonsense? Because of the response of an unsmiling senior German colleague whose opinion I requested when the session was mercifully over. He had clearly regarded the performance as neither entertaining nor nonsensical and he remarked with some feeling: 'Herr Zubin should not have called him Emil.' 'What should he have called him?' I asked. 'Professor Kraepelin' was the immediate reply. It brought to my mind two aphorisms that serve to introduce this lecture. The first is Nietzsche's saying that in the German-speaking world an ordinarius professor takes second place only to God. The second is the comment of the great French painter, Georges Braque, that every man has at least two faces, a view that he illustrated so well in his analytical Cubist portraits. It is the distinction between the two faces of Emil Kraepelin and Professor Kraepelin that constitutes my theme. An historical study may be undertaken either as a self-contained inquiry in its own right or with the aim of having the past illuminate the present. This one belongs to the second of these two categories.

Biographical note

First, a brief biographical note. Kraepelin was born in 1856, one of a tightly-knit bourgeois family in Neustrelitz in northern Germany. He was a diligent but not intellectually outstanding child with a keen interest in the natural world, especially botany. He contemplated a research career in biological science but eventually settled for a medical training, supplemented by a spell of experimental psychology in Wundt's laboratory which greatly influenced his subsequent outlook and research. On entering the field of psychiatry he quickly acquired a reputation for combining detailed clinical observation with an interest in classification. In 1887 he was appointed to a chair in the Baltic university of Dorpat, then moved to Heidelberg in 1891. He left Heidelberg for Munich in 1903, first to the university clinic and then to the Research Institute which he founded in 1916 and directed until the end of his career. There he confirmed his place as *primus inter pares* among the large group of outstanding German psychiatrists whose work laid the scientific foundations of the discipline as we know it today.

Research method and results

To evaluate the significance of Emil Kraepelin's long, productive life-time of clinical research and organizational activities in the field of mental disorder it is helpful first to establish the major contributions by which he is best known, namely his clinical method and its application to the field of classification. Here he was very much a man of his time. As Zilboorg has pointed out:

> The history of German psychiatry of the nineteenth century is the history of psychiatric somatisation... in the middle of the century German psychiatry asserted the supremacy of the brain over any other structure and proceeded systematically to produce a psychiatry without a psychology.[3]

When it became apparent that the physical substrate of many psychotic states was not readily identifiable, increasing attention was paid to the clinical delineation of the onset, course and outcome of these disorders. Kraepelin borrowed and elaborated Kahlbaum's notion of symptom-complexes but, unlike Kahlbaum, he posited the existence of disease-entities, with general paresis as the paradigm. Pending the discovery of the pathological basis of these disorders he directed his work towards the construction of a series of defined syndromes by means of careful observation of the clinical phenomena and their natural history. Studying many thousands of cases he attempted to delineate the form and content of the psychoses, abetted in this task by the virtual absence of effective treatments. In this endeavour he was less concerned with the mechanisms of disease than with the pattern of symptoms construed as biological facts. The work was conjoined to studies based principally on Wundt's objective psychology, with particular regard to laboratory experimentation. Subjective experience was minimized. Thus, in Kraepelin's opinion, 'so-called psychic causes – unhappy love, business failure, overwork – are the product rather than the cause of the disease; they are merely the outward manifestation of a pre-existing condition; their effects depend for the most part on the subject's Anlage.' So much for 'life events' and the whole concept of reactivity.

The evolution of Kraepelin's nosological thinking is best traced in the successive editions of his textbook, which grew from a brief conventional compendium of 385 pages in 1883 to a two-volume *Lehrbuch* of 2425 pages in the ninth edition of 1927. Changes were introduced in each edition, most radically in the fifth edition (1896), when the combined study of symptoms and outcome had come centre stage, and psychological speculation was virtually jettisoned. Traditionally accepted categories like secondary dementia, Wahnsinn and degeneration were discarded and a much simplified schema of disease-groupings was proposed, leading to the fertile suggestion of two major groups of functional mental disorders, the older notion of dementia praecox and the new rubric of manic-depressive psychosis. The latter appears first in the sixth (1899) edition of the textbook and is distinguished from the former by its clinical features and its relatively favourable outcome.

What did he actually do? Essentially, he recorded clinical and demographical information systematically on index cards, treated the data numerically and subjected them to personal interpretation. He described his method of procedure as follows:

I went through all the available index cards relating to the different pathological forms I had to refer to. The index cards contained a very condensed résumé of all information on each case. Then, I excluded all those cases which seemed to be incomplete or questionable and began to group them under different aspects. The most similar cases were collected into larger or smaller groups and the clinical characteristics of these subtypes were defined more precisely. Thereby, the hereditary behaviour, proven external causes, the distribution of age, sex and profession were ascertained. Furthermore, genetic development, individual physical and mental symptoms, the course and outcome were taken into consideration.

By examining the numbers, I gained criteria to judge whether the trial group arrangement was justified or should be altered.[4]

Seemingly unaware of the problems associated with sampling, observer bias and statistical analysis, Kraepelin conceded that despite his emphasis on objectivity there was a strong subjective element in his procedure. He wrote:

I must admit that one could have serious objections to my form of procedure not to represent the progress of my clinical findings in scientific individual accounts accompanied by the other relating documents and observations but rather to present it as the current state of knowledge in successive editions of my textbook. My expressed opinions often changed over a few years and I could not be sure that my colleagues would agree with me, especially as I did not inform them of the observations that formed the basis of my opinions. With these extensive studies I simply could not spare the time to substantiate my opinions, and although I tried to encourage my pupils to do so they could, unfortunately, only fill the gap incompletely. I decided not to give those opinions which were generally accepted at the time, but I felt that I should write what seemed to me to be the nearest to the truth based on the recent scientific point of view.[5]

Serious objections, indeed! Nowadays, such work would be viewed as a primitive exercise in clinical epidemiology, but with so many methodological flaws as to render it unacceptable to any editor of a peer-review journal. The weaknesses of the approach were not lost on his contemporaries. Wernicke, for example, advanced an altogether different schema of classification founded on cerebral localization;[6] Hoche pointed out the need to pay attention to symptom-complexes rather than to individual symptoms as the elements of clinical investigation;[7] Bumke took issue with the over-inclusiveness of the whole dementia praecox concept.[8] More recently, the whole binary division of the functional psychoses has been challenged radically by sophisticated empirical research.[9] But perhaps the most searching assessment of Kraepelin's clinical work was made by Adolf Meyer who urged that much

safer clinical methods should be used than the largely prognostic considerations of Kraepelin and that dynamic formulations came closer to the needs of both physician and patient than the formal and peremptory dichotomy claimed by those who see but one of two fates, either manic-depressive disorder or dementia praecox.[10]

Towards the end of his career Kraepelin acknowledged that his efforts to delineate two separate functional psychoses had failed, but he did not relinquish his belief in the existence of the disease-entities which, he asserted, would eventually be established.[11] To evaluate his claim Jablensky and his colleagues have recently re-examined the clinical data on the original count- ing-cards relating to all 721 patients admitted to the Munich University Psychiatric Clinic in 1908, when Kraepelin himself supervised the diagnostic procedure. All the cards were assessed independently by two experienced clinicians: the information was rated by means of standardized diagnostic instruments and subjected to sophisticated statistical analysis. The analysis of the data on the 63 patients diagnosed originally as 'dementia praecox' and the 134 patients with 'manic-depressive insanity' demonstrated some degree of concordance between the original diagnostic groups and current diagnos- tic concepts, but the more significant findings ran counter to Kraepelin's expectations, for the clinical pictures proved to be more important than the longitudinal patterns of disease.[12]

Clinical science

Kraepelin's credo is developed most clearly in his late paper, 'Ends and means of psychiatric research'.[13] Here, re-affirming the role of general paresis as his prototype, he declared his central objective to be a 'search for unitary morbid processes' which, he states, 'always arise from similar definite causes. Apart from certain clinical features often difficult to appre- hend, the data for the recognition of such a process are chiefly the course and result, and, in certain groups, the post-mortem appearances.' Ultim- ately, for him the final common path of all such research was an under- standing of cerebral function and the relationship of dysfunction to mental symptoms.

> For a final decision one must be guided by the upshot of the case and, in the event of death, by the finer post-mortem appearances of the brain; also, in certain circumstances, by the history of onset, but only in a minor degree by the details of the clinical picture.... What we require above all is a clear characterization of the post-mortem appearances of the brain in as many morbid processes as possible.[14]

Along with neurobiological study of the brain and the influences on it, especially endocrinological, went animal experiments and psychological research on man:

> By the elaborate methods of experimental psychology we can obtain a more exact picture of the change produced in the mental life by natural processes of disease. So far as the patient is at all amenable to such experiment, we may be able to make out whether and in what degree the perception and understanding of external impressions, their retention in the memory, the rapidity of processes of thought, the content of ideas,

the aptitude for improvement through practice, the susceptibility to fatigue, the release of voluntary impulses, the execution of simple movements, and the finer performances of speech and writing, are affected and altered by morbific influences.[15]

To help investigate these phenomena Kraepelin included the study of the effects of drugs, and his work on 'pharmacopsychology' constitutes an early attempt to foreshadow an important aspect of psychopharmacological inquiry. He also acknowledged the need to study the key concept of personality in his approach to mental disorder, always emphasizing objective inquiry into noxious influences on the life-cycle, e.g. genetic and developmental insults, injuries, toxins, degenerative change, infection, drugs and adverse environmental factors. In addition, he strongly advocated the sub-discipline of what he called 'comparative psychiatry' as a means of elucidating the causes of mental disorders and of determining the influences on their forms of presentation. In 1904 he visited the asylum of Buitenzorg in Java to examine the similarities and differences between European patients and those from an alien culture. And with the passage of time comparative psychiatry was to become more than a forerunner of the transcultural study of psychosis. It was to extend beyond institutional illness to the population at large:

The ultimate problem of comparative psychiatry is the determination of the influence of personal disposition or liability to insanity and on the forms that insanity assumes. Of prime importance in both these respects is the original mental make-up of the individual, his intellectual development, his temperamental disposition and the qualities of his will, which to some extent, however, can be altered by his conditions of life. For characterising the personality in all these aspects we must invoke the analytical and mensural resources of psychological experiment. This enables us, in some directions at any rate, to resolve our general impressions into clearly defined details. Least accessible by such means are the emotional processes, though even here, by examination of the various kinds of expressive movement, of speech and writing, and of involuntary expressions, as well as of the pulse, the blood-pressure and the respiration, there is some prospect of obtaining valuable results. Such investigations will help to provide a survey of the various modes of composition of healthy personalities. By so determining the range of normal variation, we shall obtain a standard for measuring morbid deviations – a standard that will be of value, not merely for pure science, but for many practical purposes, as for estimating school capacity, military fitness, business talent and responsibility. A first attempt in this direction is seen in the procedure devised by Binet and Simon for gauging the mental efficiency of children of different ages...[16]

In statements of this type Kraepelin shows himself to be aware of the need for a much broader research framework than that with which his name is usually associated.

Thus far his viewpoint could reasonably be viewed as a logical extension of his own clinical experience. His outlook, however, embraced a much wider spectrum of mental disease:

> The effect of injuries apt to influence unfavourably the mental disposition of man expresses itself, as we may well understand, not exclusively, nor even perhaps most seriously in the occurrence of pronounced mental illness, but much rather in the numberless more or less shocking phenomena of everyday life in which the mental constitution of the members of the community is manifested. Important among these are suicide, crime, vagrancy and prostitution, the frequency and the motives for marriage, the tendency to produce and rear offspring, and the results of education in elementary and higher schools; to some extent military fitness, certain manifestations of political and religious life, migration from rural areas into towns, business enterprise, and much else... The investigation of such phenomena affords insight therefore into the metamorphoses of the popular mind. The study of such manifestations of the popular mind furnishes a means of recognising betimes and so perhaps of counteracting, untoward and dangerous changes in its behaviour.... A mass psychiatry, having at its disposal statistics in their widest scope, must provide the foundations of a science of public mental health – a preventive psychological medicine for combating all those mischiefs that we group under the head of mental degeneracy.[17]

Nowadays this would be regarded as the province of psychiatric epidemiology. Kraepelin himself did not engage in epidemiological work along these lines, but the research programme at the Institute that he founded in the last decade of his life included biometrics and epidemiology along with neurobiology and physiological psychology to demonstrate the importance of a multidisciplinary approach for mental illness. This achievement was arguably his most durable contribution, as testified by the subsequent creation of similar institutions in other European and North American centres, and it underpins the verdict of Jablensky *et al.*, that

> Kraepelin's approach to the study of mental disorders was essentially a natural scientist's approach of an astonishing breadth. He relied on objective observation but was fully aware of the problems of observer bias and reliability; he introduced the psychological and pharmacological experiment as well as statistics, in clinical research; maintained a keen interest in technological innovation; and regarded nosological groupings as working hypotheses in continual need of testing and reformulating.[18]

This judgement has been widely endorsed, often without reservation, by Kraepelin's many admirers. The statement that 'Modern psychiatry begins with Kraepelin' which appears in a weighty English textbook[19] accords with most contemporary opinion. It has received powerful support from many 'biological' psychiatrists worldwide; and it is explicitly acknowledged by the so-called neo-Kraepelinian movement in North America where it is embodied in the systems of classification developed in the third and fourth editions of the *Diagnostic and Statistical Manual*.

The man and his outlook

This is the familiar professional face of Emil Kraepelin. It is, however, a one-sided picture. His other face belongs to the man whom my colleague at Heidelberg preferred to term Professor Kraepelin, a man whose contributions were rather different and have been much less publicized. They are of some interest both in their own right and for their wider implications but to put them in perspective demands a little more knowledge about the man and his background in time and place.

During his lifetime Kraepelin was well-known for his personal reserve and his distaste for any invasion of privacy. Contemporary accounts portray him as an energetic, determined, kindly man, with an unshakeable belief in his own capacity and in natural science, revered by his family and friends and respected by his opponents. He quotes with approval Heinroth's rules of professional conduct for the physician:

> ...he must possess good health and physical endurance.... He must be fearless and not shun toil.... His profession must interest him and take first place in his life; he must practice it with fervour and with love. He must be sincere, trustworthy and sympathetic.... He must have the power to be firm as well as gentle.... He must be not only a man of science and art but also a doctor in the broad sense of the word – one educated through study and skilled through practice. He must be neither a rank empiricist nor an idle speculator. He must adhere to the world of nature and live in the world of ideas. He must be guided by reason in his struggle against the absence of reason. He must be experienced in the ways of the world and know how to treat men as individuals. Finally, he must thoroughly understand from both the theoretical and the practical viewpoint the psychic methods of treatment of every expert, not just one therapeutic practice. He must have the capacity to experiment and to observe. If he is to advance the science of psychiatry, he must exhibit intelligence, not fanaticism; true genius is methodical but not mechanical.[20]

While this may correspond to some sort of ideal of a psychiatric registrar or consultant, to me it exhibits a touch of what Coleridge, who knew and admired the German nation, regarded as its besetting fault – what he called nimiety or too-muchness. And it does not need speculation or psychological theorizing to show that it is a misleadingly superficial picture which conceals the complex inner world emerging from Kraepelin's memoirs, his autobiography, his lesser-known writings and his poetry. These depict a restless, solitary spirit without a formal religious faith but with the quasi-mystical yearnings so often associated with German Romanticism. His internal conflicts are apparent. Not every self-professed atheist, for example, would admit that 'I consider the dogma of Buddha to be the greatest religious philosophical achievement of the human intellect'; on the authority of his daughter, Frau Dr Schmidt-Kraepelin, we know that during the last year of his life he was preoccupied with Buddhist teachings and was planning to visit Buddhist shrines in India at the time of his death. Nor can the image of the detached natural scientist be readily reconciled with a long-standing identification with the prophet Moses who so gripped his imagination as to impel him to stand before the statue of Moses in the library of Congress in Washington, DC and remark: 'I shall meet the fate of Moses. I too shall see the Promised Land from afar and then lay myself down and die.' The inner tension between a love of order and a longing for unrestrained freedom constitutes a major theme of his published poems. While these are totally devoid of literary merit they are of some autobiographical interest. Here, for example, is a quotation from a poem entitled 'Freedom':

The torment of his discord who can tell?
How brims life's chalice oft with gall before me!
And yet, my deepest nature loves it well,
This rebel's strife! Without it I abhor me.

But there was one lode-star in Professor Kraepelin's troubled firmament. 'I have', he affirmed, 'felt myself more or less lonely all through my life ... I had, however, a strongly marked feeling of race and stock and also felt my inner independence as an essential trait of the German character. My whole heart belonged to my fatherland and I willingly flung away cool objectivity of judgement when it was a matter of defending German interests.'[21]

Germany and politics

To appreciate what he understood by the 'fatherland' and by 'German interests' calls for a brief reference to modern German history. Kraepelin came to maturity during the epoch which followed his country's victory in the Franco-Prussian war of 1870 and its subsequent unification. Under the chancellorship of Otto von Bismarck Germany rapidly became a mighty military power and a leading nation in every sphere of economic, material and intellectual activity. Great importance was attached to the natural sciences and their potential contribution to the Bismarckian state, which was originally conceived as a form of liberal autocracy. By the year 1900 it was possible for a German statesman to remark that Germany would be either the hammer or the anvil of the twentieth century, a metaphorical prediction of two world wars and a death toll of some 50 million people.

Medicine shared in these expanding developments and psychiatry was a major beneficiary. In the course of one generation the foundations of academic and institutional psychiatry had been laid by the end of the nineteenth century. Kraepelin himself sketched its evolution in his book, *One Hundred Years of Psychiatry* (1962).[22] By 1911 he calculated that some 500 institutions for the mentally ill had been constructed, and all German medical schools contained university departments of psychiatry. 'We are', he commented, 'in this respect superior to all other nations of the world.'

And not only in this respect. In Germany for a whole generation the notion of superiority, of national and racial superiority, had been supported by attempts to apply the biological sciences to socio-political issues. The whole tangled story has been unravelled by Paul Weindling in his monograph, *Health, Race and German Politics between National Unification and Nazism, 1870–1945*.[23] From the 1880s onwards the academic medico-scientific community, led by its professoriate, was increasingly preoccupied with human genetics, eugenics, 'racial hygiene', theories of degeneration, and monism, and with the adoption of such measures as abortion, sterilization, selective breeding and the prevention of alcohol consumption and venereal disease, all with the aim of improving racial purity. The physician, in Weindling's phrase, became 'the hygienic Führer of the Volk'. Psychiatrists played a major role in this movement and Kraepelin was prominent among them.

Just how far he was prepared to discard 'objectivity of judgement' in pursuit of his patriotic ideals emerges from the development of his medical and political work in the public domain. While still at Heidelberg he had formed the opinion that mental illnesses were above all social disorders and his views on the body politic (*Volkskorper*) are set out in his early paper on 'Crime as a social disease', in which he extrapolated from his clinical experience and attributed most criminal behaviour to what he called a 'congenitally inferior predisposition'.[24] In contrast to the fatalistic determinism which characterized his view of mental illnesses as essentially degenerative disorders, his approach to mental hygiene was altogether more positive. Basing his stand on his extensive experience of institutional psychiatry, he expressed himself forcibly on the prevention of alcoholism and syphilis, two of the indisputable causes of severe psychosis. In 1895 he advocated total abstinence from alcohol and thenceforward was a tireless, even a fanatical supporter of anti-alcohol campaigns.

On the outbreak of the First World War Kraepelin's nationalism became more intense and steadily grew as the outcome of the conflict became increasingly uncertain. Viewing venereal disease as a major threat to the health of the German army, he launched a personal campaign to establish a national screening programme which involved him in a tenacious but ultimately unsuccessful struggle with the Ministry of War. Frustrated by failure, he took up active politics. He joined the People's Committee for the Rapid Subjugation of England, a body dominated by right-wing members of the academic community. He helped to draw up the annexationist *Guidelines for Paths to Lasting Peace*. And he campaigned for the overthrow of the Chancellor and the introduction of a more authoritarian rule in Germany.

None of these projects came to fruition, as he admitted in a revealing poem:

Trusting in the wings of my will
I swore to dispatch the misery of my people,
To drive us through peril and danger
And fulfil the promise of their prosperity.
Arduous and long the journey. In bloody victories
And with an ardent heart did I execute my mission
To but one enemy was I to succumb:
The thanklessness and delusion of my own people.

The defeat of Germany left him an embittered man who devoted his post-war years to building up the German Research Institute for Psychiatry, of which he wrote in 1921:

Of course our institute should be the home of vigorous science. But at the same time we never want to lose sight of the ultimate goal envisioned by our patrons: to serve the nation's health and to work toward healing the deep wounds which bitter fate has inflicted upon our fatherland.[25]

What Kraepelin failed to realize, however, was that his fatherland was already a thing of the past. His fatherland was Bismarck's Germany, based originally on a liberal authoritarianism allied to military power and material prosperity which Max Weber had scornfully dismissed as a short-term political episode. 'What is truly German', said Weber, 'is held together only by the German language and by the spiritual life which manifests itself in it. ... The political aspect is merely one dimension, and an unhappy one at that, a history that proceeds from one catastrophe to another.' Kraepelin preferred Bismarck. In a paper on Bismarck's personality and achievements, written in 1920, he expressed unbounded admiration of the Iron Chancellor without appearing to appreciate that the dismissal of Bismarck and the ascendancy of Wilhelm II had heralded a new, aggressive chauvinism which was to be exacerbated by the defeat in the First World War.[26] In company with most like-minded members of the educated classes whose outlook had been formed in the heyday of Bismarck's era, Kraepelin interpreted the disastrous political and military consequences of pan-Germanic nationalism as the result of an unfortunate disease of the body politic which called for prompt treatment and rehabilitation. He was, in effect, assuming the role of a psycho-hygienic Führer, applying his own brand of biologically-based medical expertise to the political and social problems of the day. And in 1919 he made his views explicit in a paper entitled 'Psychiatric observations on contemporary issues', in which he declared himself to be 'a psychiatrist who takes a stand on contemporary issues, reporting from the perspective of his professional experience'.[27] A few extracts illustrate his conclusions:

On war:

> ...there can be absolutely no talk whatsoever of a morbid disorder. The drive of self-assertion is the primal and most powerful force behind all individual and group action.

On the German emperor, William II:

> ...it is simply impossible in the case of William II to posit the existence of an acute mental disorder.

On sex differences:

> Based upon broad experience I believe we can view these apparently arbitrary upheavals of the will as the response of primal defence mechanisms to the dangers of life.... In the case of the mature and emotionally well-anchored male, these antiquated defence mechanisms against overwhelming external pressures no longer have a role to play... it was the women who proved to be ill-prepared for the prolonged state of war and who tormented their sons and husbands at the front with their complaints and who at times breached the trust of those in the field.

On 'individuals with distinctly hysterical traits':

> among the leaders of current and past upheavals one also finds a surprising number of people who in one way or another fall outside the bounds of normality.

In this latter category he includes 'dreamers and poets, swindlers and Jews':

> The active participation of the Jewish race in political upheavals has something to do with this [morbidity]. The frequency of psychopathic

predisposition in Jews could have played a role, although it is their harping criticism, their rhetorical and theatrical abilities, and their doggedness and determination which are most important.

On the causes of social unrest:

What struck the informed observer was the wholesale ignorance of the collective psyche.... Experience with accident neurosis has shown that providing pensions to those unwilling to return to work breeds an artificial work-disability which under certain circumstances can result in lasting mental decrepitation.... The government measures presume that humans by nature tend to perform their duties, to work hard and to commit themselves to the common good. The development of every child teaches us that this conviction is false ... we cannot escape the fact that the natural and self-evident drive behind all actions is selfishness and that in the case of popular rule this selfishness will seek its due with violent force as soon as the powers of the state designed to hold it in check are destroyed.... It must be made absolutely clear that the stratification of human society is certainly far more the expression than the cause of the immeasurable inequality among humans. Accordingly, the emergence of classes of people would very much depend, if not for the individual then certainly for the succession of the lineages, on those abilities which come to be developed in them. And the proletariat would be chiefly a conglomeration of those countrymen whose ancestors could not, over the centuries, rise to the top ... true popular rule is entirely impossible. Invariably the masses submit to individual leaders who by virtue of certain qualities have risen to the top. They are true leaders; those led by them are left with only the appearance of sovereignty. It is not they who decide, but rather the superior leaders who understand how to force the others to follow.

On future measures:

We will have to work systematically and employ all of our resources in the physical, mental and moral regeneration of our people. The essential framework has already been explicated numerous times during the course of the war, especially by doctors. Attention must be focused above all on the fight against all those influences threatening to destroy future generations, in particular hereditary degeneration and genetic influences resulting from alcohol and syphilis. Furthermore, the following will be necessary: the greater possible encouragement of early marriage, the fostering and strengthening of the joys of parenthood, the protection of the younger generation from the changes of physical, mental and moral neglect, the strengthening of the body, of the mind, and in particular of the will, by means of their regular and appropriate engagement.

This is not merely the language of pseudo-science. In its historical context it carries the disturbing political overtones of proto-fascism. It gives more sophisticated expression to the rhetoric being fed to the brown-shirted ruffians who were then congregating in the nearby Munich beer-cellars to form the nucleus of the National Socialist party, and at first sight it is difficult to reconcile with the objective outlook and independence of mind exhibited by Emil Kraepelin, the clinician and natural scientist. But Professor Kraepelin belonged to a different thought-collective, one which incorporated ideas and sentiments that led to an implacable opposition to the Weimar Republic and which contributed to the demise of democratic government in 1932.

The historian A.J.P. Taylor has summarized the tragic outcome succinctly:

> The defeat of Germany and the fall of the monarchy in 1918 threw the admirers of Bismarck into confusion.... The great majority of the Bismarckians, with the university professors at their head, remained faithful to the dead monarchy.... They still prized the Rechtstaat, the rule of law, but they supposed it would survive the overthrow of the republic.... The Bismarckians got their way. The republic was overthrown by Hitler in 1933.... Then the Bismarckians discovered to their horror that, while they had got everything they wanted, they had also lost everything that they prized. The Rechtstaat, the rule of law, had vanished. The Nazi barbarians ruled.... Once more, as in 1914, the respectable Germans of all classes tried to present the war (1939–45) as one of defence, and they clung desperately to the hope that the Rechtstaat would be restored when the war was over.[28]

Their hopes were to be sadly disappointed.

Implications and conclusion

Dying as he did in 1926, Kraepelin was spared involvement in these terrible events. We cannot know whether, like the overwhelming majority of German professors, he would have voted for Hitler in 1932. Or what he would have made of the version of his fatherland adopted by the Third Reich. Or how he would have responded to developments within his own Institute in the 1930s, when his close associate and successor – the psychiatric geneticist Ernst Rüdin – joined the Nazi party and participated actively in the racial hygiene programme that was to lead to a policy of genocide and the nimiety of the gas chambers. Or if he could ever have accepted Fritz Stern's considered verdict that from 1933 to 1945 the German academic profession, with medicine and psychiatry in the vanguard, furnished 'the most flagrant example of a *trahison des clercs* in the twentieth century'.[29]

What general lessons can be learnt from this brief scrutiny of Kraepelin's two faces? I would suggest that there are two major conclusions of contemporary relevance, one negative and the other positive.

The first of these is simple. Kraepelin's reputation, derived from a partial knowledge of the man and his work, is iconic. Icons exist to be worshipped, but a touch of iconoclasm is a safer bet. Histographical research is making it clear that, with a handful of exceptions, the leading figures in the history of psychiatry exhibit far too much clay below the ankles. Kraepelin is one among many.

The second, more complex issue has to do with ethics. Sir Aubrey Lewis always insisted on posing the question: 'How far can the psychiatrist keep his *Weltanschauung*, his general philosophy of life, apart from his scientific medical work?'.[30] He concluded:

> Nobody in psychiatry can do without a philosophical background, but very often it is an implicit and not an explicit one....This matter has received much less attention than it deserves. Philosophical influences, social influences, religious influences, ideological influences, all play their part in moulding the mental outlook of psychiatrists. We need to acknowledge and reckon with this when we are trying to establish a truly sound scientific discipline of psychiatry.

Kraepelin would have disagreed. He equated the true beginnings of his discipline with what he called 'the victory of scientific observation over philosophical and moral meditation'. The weaknesses of his position, however, were searchingly exposed by Karl Jaspers, a more profound German psychiatrist/philosopher, who pointed out that the supposedly atheoretical Kraepelinian system is replete with such implicit philosophical concepts as Kantian disease-entities, the cloudy notion of the 'will' and an idealistic version of the mind–brain nexus. And while acknowledging its heuristic value in providing testable biological hypotheses Jaspers observed that

> ...the biology of this so-called 'biological psychiatry'...expresses the drive of an idea, a philosophical tendency, which perhaps does not quite understand itself but as an object for scientific research it appears quite baseless...Science is wrongly identified with natural science...Natural science is indeed the groundwork of psychopathology and an essential element in it but the humanities are equally so and, with this, psychopathology does not become in any way less scientific but scientific in a different way.[31]

This critique raises the crucial question of precisely what philosophical position should be adopted by psychiatrists. That large topic goes far beyond my remit, but its shadow falls on the two faces of Professor Emil

Kraepelin. Three contemporary observers have justly concluded that probably his greatest and longest-lasting influence lies in 'the impetus that he gave to psychiatric research'.[32] It detracts in no way from his achievements as a clinical scientist to point out that his philosophical amblyopia, allied to the ineradicably chauvinistic elements in his outlook – formed in his youth and shared by many others as part of a national consciousness – resulted in a failure to demarcate the boundaries of his professional expertise and seriously distorted his judgement on the wider implications of his own contributions. He was guilty of what medieval scholastics termed *ignoratio elenchi* and modern logicians call category error. Taken as a whole his work illustrates not only the potential value but also the evident limitations of natural science, *Naturwissenschaft*, in the study of human behaviour. Both lessons are highly relevant to the theory and practice of psychological medicine today.

References

1   A. Lewis, 'Edward Mapother and the making of the Maudsley Hospital', *British Journal of Psychiatry*, 1969, 115: 1349–66.
2   J. Zubin, 'Closing comments', in H. Häfner, W.F. Gattaz, and W. Janzarik (eds) *Search for the Causes of Schizophrenia*, Berlin, Springer-Verlag, 1987, p. 359.
3   G. Zilboorg, *A History of Medical Psychology*, New York, Norton, 1941, pp. 434–5.
4   E. Kraepelin, *Memoirs*, trans. C. Wooding-Deane, Berlin, Springer-Verlag, 1987.
5   ibid.
6   C. Wernicke, *Fundamentals of Psychiatry*, Leipzig, Thieme, 1906.
7   A. Hoche, 'The significance of symptom complexes in psychiatry', trans. R.G. Dening and T.R. Dening, *History of Psychiatry*, 1991, 2: 334–43.
8   O. Bumke, 'The dissolution of dementia praecox', trans. Per Halen, *History of Psychiatry*, 1993, 4: 133–9.
9   T.J. Crow, 'Psychosis as a continuum and the virogenic concept', *British Medical Bulletin*, 1987, 43: 754–67.
10 A. Meyer, 'Constructive formulation of schizophrenia', *American Journal of Psychiatry*, 1922, 1: 355–62.
11 E. Kraepelin, 'Patterns of mental disorder', trans. H. Marshall, in S.R. Hirsch and M. Shepherd, *Themes and Variations in European Psychiatry*, Bristol, John Wright, 1974, pp. 7–30.
12 A. Jablensky, H. Hagler, M. von Cranach *et al.*, 'Kraepelin revisted: a reassessment and statistical analysis of dementia praecox and manic-depressive insanity in 1908', *Psychological Medicine*, 1993, 23: 848–58.
13 E. Kraepelin, 'Ends and means of psychiatric research', trans. Sydney J. Cole, *Journal of Mental Science*, 1922, 68: 115–43.
14 ibid.
15 ibid.
16 ibid.
17 ibid.
18 Jablensky *et al.*, op. cit.
19 E. Slater and M. Roth, *Clinical Psychiatry*, 3rd edn, London, Baillière, Tindall & Cassell, 1969, p. 10.

20 E. Kraepelin, *One Hundred Years of Psychiatry*, trans. W. Baskin, New York, The Citadel Press, 1962, pp. 107–8.
21 L. Brink and S.E. Jolliffe, 'Emil Kraepelin, psychiatrist and poet', *Journal of Nervous and Mental Disease*, 1932, 66: 274–82.
22 Kraepelin, *One Hundred Years*, op. cit.
23 P. Weindling, *Health, Race and German Politics between National Unification and Nazism, 1870–1945*, Cambridge, Cambridge University Press, 1989.
24 E. Kraepelin, 'Verbrechen als soziale Krankheit' (Crime as a social illness), *Monatschrift K/S*, 1906/7: 258–65.
25 E. Kraepelin, 'German Research Institute', *Journal of Nervous and Mental Disease*, 1922, 56: 209–14.
26 E. Kraepelin, 'Bismarcks persönlichkeit. Ungedrukte persönliche erinnerungen' (Bismarck's personality. Unpublished personal memories), *Süddeutsche Monatshefte*, 1921, 19: 105–22.
27 E. Kraepelin, 'Psychiatric observations on contemporary issues', trans. E.J. Engstrom, *History of Psychiatry*, 1992, 3: 259–69.
28 A.J.P. Taylor, *Bismarck*, London, Hamish Hamilton, 1955.
29 F. Stern, 'Analysts without resistance: psychotherapy and psychologists under National Socialism, *New York Review of Books*, 1986, 25: 172–90.
30 A. Lewis, 'Dilemmas in psychiatry', *Psychological Medicine*, 1991: 581–5.
31 K. Jaspers, *General Psychopathology*, trans. J. Hoenig and M.W. Hamilton, Manchester, Manchester University Press, 1963, p. 591.
32 H. Hippius, G. Peters, and D. Ploog, 'Foreword', in Kraepelin, *Memoirs*, op. cit., p. xi.

Select bibliography

Books

1 *A Study of the Major Psychoses in an English County.* Maudsley Monograph Series, No. 3, Chapman and Hall, 1957.

2 *The Teaching of Psychiatry in the United States.* Pitman Medical, 1963.

3 *Psychiatric Education* (joint editor with D.L. Davies). Pitman Medical, 1964.

4 *Psychiatric Illness in General Practice* (with B. Cooper, A.C. Brown, and G.W. Kalton). Oxford University Press, 1966, 2nd edition (additional material jointly with A.W. Clare), 1981.

5 *Studies in Psychiatry* (joint editor with D.L. Davies). Oxford University Press, 1968.

6 *Clinical Psychopharmacology* (with M.H. Lader and R. Rodnight). English Universities Press, 1968.

7 *An Experimental Approach to Psychiatric Diagnosis* (with E.M. Brooke, J.E. Cooper, and T.Y. Lin). *Acta Psychiatrica Scandinavica* Supplement 201, 1968.

8 *Childhood Behaviour and Mental Health* (with A.N. Oppenheim and S. Mitchell). London University Press, 1971.

9 *Themes and Variations in European Psychiatry* (joint editor with S.R. Hirsch). Bristol, John Wright, 1974.

10 *A Multi-axial Classification of Child Psychiatric Disorders* (with M. Rutter and D. Shaffer). World Health Organization, 1975.

11 *The Career and Contributions of Sir Aubrey Lewis.* The Bethlem Royal and Maudsley Hospitals, 1977.

12 *Psychotropic Drugs in Psychiatry.* Jason Aronson, 1981.

13 *Psychiatrists on Psychiatry* (editor). Cambridge University Press, 1982.

14 *Handbook of Psychiatry*, 5 vols (general editor). Cambridge University Press, 1982–4.

15 *The Psychosocial Matrix of Psychiatry: Collected Papers.* Tavistock, 1983.

16 *The Spectrum of Psychiatric Research.* Cambridge University Press, 1984.

17 *Sherlock Holmes and the Case of Dr Freud.* Tavistock, 1985.

18 *The Anatomy of Madness* (joint editor with W.F. Bynum and R. Porter). *Vol. I: People and Ideas.* Tavistock, 1985. *Vol. II: Institutions and Society.* Tavistock, 1985.

19 *Mental Illness in Primary Care Settings* (joint editor with G. Wilkinson and P. Williams). Tavistock, 1986.

20 *The Clinical Roots of the Schizophrenia Concept* (joint editor with J. Cutting). Cambridge University Press, 1986.

21 *Minor Psychiatric Morbidity and General Practice Consultations: the West London Survey* (with P. Williams, A. Tarnopolsky, and D.J. Hand). Psychological Medicine Monograph Supplement, No. 9. Cambridge University Press, 1987.

22 *A Representative Psychiatrist: The Career, Contributions and Legacies of Sir Aubrey Lewis.* Psychological Medicine Monograph Supplement, No. 10. Cambridge University Press, 1987.

23 *The Classification of Mental Disorder in Primary Care* (with R. Jenkins and N. Smeeton). Psychological Medicine Monograph Supplement, No. 12. Cambridge University Press, 1988.

24 *The Anatomy of Madness* (joint editor with W.F. Bynum and R. Porter) *Vol. III: The Asylum and its Psychiatry.* Routledge, 1988.

25 *The Natural History of Schizophrenia* (with D.C. Watt, I. Falloon, and N. Smeeton). Psychological Medicine Monograph Supplement, No. 14. Cambridge University Press, 1989.

26 *Non-specific Aspects of Treatment* (joint editor with N. Sartorius). Huber, 1989.

Contributions to books

1 Reserpine and clinical trials. In *Psychotropic Drugs* (eds S. Garattini and V. Ghetti). Elsevier, p. 565, 1957.

2 Reserpine use in the schizophrenias. In *Psychopharmacology Frontiers.* Proceedings of the Psychopharmacology Symposium of the 2nd International Congress of Psychiatry, Zurich. Boston, Little, Brown and Co. p. 57, 1959.

3 Methods and analysis of drug-induced abnormal mental states in man. In *Neuro-Psychopharmacology* (ed. P.B. Bradley). Elsevier, p. 91, 1959.

4 The influence of specific and non-specific factors on the clinical effects of psychotropic drugs. In *Neuro- Psychopharmacology* (ed. E. Rothlin). Proceedings of the 2nd International Meeting of the Collegium Internationale Neuro-Psychopharmacologicum, Basle. Elsevier, p. 183, 1961.

5 Pharmacological aspects of psychiatry (with L. Wing). In *Advances in Pharmacology* (eds S. Garattini and P.A. Shore). New York, Academic Press, p. 277, 1962.

6 Clinical and social factors relevant to outcome. In *The Burden on the Community: The Epidemiology of Mental Illness.* Nuffield Provincial Hospitals Trust Symposium. Oxford University Press, p. 60, 1962.

7 Comparative psychiatric treatment in different countries. In *Aspects of Psychiatric Research* (eds D. Richter, J.M. Tanner, Lord Taylor, and O.L. Zangwill). Oxford University Press, p. 110, 1962.

8 The effectiveness of drugs in relationship to psychological and social forms of treatment. In *Neuropsychopharmacology* (eds P.B. Bradley, F. Flugel, and P. Hoch). Elsevier, p. 139, 1964.

9 Psychiatric education: general review and future needs. In *Psychiatric Education* (eds M. Shepherd and D.L. Davies). Pitman Medical, 1964.

10 The tutorial system of teaching in psychiatry. In *Psychiatric Education* (eds M. Shepherd and D.L. Davies). Pitman Medical, 1964.

11 Centrally acting drugs. In *Evaluation of New Drugs in Man* (ed. E. Zaimis). Pergamon, p. 111, 1965.

12 The method of the multi-centred clinical trial. In *Proceedings of the V International Congress of the Collegium Internationale Neuropsychopharmacologicum.* Excerpta Medica, p. 51, 1966.

13 Implications of a multi-centred clinical trial of treatments of depressive illness. In *Anti-Depressant Drugs* (ed. S. Garattini). Excerpta Medica, p. 332, 1967.

14 Some aspects of clinical trials in psychiatry. In *Practical Treatment in Psychiatry* (ed. J.L. Crammer). Blackwell Scientific, p. 145, 1969.

15 Life change, stress and mental disorder: the ecological approach (with B. Cooper). In *Modern Trends in Psychological Medicine* (ed. J.H. Price). Butterworths, p. 102, 1970.

16 Evaluation of psychotropic drugs in the treatment of depression: 1959–1969. In *The Principles and Practice of Clinical Trials* (eds E.L. Harris and J.D. Fitzgerald). Livingstone, p. 199, 1970.

17 Some teaching methods at the Institute of Psychiatry. In *The Training of Psychiatrists*, (eds G.F.M. Russell and H.J. Walton). Headley Bros., p. 70, 1970.

18 Programme formation (curricula). In *The Training of Psychiatrists* (eds G.F.M. Russell and H.J. Walton). Headley Bros., p. 82, 1970.

19 Clinical outcome and the teaching of psychiatry. In *Clinical Tutors in Psychiatry* (eds D.C. Watt and B. Barraclough). Royal Medico-Psychological Association, p. 56, 1970.

20 A critical review of clinical drug trials. In *Depression in the 1970s* (ed. R.R. Fieve). Excerpta Medica, p. 105, 1971.

21 Childhood behaviour, mental health, and medical services. In *Problems and Progress in Medical Care* (ed. G. McLachlan). Oxford University Press, p. 89, 1971.

22 Psychological medicine. In *Price's Textbook of the Practice of Medicine*, 11th edition (ed. R. Bodley Scott). Oxford University Press, p. 1331, 1972.

23 Clinical psychopharmacology (with R.H.S. Mindham). In *Recent Advances in Medicine* (eds D.N. Baron, N. Compston, and A.M. Dawson). Churchill Livingstone, p. 293, 1973.

24 Epidemiology and abnormal psychology (with B. Cooper). In *Handbook of Abnormal Psychology* (ed. H.J. Eysenck). Pitman, p. 34, 1973.

25 A study of psychiatric disorders of old age identified in general practice. In *Portfolio for Health: 2.* Oxford University Press, 49, 1973.

26 Progress and problems in mental health. In *Benefits and Risks in Medical Care* (ed. D. Taylor). Office of Health Economics, p. 43, 1974.

27 Continuation treatment with antidepressant medication. In *Psihofarmakologija 3* (eds N. Bohacek and M. Mihovilovic). Zagreb, Medicinska Naklada, p. 227, 1974.

28 The evaluation of treatment in psychiatry. In *Methods of Psychiatric Research*, 2nd edition (eds P. Sainsbury and N. Kreitman). Oxford University Press, p. 88, 1975.

29 Epidemiologische Psychiatrie. In *Psychiatrie der Gegenwart*, Vol. III, 2nd edition (eds K.P. Kisker, J.-E. Meyer, C. Müller, and E. Strömgren). Springer, p. 119, 1975.

30 Impact of long-term neuroleptics on the community: advantages and disadvantages (with D.C. Watt). In *Neuropsychopharmacology* (eds J.R. Boissier, H. Hippius, and P. Pichot). Excerpta Medica, p. 379, 1975.

31 Neurosis: the epidemiological perspective. In *Research In Neurosis* (ed. H.M. van Praag). Bohn, Scheltema, Holkema, and Netherlands, 1976.

32 Definition, classification and nomenclature: a clinical overview. In *Schizophrenia Today* (eds D. Kemali, G. Bartholini, and D. Richter). Pergamon, p. 3, 1976.

33 Beyond the layman's madness: the extent of mental disease. In *Developments in Psychiatric Research* (ed. J.M. Tanner). London, Hodder & Stoughton, 1977.

34 Long-term treatment with neuroleptics in psychiatry (with D.C. Watt). In *Current Developments in Psychopharmacology*, Vol. 4, 1977.

35 Psychiatry and family practice (with A.W. Clare). In *Scientific Foundations of Family Medicine* (eds J. Fry, E. Gambrill, and R. Smith). Heinemann, 1978.
36 Psychological Medicine. In *Price's Textbook of the Practice of Medicine*, 12th edition (ed. R. Bodley Scott). Oxford University Press, p. 1405, 1979.
37 Epidémiologie et limites des maladies mentales. Symposium *Biologie du Cerveau et Maladies Mentales*, Paris, Psychologie Médicale 11:6, 1976.
38 Mental health and primary care in the seventeenth century. *Acta Psychiatrica Scandinavica*, Supplement 285, Vol. 62: 121, 1980.
39 Reluctance to go to school (with S. Mitchell). In *Out of School* (eds L. Hersov and I. Berg). John Wiley, p. 7, 1980.
40 Psychosocial disorder in primary medical care (with P. Williams). In *Symptoms, Illness Behaviour and Help-seeking* (ed. D. Mechanic). Prodist, p. 115, 1982.
41 The application of the epidemiological method in psychiatry. In *Epidemiology and Mental Health Services: Principles and Applications in Developing Countries* (eds T.A. Baasher, J.E. Cooper, H. Davidian, A. Jablensky, N. Sartorius, and E. Strömgren). *Acta Psychiatrica Scandinavica*, Suppl. 296, Vol. 265, p. 9, Copenhagen, Munksgaard, 1982.
42 The sciences and general psychopathology. In *Handbook of Psychiatry*, Vol. 1 (eds M. Shepherd and O.L. Zangwill), p. 1. Cambridge, Cambridge University Press, 1983.
43 Mental illness and general practice (with R. Jenkins). In *Mental Illness: Changes and Trends* (ed. P. Bean). Chichester, Wiley, p. 379, 1983.
44 Social criteria of the outcome of mental disease. In *Measuring the Social Benefits of Medicine* (ed. G. Teeling- Smith). Office of Health Economics, London, 1983.
45 Epidemiology of mental disorder in the elderly. In *Book of Proceedings I. 3rd European Symposium on Social Psychiatry*, 12–15 Sept. 1982. Finnish Association for Mental Health.
46 Promotion of research in psychiatry. In *Training and Education in Psychiatry* (eds J.J. López Ibor Alino and G. Lenz). Facultas-Verlag, Vienna, pp. 201–4, 1984.
47 The application of public health methods to control: psychiatric. In *Oxford Textbook of Public Health, vol. 4* (eds W.W. Holland, R. Detels, and G. Knox). Oxford Medical Publications, Oxford University Press, pp. 102–11, 1985.
48 Contribution of epidemiological research to the classification and diagnosis of mental disorders. In *Mental Disorders: Alcohol- and Drug-related Problems*. Excerpta Medica, International Congress Series 669, pp. 337–41, 1985.
49 Epidemiologica psichiatrica e psichiatria epidemiologica. In *L'Approccio Epidemiologico in Psichiatria* (ed. M. Tansella). Boringhieri, Turin, 1985.
50 Formulation of new research strategies in schizophrenia. In *Search for the Causes of Schizophrenia* (eds H. Häfner, W.F. Gattaz, and W. Janzarik). Berlin, Springer Verlag, pp. 29–38, 1987.
51 Introduction to *The Natural History of Disease* by John Ryle. The Keynes Press, British Medical Association, London, pp. xi–xix, 1988.
52 The primary care of mental health in the community. In *Proceedings of the Regional Symposium on Mental Health Community Services*. World Psychiatric Association and Spanish Neuropsychiatric Association, Granada, pp. 19–25, 1989.

Contributions to journals

1 Reserpine in the treatment of anxious and depressed patients. *Lancet* 2: 117, 1955.
2 Unusually severe lesions in the brain following Status Epilepticus, *Journal of Neurology, Neurosurgery and Psychiatry* 18: 24, 1955.

3   Report of a family suffering from Friedreich's Disease, personal muscular atrophy and schizophrenia. *Journal of Neurology, Neurosurgery and Psychiatry* 19: 297, 1955.

4   Chlorpromazine and reserpine in chronic schizophrenia: a controlled clinical study (with D.C. Watt). *Journal of Neurology, Neurosurgery and Psychiatry* 19: 232, 1956.

5   Reserpine: problems associated with the use of a so-called 'tranquillizing agent'. *Proceedings of the Royal Society of Medicine* 49: 849, 1956.

6   An English view of American psychiatry. *American Journal of Psychiatry* 114: 417, 1957.

7   Alcoholism: a medical and social problem. *Medical World* 87: 246, 1957.

8   The age for neuroses (with E.M. Gruenberg). *Milbank Memorial Fund Quarterly* 35: 258, 1957.

9   The social outcome of early schizophrenia. *Psychiatria et Neurologia* 137: 224, 1958.

10 Public health and psychiatry in Great Britain. *Medical Officer* 100: 141, 1958.

11 Evaluation of drugs in the treatment of depression. *Canadian Psychiatry Association Journal* 4: Special Supplement, 1959.

12 Psychiatric morbidity in an urban group practice. *Proceedings of the Royal Society of Medicine* 52: 269, 1959.

13 Psychiatric illness in the general hospital (with B. Davies and R.H. Culpan). *Acta Psychiatrica Neurologica Scandinavica* 35: 518, 1960.

14 Purines in the urine of normal and schizophrenic subjects (with B.M. Ballard, R.H. Culpan, N. Monks, and H. McIlwain). *Journal of Mental Science* 106: 1,250, 1960.

15 The epidemiology of neurosis. *International Journal of Social Psychiatry* 5: 276, 1960.

16 Morbid jealousy: Some clinical and social aspects of a psychiatric symptom. *Journal of Mental Science* 107: 687, 1961.

17 Neurosis in hospital and general practice (with W.I.N. Kessel). *Journal of Mental Science* 108: 159, 1962.

18 The teaching of undergraduate psychiatry in North America: its implications for the United Kingdom. *Lancet* 1: 457: 1963.

19 Epidemiology and mental disorder: a review (with B. Cooper). *Journal of Neurology, Neurosurgery and Psychiatry* 27: 277, 1964.

20 The health and attitudes of people who seldom consult a doctor (with W.I.N. Kessel). *Medical Care* 3: 6, 1965.

21 A study of the interaction between desmethylimipramine and tetrabenazine in normal man (with P. Dick). *Psychopharmacologia* 8: 32, 1965.

22 Interaction between centrally acting drugs in man: some general considerations. *Proceedings of the Royal Society of Medicine* 58: 964, 1965.

23 Childhood behaviour disorders and the child-guidance clinic: An epidemiological study (with A.N. Oppenheim and S. Mitchell). *Journal of Child Psychology and Psychiatry* 7: 39, 1966.

24 A comparative study of children's behaviour at home and at school (with S. Mitchell). *British Journal of Educational Psychology* XXXVI: 248, 1966.

25 The child who dislikes going to school (with S. Mitchell). *British Journal of Educational Psychology* XXXVII: 32, 1967.

26 Early evaluation of psychotropic drugs in man (with B. Blackwell). *Lancet* 2: 819, 1967.

27 Prophylactic lithium: another therapeutic myth? (with B. Blackwell). *Lancet* 1: 968: 1968.

28 Therapeutic problems with psychotropic drugs: some epidemiological considerations. *Psychiatria, Neurologia, Neurochirurgia* 72: 513, 1969.

29 The use and abuses of drugs in psychiatry. *Lancet* 1: 31, 1970.

30 Neuropsychiatric illness and neuropathological findings in a case of Klinefelter's syndrome (with I. Janota and A. Jablensky). *Psychological Medicine* 1: 18, 1970.

31 Research in the field of psychiatry. *Bulletin of the Swiss Academy of Medical Sciences* 25: 111, 1970.

32 A critical appraisal of contemporary psychiatry. *Comprehensive Psychiatry* 12: 302, 1971.

33 The classification of psychotropic drugs. *Psychological Medicine* 2: 96, 1972.

34 The benzodiazepines. *Prescribers' Journal* 12: 144, 1972.

35 Psychiatric education and the social function of the psychiatrist. *Social Science and Medicine* 7: 95, 1973.

36 An evaluation of continuation therapy with tricyclic antidepressants in depressive illness (with R.H.S. Mindham and C. Howland). *Psychological Medicine* 3: 5, 1973.

37 The prevalence and distribution of psychiatric illness in general practice. *Journal of the Royal College of General Practitioners* 23, Suppl. 2: 16, 1973.

38 General practice, mental illness, and the British National Health Service. *American Journal of Public Health* 64: 230, 1974.

39 Pollution and mental health, with particular reference to the problem of noise. *Psychiatria Clinica* 7: 226, 1974.

40 The case of Arise Evans: A historico-psychiatric study (with Christopher Hill). *Psychological Medicine* 6: 1976.

41 The extent of mental disorder. *Canadian Psychiatric Association Journal* 21: 401, 1976.

42 A representative psychiatrist: the career and contributions of Sir Aubrey Lewis. *American Journal of Psychiatry* 134: 1, January, 1977.

43 Aubrey Lewis: The making of a psychiatrist. *British Journal of Psychiatry* 131: 238, 1977.

44 Schizophrenia succeeded by affective illness: catemnestic study and statistical enquiry (with C. Sheldrick, A. Jablensky, and N. Sartorius). *Psychological Medicine* 7: 1977.

45 Increased brain dopamine and reduced glutamic acid decarboxylase and choline acetyl transferase activity in schizophrenia and related psychoses (with E.D. Bird, J. Barnes, L.L. Iversen, E.G. Spokes, and A.V.P. Mackay). *Lancet*, 3 Dec. 1977.

46 A comparative controlled trial of pimozide and fluphenazine decanoate in the continuation therapy of schizophrenia (with I. Falloon and D.C. Watt). *Psychological Medicine* 8, 1978.

47 The social outcome of patients in a trial of long-term continuation therapy in schizophrenia: pimozide vs. fluphenazine (with I. Falloon and D.C. Watt). *Psychological Medicine* 8: 265–74, 1978.

48 Epidemiology and clinical psychiatry. *British Journal of Psychiatry* 133: 289–98, 1978.

49 Epidemiological perspective: psychosomatic medicine. *International Journal of Epidemiology* 7: 3, 1978.

50 The psychohistorians. *Encounter*, March 1979.

51 Social work and the primary care of mental disorder (with B. Harwin, C. Depla, and V. Cairns). *Psychological Medicine* 9: 661–9, 1979.

52 Psychoanalysis, psychotherapy, and health services. *British Medical Journal* 2: 1,557–9, 1979.

53 Psychotropic drugs and taxonomic systems. *Psychological Medicine* 10: 25–33, 1980.
54 Medico-social evaluation of the long-term pharmacotherapy of schizophrenia. *Prog. Neuro-psychopharmacol.* 3: 383–9, May 1979.
55 From social medicine to social psychiatry: the achievement of Sir Aubrey Lewis. *Psychological Medicine* 211–18, 1980.
56 Continuation therapy with lithium and amitriptyline in unipolar and depressive illness: a controlled clinical trial (with A.I.M. Glen and A.L. Johnson). *Psychological Medicine* 11: 409–16, 1981.
57 Psychiatrie in England: Psychologische Medizin. *Psycho* 8, 1982.
58 The epidemiological approach to psychotropic medication. *Journal of the Royal Society of Medicine* 75, April 1982.
59 Who should treat mental disorders? *Lancet*, 22 May 1982.
60 Psychiatric research and primary care in Britain – past, present and future. *Psychological Medicine* 12: 493–9, 1982.
61 Karl Jaspers: General Psychopathology. *British Journal of Psychiatry* 141: 310, 1982.
62 Nosographie psychiatrique et psychotropes. *Psychologie Médicale* 14: 1963, 1982.
63 Psychiatric epidemiology and the classification of mental disorder. *International Journal of Epidemiology* 11: 312, 1982.
64 Psychogeriatrics and the neo-epidemiologists. *Psychological Medicine* 13: 697, 1983.
65 Social psychiatry and epidemiology. *The Practitioner*, Jan. 1983, Vol. 227, pp. 148–50.
66 Psychiatric research in medical perspective. *Archiv. für Psychiatrie und Nervenkrankenheiten* 232: 501–6, 1982.
67 Die Bedeutung des Hausarztes ist so gross wie noch nie. *Psycho* 9: 59–60, 1983.
68 Mental disorder and primary care in the United Kingdom. *Journal of Public Health Policy* 14, 1, March 1983.
69 Sleeping and dreaming. *British Medical Journal* 287, 1983.
70 The origins and directions of social psychiatry. *Integrative Psychiatry*, Sept./Oct. 1983, 86–8.
71 The natural history of schizophrenia: a prospective 5-year follow-up of a representative sample of schizophrenics by means of a standardized clinical and social assessment (with D.C. Watt and K. Katz). *Psychological Medicine* 13: 663–70, 1983.
72 La recherche en psychiatrie dans une optique médicale. *L'Évolution Psychiatrique* 48: 3, 1983.
73 Ursprunge und Richtungen der Sozialpsychiatrie. *Psycho* 9: 845–9, 1983.
74 Continuation therapy with lithium and amitryptiline in unipolar depressive illness: a randomised, double-blind controlled trial (with A.I.M. Glen and A.L. Johnson). *Psychological Medicine* 14: 37–50, 1984.
75 La découverte de la nature de la pellagre. *Acta Psychiatrica Belgica* 83: 295–303, 1984.
76 What price psychotherapy? *British Medical Journal* 288: 809–10, 1984.
77 Urban factors in mental disorders – an epidemiological approach. *British Medical Bulletin* 40(4): 401–4, 1984.
78 Biological markers in mental disorders. *Journal of Psychiatric Research* 18(4): 555–6, 1984.
79 The contribution of epidemiology to clinical psychiatry. *American Journal of Psychiatry* 141: 1,574–6, 1984.

80 Psychiatric epidemiology and epidemiological psychiatry. *American Journal of Public Health* 75(3): 275–6, 1985.

81 A study of the classification of mental ill-health in general practice (with R. Jenkins, M. Marinker and N. Smeeton). *Psychological Medicine* 15: 403–9, 1985.

82 Sozialpsychiatrie: die Geschichte eines Begriffs. *Gesnerus* 42: 425–31, 1985.

83 Healing in perversion. *Nature* 1985, 318, p. 515.

84 Gli Orizzonti della Psichiatria. Conversazione con Michael Shepherd, by G. de Girolamo. In *Rivista Sperimentale di Freniatria*, Vol. CX, 1986, pp. 3–28.

85 Whither psychiatry in the UK? *World Hospitals* 22(1): 17–19, 1986.

86 Psychological medicine redivivus: concept and communication. *Journal of the Royal Society of Medicine* 79: 639–45, 1986.

87 Jean Starobinski. *Lancet*, 1987, p. 798.

88 New drugs for mental diseases? *Journal of the Royal Society of Medicine*, 401–2, 1987.

89 The classification of mental disorders. *The Practitioner*, July 1987, vol. 231, p. 9.

90 Psychiatry and its historians. *Journal of the Royal Society of Medicine* 81: 63–4.

91 The logic of a myth. *Semiotica* 68: 155–7, 1988.

92 Primary care as the middle ground for psychiatric epidemiology (with G. Wilkinson). *Psychological Medicine* 18: 263–7, 1988.

93 Changing disciplines in psychiatry. *British Journal of Psychiatry* 18: 737–45, 1988.

94 Lectures and lecturers. *British Medical Journal* 297: 1,682–3, 1988.

95 The development of a computerized assessment for minor psychiatric disorder (with G. Lewis, A.J. Pelosi, E. Glover, G. Wilkinson, S.A. Stansfeld, and P. Williams). *Psychological Medicine* 18: 737–45, 1988.

96 Sir Aubrey Lewis, 1900–1975. *L'Évolution Psychiatrique* 53: 993–6, 1988.

97 Hinweis auf Jean Starobinski. *Nervenarzt* 60: 120, 1989.

98 Psychotherapy vs. pharmacotherapy. *Transmission* 1, 7: 4–7, 1989.

99 Primary care of patients with mental disorder in the community. *British Medical Journal* 299(6700): 666–9, 1989.

100 Twenty years on (editorial). *Psychological Medicine* 20: 1–2, 1990.

101 The hidden victims of disaster: helper stress. *Stress Medicine* 6(1): 29–35, 1990.

102 The 'neuroleptics' and the Oedipus effect. *Journal of Psychopharmacology* 4(3): 1990.

103 The management of psychiatric disorders in the community. The research magnificent. *Journal of the Royal Society of Medicine* 83: 219–22, 1990.

104 Primary care psychiatry: the case for action. *British Journal of General Practice* 41(347): 252–5, 1991.

105 Psychiatric journals and the evolution of psychological medicine. *Psychological Medicine* 22(1): 15–25, 1992.

106 Comparing need with resource allocation. *Health Visitor* 65(9): 303–6, 1992.

107 Historical epidemiology and the functional psychoses. *Psychological Medicine* 23(2): 301–4, 1993.

108 The placebo: from specificity to the non-specific and back. *Psychological Medicine* 120: 94–100, 1993.

109 Kraepelin and modern psychiatry. *European Archives of Psychiatry and Clinical Neuroscience* 245(4–5): 189–95, 1995.

Note: numerous book reviews, unsigned editorals, etc. have not been included in this selected list.

Name index

Alarcón, J. de 180
Anthony, E.J. 134–5, 136–7, 141
Auden, W.H. 15, 23

Babcock 174–5
Bell, J. 7, 16, 24
Berlin, I. 17
Blacker, C.P. 137
Bleuler, E. 31, 49, 81
Bowen, Stella 123–4
Brock, L. 77
Brophy, B. 23
Brown, G.W. 183
Bucknill, J. 91–2

Cairns, Sir Hugh 124–5
Chesterton, G.K. 3

Diderot, D. 96
Doyle, A. Conan 4, 5, 11, 13, 14, 15, 16
Dunham, D. 204, 205

Evans, A. 161; clinical status of 167–70; life of 165–7

Farr, W. 74, 76
Febvre, L. 161
Fleck, L. 101
Florey, Sir Howard 124, 126, 138
Frank, J. 217
Freud, S. 1–23, 50, 189, 302–3, 215
Fry, J. 199

Goldberger, J. 174–9
Gordon, M. 102–4
Gregg, A. 143, 144, 198
Griesinger, W. 27, 31, 86, 179, 189
Grotjahn, A. 74, 85
Gruhle, H.W. 27, 46, 49

Hauser, A. 12
Herrington, J.C. 175
Hill, A.B. 78, 83
Himmelfarb, G. 72
Holmes, Sherlock 1–23

Isherwood, C. 16

Janet, P. 218
Jaspers, K. 27, 41, 107–19, 160, 187–90
Jones, E. 5
Jortin, J. 168–9
Jung, C.G. 4, 19

Kardiner, A. 4
Kleist, K. 169–70
Kraepelin, E. 3, 27, 46, 49, 143, 144, 183, 221–37, 278; *see also* Subject index

Lewis, Sir Aubrey 44, 79, 122–50, 155; *see also* Subject index

Mairet, A. 42, 49
Malcolm, J. 215
Mapother, E. 136
Marcus, S. 21–2
Marshall, H. 97
Maudsley, H. 54–5, 71–2, 73, 97, 143, 145, 148
Medawar, P. 17
Meyer, J.E. 28
Meyer, N. 1, 5
Molière 184
Morelli, G. 9–12
Moriarty, Professor 1
Mumford, L. 201
Musto, D. 5–6

Oakeshott, M. 85, 108

Rank, O.   212–15
Rows, R.G.   76
Ryle, J.A.   74–5, 78, 83, 192–9

Shaw, G.B.   72
Steiner, G.   18
Stengel, E.   29, 70
Stephen, L.   96–7
Sydenstricker, E.   177
Symonds, Sir Charles   198

Thomas, D.M.   19–20
Tuke, H.   54–5
Tuke, T.D.   91, 218

Vico, G.   18
Virchow, R.   172–3

Voltaire   8, 17, 157, 158
von Feuchtersleben, E.   95

Watson, Dr J.H.   1, 5, 6, 22, 23
Watt, D.C.   79
Weber, M.   189, 199, 202
Webster, F.D.   197
White, W.A.   203
Wind, E.   11–12
Winslow, F.B.   92–4, 97, 105
Wolf Man, the (Pankeyev, S.K.)   3–4, 20–1
Woolf, V.   69–70

Young, G.M.   71–2, 73

Zadig: method of   6–9, 15, 20, 22

Subject index

actuarial assessment of illness-expectancy in relatives and in patients 184
Adelaide, in early twentieth century 123–5

behaviour disorder in childhood 84

causation of mental disorder 86; of schizophrenia 34–8
century: nineteenth 71–4; seventeenth 161–5
classification, and epidemiology of schizophrenia 28–31
cocaine 5–6
comparative anatomy 277

depression and 'learned helplessness' 118–19
detective fiction 1–4, 13–16; and myth 23
disposition, congenitally inferior criminal behaviour attributed to 231
distress, epidemiological studies of, and sub-clinical mental disorder 207–9

editors, medical 100–1, 104–5
endemiology 75
epidemiology 75, 114, 153, 155; controlled clinical trial 184; definition 172–3; diagnosis and classification 184; environmental factors 180–1; and genetics 180; host 180; 'illness-proneness' 182–3; investigating causation 178–9; in psychiatry 179–85; outcome and prognosis 183; spectrum of disease completion 182–3; transmission of mental disorders 179–80; Tristan da Cunha, volcanic eruption 180–1

existentialism 111
experimental psychology 226–7

General Psychopathology (K. Jaspers) 107–19, 187–90
genetics 116–17

Heidelberg University, anniversary celebration 221
history and mental disorder 160–1
Hutterites 20–4, 207

institutes of research 142–5

jealousy, morbid 39–58; associated disorders 44–9; concept of 39–40; forensic aspects of 53–7; management and outcome of 57–8; phenomenology of 42–4; psychopathology and social aspects of 49–53
Journal of Mental Science 76–7, 97, 98
Journal of Neurology and Psychopathology, Journal of Neurology, Neurosurgery and Psychiatry 98, 99
Journal of Psychological Medicine and Mental Pathology 91, 92
journals, medico-scientific 96–7, 101–5; psychiatric 97–9; *see also* *Psychological Medicine*

Kraepelin, E.: anti-alcoholism, his campaign for 231; his career 223–5; dementia praecox and manic-depressive psychosis, his separation of 224–6; degenerative disorders, mental illness as 231; his inner world 229–30; interviewed by Dr Joseph Zubin 222; his method and

weakness of, assessed by Jablensky
  et al. 225–6; his nationalism 231–2;
  pharmacopsychology 227;
  psychiatric epidemiology 228;
  psychiatry, his somatization of
  223–4; venereal disease, believed a
  threat to German army 232

law of scatter 101–2
lectures 69–71
Lewis, Sir Aubrey 122–50;
  anthropology, his view of 128–9;
  breakthrough in psychiatry 131–3;
  British Association of Teachers of
  Psychiatry, appreciation by 131;
  integrity of 132; Maudsley
  psychiatry, his views on 129;
  medicine, his choice of 125;
  psychiatry, his choice of
  128–9; scepticism of 131–2; at
  school 125; social psychiatry, his
  views on 130; undergraduate, period
  as 126–8

Maudsley Hospital, Mapother's making
  of 221
myth and reason 15–16; and
  imaginative understanding 17–19;
  and literature 19–23; and
  psychoanalysis 17–19

natural history of mental disorders 82;
  of schizophrenia 32–4
neurology 98–9
neuroses and personality disorders,
  epidemiological studies of 205–7
non-specific treatment 174–5

peer review 102–4
primary care, and epidemiology
  205–6
psychoanalysis 11–12, 212–13, 215;
  and literature 19–23; and morbid

jealousy 50–1; and myth 16–17,
  18–19, 23; theory of 122–3
psychological medicine, concept of
  94–5
Psychological Medicine (journal)
  99–100, 102
psychological understanding 109
psychopathology 95–6
psychotherapy 189–90, 217–19
psychotropic drugs, efficacy of 81, 83
public health 74, 76, 77–8, 79

racial purity 231
Royal Medico-Psychological
  Association 76–7

schizophrenia 27–37; causation of
  34–6, 115–16; definition of 28–31;
  and morbid jealousy 46–7; outcome
  of 32–4, 205
science: behavioural 116–18;
  clinical 111–12; and general
  psychopathology 107–19; methods
  of 8–9, 17; and models 114–15;
  neurobiological 211
social hygiene 74
social medicine 75, 195–6
social psychiatry 152–6
social psychology, historical 161
social statistics 73–4
sociology 74, 15, 204–5
St John's Hospital, Stone, Bucks 79,
  81, 82, 83

torture 157–9
treatment: and clinical trials 83; of
  mental disorders 80–2, 113; of
  morbid jealousy 57–8; and
  psychoanalysis 16–17

understanding, metaphysical 109–10
urbanization, and mental
  disorders 201–10